PENGUIN BOOKS
FOOD FACTS

Dr David Briggs is a food scientist and Senior Lecturer in the Department of Human Nutrition at Deakin University. He is the author of many scientific publications, a contributor to the book *Food and Nutrition in Australia* (Methuen, 1982) and a member of several professional associations including the Nutrition Society of Australia, the Australian Nutrition Foundation and the Australian Institute of Food Science and Technology. He has worked in Europe and South-east Asia. He now lives in Geelong with his wife and three children.

Dr Mark Wahlqvist is Professor of Human Nutrition at Deakin University and a consultant physician at Prince Henry's Hospital, Melbourne. He has held various clinical, teaching and research appointments in Australia and Sweden. Besides numerous scientific publications he is the joint author with his wife, Soo Huang, of *Use and Abuse of Vitamins* (Sun Books, 1983) and is editor of *Food and Nutrition in Australia* (Methuen, 1982). He is responsible for dietetic training in the state of Victoria and is a member of several international committees related to health and nutrition including the International Union of Nutritional Sciences. He was a member of the Working Party that devised national dietary guidelines in Australia. He is familiar in Australia for his frequent appearances on television and radio and in newspaper articles. Born in Adelaide, his home is now Melbourne where he lives with his wife and two children.

David Briggs & Mark Wahlqvist

FOOD FACTS

the complete no-fads-plain-facts guide to healthy eating

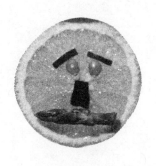
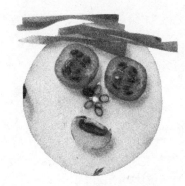
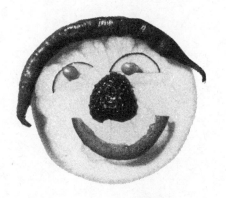
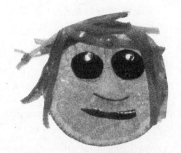
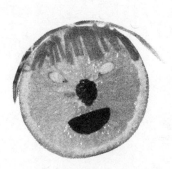
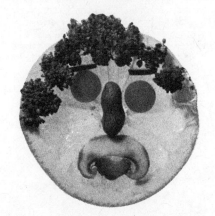

We express our gratitude to Jackie Yowell for her
inspiration, support and criticism of the manuscript,
to Helen Semmler for her design, and to her and
Bill Farr for their artwork.

Penguin Books Australia Ltd,
487 Maroondah Highway, P.O. Box 257
Ringwood, Victoria, 3134, Australia
Penguin Books Ltd,
Harmondsworth, Middlesex, England
Penguin Books,
40 West 23rd Street, New York, N.Y. 10010, U.S.A.
Penguin Books Canada Ltd,
2801 John Street, Markham, Ontario, Canada,
Penguin Books (N.Z.) Ltd,
182-190 Wairau Road, Auckland 10, New Zealand

First published by Penguin Books Australia, 1984

Copyright © D. Briggs & Mark Wahlqvist, 1984

Typeset in Concorde by Dovatype, Melbourne

Made and printed in Australia by
The Dominion Press — Hedges and Bell, Victoria

CIP

Wahlqvist, Mark L.
Food facts

Includes index.
ISBN 014 046542 1

1. Nutrition. I. Briggs, David. II. Title.

641.1

To Heather and Soo, for believing in and sustaining us,
and to Michael, James, Alexandra, Ingmar and Kerstin for
giving us perspective and hope for the future.

CONTENTS

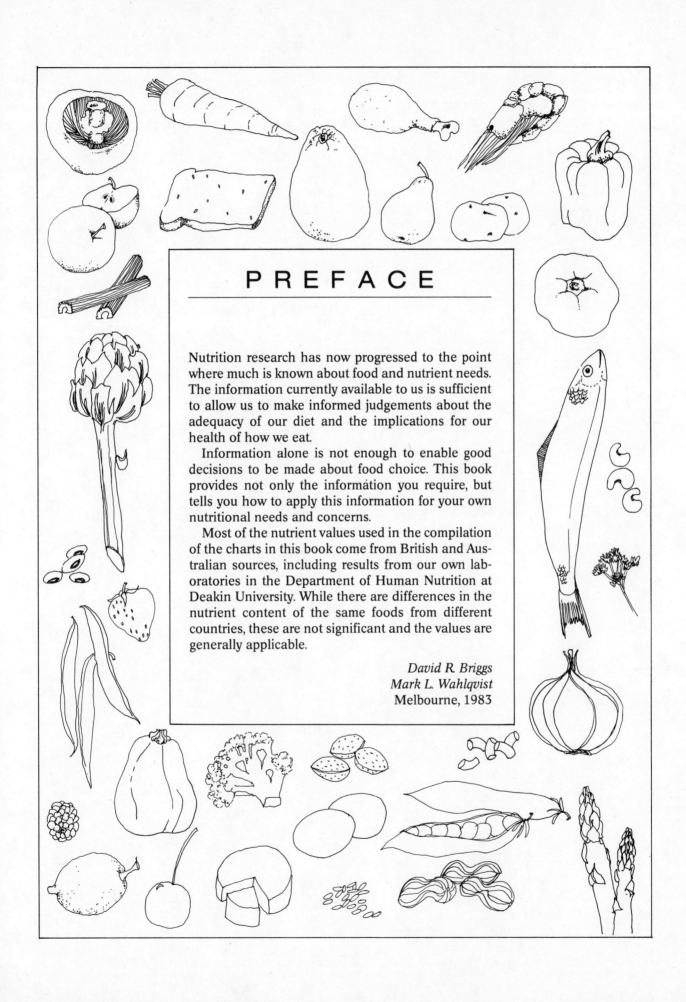

PREFACE

Nutrition research has now progressed to the point where much is known about food and nutrient needs. The information currently available to us is sufficient to allow us to make informed judgements about the adequacy of our diet and the implications for our health of how we eat.

Information alone is not enough to enable good decisions to be made about food choice. This book provides not only the information you require, but tells you how to apply this information for your own nutritional needs and concerns.

Most of the nutrient values used in the compilation of the charts in this book come from British and Australian sources, including results from our own laboratories in the Department of Human Nutrition at Deakin University. While there are differences in the nutrient content of the same foods from different countries, these are not significant and the values are generally applicable.

David R. Briggs
Mark L. Wahlqvist
Melbourne, 1983

INTRODUCTION

WHY YOU NEED THIS BOOK

Food has many functions, not the least of them social. There is no good reason why healthy eating should not be enjoyable.

While books about diet and food fads abound in Britain, the United States and Australia, it is still difficult for the individual to find the basic facts about food that will enable him or her to plan and follow a healthful diet geared to particular needs.

The purpose of this book is to provide such information. It answers many questions that arise every day, such as 'are there any vitamins in the frozen peas I'm eating?'. It is also designed to help readers understand the principles of good nutrition for themselves and their families. They can then plan, in an informed and intelligent way, their food intake under different circumstances.

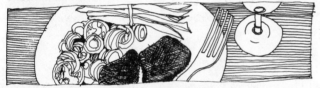

WHY IS NUTRITION IMPORTANT?

There is considerable truth in the adage 'You are what you eat'. The state of your body and how well it works depends to a large extent on how appropriately it is nourished.

Malnutrition can be found in contemporary Western society and is not peculiar to developing countries. Malnutrition occurs when a person's body is not adequately serviced by its food intake. Each individual's needs change under different circumstances. Moreover, the foods needed by an athlete, a grandmother, a growing boy, an office worker or a pregnant woman are not the same. Nutritional needs vary even from one office-worker to another, according to genetic make-up, level of activity, general state of health and environment.

Some groups of people who are at risk from nutrient deficiencies can be generally identified. These include those who are socio-economically disadvantaged; women during the reproductive years because of the added nutritional demands of menstruation and of pregnancy; the elderly; those who have a particular health problem, such as diabetes, faulty absorption of food or who are on certain medications; those with lifestyle problems such as cigarette smoking and alcohol abuse.

Diet and health

The most significant nutritionally related problems in industrialized nations are those health conditions that are the result of, or are made worse by, a diet that is not prudent:

- overweight (obesity)
- hardening of the arteries (atherosclerosis), leading to reduced blood flow to the heart (coronary heart disease), brain (strokes), legs (pain on walking) and other organs
- certain tumours, especially of the large bowel.

Diet can increase the risk of heart disease in several ways. Eating foods that are high in saturated fat, low in polyunsaturated fat and high in cholesterol can raise the level of cholesterol in the blood. When the blood cholesterol level is increased the risk of coronary heart disease is increased. Another kind of blood fat (lipid) known as triglyceride can also be elevated and increase the risk of heart disease. Conversely, when relatively more fruits, vegetables and wholegrain cereals are eaten the blood fats are lower.

High blood pressure (hypertension) also increases the risk of heart disease, strokes and kidney failure. Blood pressure is higher when sodium intake is high, potassium intake (an element obtained mainly from plant foods) is low, alcohol intake is high and there is excess body weight. Eating too much, with consequent obesity, increases the risk of heart disease by increasing the work of the heart, increasing blood pressure, and increasing blood fats; obesity also increases the risk of diabetes. Nutritional factors can also alter the 'stickiness' of some blood cells, called platelets; this contributes to hardening of the arteries and may result in a blockage of the artery. Some polyunsaturated fish oils reduce the stickiness of platelets and may account for the rarity of heart disease amongst fish-eating communities, such as the Eskimos.

As far as tumours or cancers are concerned, a number of interesting food factors are emerging from research. A food intake low in fat and cholesterol, high in dietary fibre from wholegrain cereals, with plenty of vegetables and little alcohol seems protective against large bowel (colon and rectum) cancer. The reasons for this are not yet known. The same kind of dietary pattern may also reduce the risk of tumours of lung, breast, uterus, prostate and pancreas. There is little evidence so far to suggest that food additives are significant in the development of cancer.

Diabetes is a condition where the blood sugar (glucose) is too high because not enough insulin is produced by the pancreas for the body's needs. The glucose spills from the blood into the urine, leading to a large loss of water as urine; thirst then follows. Broadly there are two types of diabetes, one where it is necessary to administer insulin from the time of diagnosis and the other where it is not. Amongst Caucasians in industrialized nations two to three people in every 100 are affected. When non-Caucasians adopt the food habits of affluent society, they appear to be particularly susceptible to diabetes; from 15 to 40 per cent of Australians of Aboriginal or Pacific-Islander descent suffer from diabetes. Being overweight is a particularly important risk factor for developing the type of diabetes where administered insulin is not usually needed. A diet with a high intake of high-carbohydrate, high-dietary-fibre foods and a low intake of fat seems protective against the development of this type of diabetes.

Since most premature deaths in affluent societies result from atherosclerotic disease of blood vessels (vascular disease), and from lung, breast and large bowel cancer, there is great potential for dietary change to increase life expectancy and, indeed, to reduce morbidity and chronic illness.

THE OPTIMAL WAY OF EATING

Because health is so closely related to diet, nutritionists and public health workers have sought to identify the optimal diet. The first principle of an optimal diet is to ensure that the amount of food is right — not too little and not too much. If a person's growth has proceeded satisfactorily and weight is appropriate, this particular goal is realized.

The second nutritional principle is to have as wide a variety of foods as possible. The greater the variety of foods you eat, the more likely you are to obtain the full range of nutrients required. Traditionally, and for most of human experience, as hunter-gatherers, people collected fruits, nuts, seeds, leaves, roots, caught small animals and fish, and hunted, with less success, larger game. This is the diet with which humans evolved; our bodies are designed to be serviced by the nutrients in such a diet. Another reason for emphasizing the importance of variety from a range of biological sources of food is that, if there is any toxic or harmful factor in a particular food, it will tend to be diluted to a level where it is not hazardous. The advent of food staples — such as potatoes, wheat and rice — is more a reflection of agricultural practice and a way of feeding a larger number of people at a lower cost than of nutritional principle. Insofar as a staple is often unavoidable, it is best to have it unrefined so that as many nutrients as possible are consumed.

The third nutritional principle, related to the first, is to balance food intake with the rate our bodies use it up. In our society the balance is often not achieved, because our level of physical activity is so much less than that of our hunter-gatherer forbears. Important concepts nutritionists use in finding what the balance should be are 'energy density' and 'nutrient density'. The average person, with an average level of physical activity, needs a certain minimum of energy every day — not less than 1200 kilocalories* (about 5000 kilojoules) per day. The more energy (kilojoules or kilocalories) there is per unit (weight or volume) of a food, the more 'energy dense' it is. The more nutrients there are for a particular amount of energy, the more 'nutrient dense' it is. Fatty foods are generally the most energy dense. Some are also nutrient poor, like butter and lard. Vegetables tend to be low in energy density and high in nutrient density. The less physically active we are, the less can we have energy-dense foods and the more we should have nutrient-dense foods.

Dietary guidelines

The pattern of disease in affluent society — obesity, vascular disease, cancers, diabetes, etc. — is associated with a high intake of fatty meat and dairy products, a high intake of alcohol, a low intake of wholegrain cereals, fruits and vegetables, and a high intake of sodium (especially as salt). It is for these reasons that several countries have now developed dietary guidelines similar to the following:

- eat a variety of foods each day
- encourage breast feeding
- prevent and control obesity
- decrease total fat intake
- decrease consumption of sugar
- limit alcohol consumption
- increase consumption of cereals, fruits and vegetables
- reduce sodium intake
- encourage water intake.

---

*The amount of energy released from the food we eat is measured in units called kilocalories or sometimes Calories spelt with a capital C. Another unit of energy commonly used is the kilojoule. It is easy to convert kilojoules to kilocalories and vice versa:

1 kilocalorie = 1 Calorie
1 kilocalorie = 4.2 kilojoules (approximately 4)
1 kilojoule = 0.24 kilocalories (approximately ¼)
1 megajoule = 1000 kilojoules

Encouragement of breast feeding is included in recognition of breast milk's unique properties, such as those protecting against infection, which cannot as yet be reproduced in infant milk formulas.

Average life expectancy in the twentieth century has increased. Yet among developed countries there is a hierarchy of life expectancy with, for example, Sweden, Greece and Japan being ahead of the United Kingdom, Australia, New Zealand and the United States. To some extent, these differences appear to relate to food intake pattern. It seems that much may be gained from analysing why this is so, identifying an optimal diet and following guidelines that promote it. Food is not the only factor that can influence health; most health problems in modern society are 'multifactorial' in origin. But nutrition is clearly a very important factor. If you can establish healthy dietary habits in conjunction with attention to other factors (such as physical activity, smoking, stress, work environment), you will give yourself the best chance against ill health and for a long and active life.

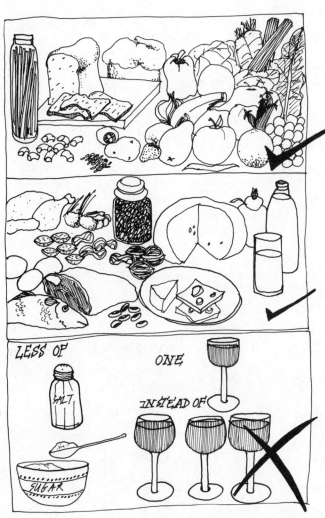

WHAT IS FOOD?

Food makes your body work, grow and repair itself. The kind of food you eat can affect the efficiency of these processes. Body function and the food that sustains it is infinitely complex. Food is in fact one of the most complicated sets of chemicals imaginable.

Getting to know which nutrients are in which foods can help you to understand something of this complex relationship between your food and your body.

Chemicals in food

Food is composed of many different chemical substances — 'macronutrients' (major nutritional components that are present in relatively large amounts, such as protein), 'micronutrients' (major nutritional components that are present in relatively small amounts, such as vitamins), water, and roughage (dietary fibre). Many other components can also be present in food (see Figure 1).

Food may contain colours (natural and synthetic), flavours, pharmacologically active substances (such as caffeine, steroids, and salicylates, which chemically affect the body), natural toxicants (naturally occurring poisons, such as cyanide), additives, and various contaminants (substances resulting from a contaminated environment, such as pesticides). Even characteristic flavours such as those of oranges and passionfruit can depend on the presence of a dozen or more chemicals.

The chemical nature of food is changed by storage, preservation and, especially, by cooking. Food chemicals can also interact amongst themselves within the body. For example, the availability to the body of iron from plant sources depends on the amount of vitamin C present in the food eaten. The way in which carbohydrate is absorbed from the bowel depends to some extent on the presence of dietary fibre, even though the fibre itself is not absorbed.

Physical form of food

Food is also more than just the chemicals it contains. Its physical characteristics are important. The size of food particles can affect the extent to which nutrients are digested and made ready for absorption by the body. For example, eating an intact apple has nutritional value different from drinking all the same chemicals in an apple purée. Ground rice is more rapidly digested than unground rice. Nutrients can be more easily absorbed from peanut butter (paste) than from peanuts eaten whole.

Acid or alkaline

The acidity and alkalinity of food are physical properties often thought to be important. In fact, they are only important insofar as they might alter the rate of emptying of the stomach, digestion in the small bowel and the acidity or alkalinity of the urine. Our bodies can cope with a wide range in food acidity and alkalinity without much problem. Acid foods are generally sour while alkaline foods often have a slightly soapy taste. The use of sodium bicarbonate (baking soda) can make foods alkaline. It can also cause loss of vitamin C and contribute to our intake of sodium.

THE TOTAL DIET

In following any diet or food fashion you should know why it recommends the eating patterns it does. The facts about food presented in this book will enable you to be more critical — to tell whether any new diet is merely a fad, or is soundly based and suitable to your particular needs.

For a safe and healthy diet, some foods should be eaten in relatively greater quantities than others, and these relationships can be represented by position in a 'pyramid'. The food pyramid in Figure 2 shows three categories of relative use:

• the category at the base represents foods we should eat most days and in greater quantity
• from the middle category, we should eat different foods on different days, and as wide a variety as possible
• we can eat the foods at the top of the pyramid in moderation or occasionally.

More information about the nutritional characteristics of these food categories can be obtained by reference to Figure 3, and Figure 21.

KNOWING THE NATURAL SOURCES OF FOOD

Foods from similar sources in nature have common nutritional characteristics. Getting to know the biological sources makes it easier to remember the main nutritional properties of various foods (Figure 3).

FIGURE 1: COMPONENTS OF FOOD IN THE TOTAL DIET

A single food or even a meal will not contain all possible components of food. The total diet will include things eaten on many different occasions. The number of chemicals found in the total diet will be large.

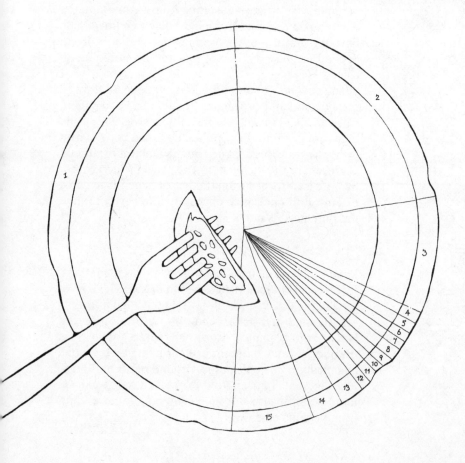

1 Water

2 Carbohydrate

3 Fat

4 Alcohol

5 Trace elements

6 Vitamins

7 Flavours (natural & added)

8 Colours (natural & added)

9 Natural poisons (e.g. cyanide)

10 Pharmacologically active substances (e.g. caffeine)

11 Additives (e.g. preservatives)

12 Contaminants (e.g. pesticides)

13 Elements (minerals)

14 Dietary fibre

15 Protein

FIGURE 2: THE FOOD PYRAMID

For a safe and healthy diet some foods should be eaten in relatively greater quantities than others.

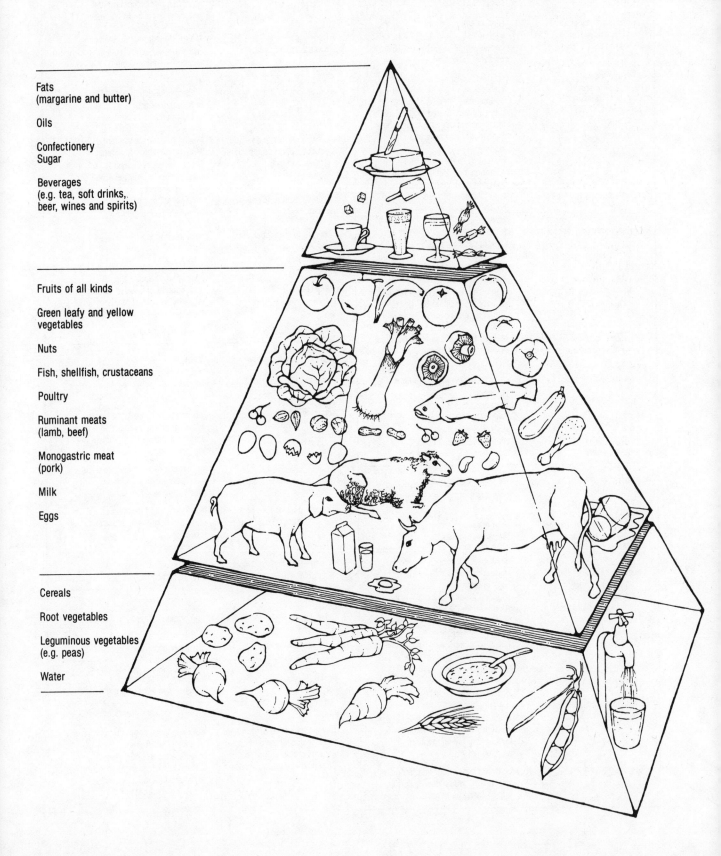

Fats
(margarine and butter)

Oils

Confectionery
Sugar

Beverages
(e.g. tea, soft drinks,
beer, wines and spirits)

Fruits of all kinds

Green leafy and yellow
vegetables

Nuts

Fish, shellfish, crustaceans

Poultry

Ruminant meats
(lamb, beef)

Monogastric meat
(pork)

Milk

Eggs

Cereals

Root vegetables

Leguminous vegetables
(e.g. peas)

Water

FIGURE 3: FOODS GROUPED ACCORDING TO BIOLOGICAL SOURCE

GROUP	NUTRITIONAL CHARACTERISTICS	GROUP	NUTRITIONAL CHARACTERISTICS
ANIMAL	High content of good-quality protein	Wheat, rye, barley	High in starch
Eggs	High cholesterol in yolk		Moderate protein content, but relatively deficient in one essential amino acid (lysine)
Milk and dairy products	High in saturated fat High in calcium (except butter) Lactose (milk sugar) is not tolerated by some individuals	Corn (e.g. sweetcorn, maize)	Relatively deficient in two amino acids (lysine and trytophan) and the B-group vitamin, niacin
Muscle meats:		Fruits:	
Fish — freshwater	Less sodium than in seawater fish	Citrus (e.g. oranges, lemons)	Dietary fibre rich in pectin, with gelling properties
Fish — seawater	Source of essential fatty acids (i.e. polyunsaturated fatty acids)		Moderate amounts of vitamin C and the B-group vitamin, folacin
Shellfish (e.g. mussels, oysters)	More cholesterol than in fish, but contribute more essential fatty acids High in trace elements and sometimes contaminated with 'heavy' metals (e.g. mercury)	Stone fruit (e.g. plums, apricots, cherries, peaches) Apples and pears	Moderate carotene content Moderate vitamin C content Mainly water, carbohydrate and dietary fibre, with little vitamin or mineral content
Crustaceans (e.g. prawns, lobster)	More cholesterol than in fish, but contribute more essential fatty acids	Tropical fruit (e.g. mango, papaya)	Rich source of carotene Rich source of vitamin C Rich source of pectin
Ruminants (e.g. sheep, cattle)	High iron content High in saturated fat	Berries (e.g. raspberries, strawberries, blueberries, blackberries)	High in vitamin C
Monogastric — domesticated (e.g. pig)	The type of fat reflects the animal's dietary intake to a greater extent than in ruminants.		
Monogastric — game (e.g. kangaroo, rabbit)	Although lean, the type of fat again reflects the animal's dietary fat intake to a greater extent than in ruminants.	Nuts (e.g. peanuts, walnuts, macadamia, hazel nuts, etc.)	High energy density High content of fat with various types of fatty acids Moderate protein content
Avian — poultry	Usually low in fat (if skin removed)	Herbs and spices	Low energy density
Avian — game birds	Low in fat		
Organ meats:		**CONFECTIONERY** (e.g. sweets)	High energy density Low nutrient density
Liver	Good source of most vitamins and elements High cholesterol content High in nucleic acids		
Brain	High cholesterol content	**MICROBIOLOGICAL**	
Other (kidneys, heart, intestine, etc.)	High cholesterol content	Soil micro-organisms	Vitamin B-12 is produced by the micro-organisms; vegans who are very hygienic may be deficient in this vitamin.
PLANT	All contain dietary fibre. Contain potassium rather than sodium.	Yeast	Wide range of vitamins and trace elements High in nucleic acids
Vegetables:		Fermented beverages (e.g. beer, wines, spirits)	Nutrient content depends on source of carbohydrate and extent of processing. Ethanol (alcohol)
Root (e.g. carrots, sweet potatoes, potatoes)	High in starch Moderate vitamin C content Carotene (forms vitamin A) content high in yellow-orange vegetables	Fermented foods (e.g. soya sauce, tempeh)	High amino acid content Sodium can be high
Green leafy (e.g. spinach, cabbage)	High in carotene High in vitamin K	**INSECT**	
Marrow-like	High in carotene (if yellow-orange)	Bodies	High protein content
Flowers (e.g. broccoli, cauliflower)	High vitamin C content	Honey	High in simple sugars (e.g. fructose, glucose and sucrose)
Stalks (e.g. celery)	Low energy density		
Onion-like (e.g. spring onions)	Low energy density	**WATER**	No energy (kilocalories) Variable element content
Tomatoes	Low energy density Moderate vitamin C content		
Peppers (e.g. capsicum)	Low energy density High vitamin C content	**SOIL** (Usually a contaminant in food, but deliberately used in cooking by some ethnic groups, e.g. Aboriginal Australians and in Iran)	Variable element and micro-organism contribution Clay-eaters can suffer element deficiencies because these nutrients are trapped by the clay, and so cannot be absorbed.
Legumes (e.g. beans, peas, lentils)	High in starch Moderate amount of protein but relatively deficient in one essential component (the amino acid, methionine)		
Cereals and grains:	Contain dietary fibre that is rich in 'pentosans', which have a particular role in bowel function.		

WHAT HAPPENS TO THE FOOD WE EAT

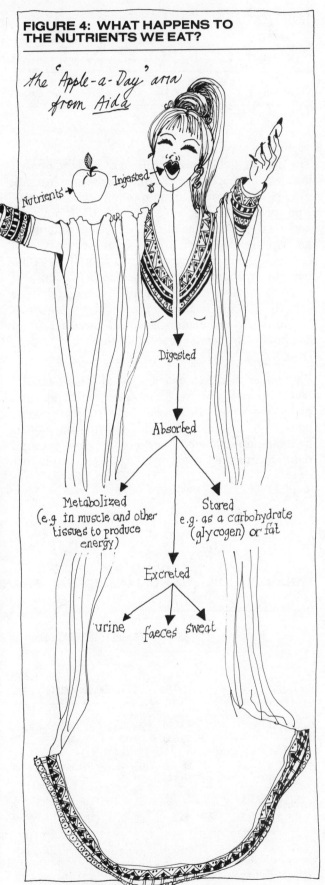

FIGURE 4: WHAT HAPPENS TO THE NUTRIENTS WE EAT?

The nutrients in food are used by our bodies in varying ways. Each nutrient plays some part in normal body function (that is, body physiology).

Not all components of food are nutrients, and not all nutrients are essential to life. Some nutrients may have important physiological functions without being absorbed from the gut, for example dietary fibre. Dietary fibre, while not being essential to life, is associated with health because of its role in the correct functioning of the bowel. Its absence may increase the risk of bowel disease.

Although recommendations about nutrient intakes are made in terms of daily intakes, not all nutrients are needed every day. Most can be stored to a lesser or greater extent in our bodies. The macronutrients that provide energy are stored in the liver and muscles in the form of a carbohydrate called glycogen, and in fatty tissues (adipose tissue) and muscles in the form of fats, known as triglycerides. The situation for micronutrients varies. Fat-soluble vitamins, such as vitamin A, tend to be stored in liver and fat and do not need to be replenished every day; they can last for weeks if the stores are good. In general, water-soluble components like vitamin C are quickly excreted in the urine. But some water-soluble nutrients such as vitamin B-12 and folacin (folic acid) can be stored for years and months, respectively, in the liver. Some nutrients, for example calcium and phosphorus, are in effect stored in bone.

How often a nutrient needs to be ingested depends on how all of the various processes shown in Figure 4 operate for the nutrient in question.

Although not every nutrient is needed every day, it is safest to 'top up' regularly through a consistent pattern of eating. Nevertheless, undue concern about particular food preferences, for example about children who seem to want one kind of food and not another for a few days, is probably unnecessary. As long as a variety of foods are eaten in the longer term, the range of essential nutrients should be provided.

OUR NUTRIENT NEEDS

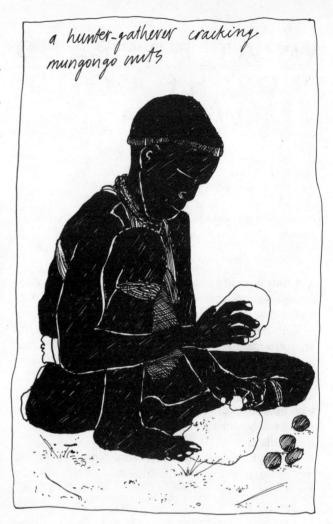

a hunter-gatherer cracking mungongo nuts

The human diet has evolved from that of the hunter-gatherer, through that of the subsistence agriculturalist, to that of the urban-dweller in an industrialized society. The differences between the former diet and the so-called 'affluent' diet of developed countries are shown in Figure 5. The increased intake of macronutrients and decreased intake of dietary fibre have been accompanied by increased incidence of diseases such as diabetes, heart disease, and some cancers. A more healthful diet, relatively higher in carbohydrate and dietary fibre, and lower in fat and alcohol, is advocated by most nutritionists.

The amounts of nutrients suggested for a healthful diet cover quite wide ranges of values, which are compatible not only with survival, but also with optimal health. Not only do individuals differ from each other in their nutrient needs, but also any one person's requirements may change with age, as shown in Figure 6.

FIGURE 5: HOW THE HUMAN DIET HAS CHANGED

		AMOUNTS OF DIFFERENT NUTRIENTS INGESTED DAILY (grams)					PROPORTION EACH NUTRIENT CONTRIBUTES TO ENERGY INTAKE (%)				
		PROTEIN	FAT	CARBOHYDRATE	DIETARY FIBRE	ALCOHOL	PROTEIN	FAT	CARBOHYDRATE	DIETARY FIBRE	ALCOHOL
Hunter-gatherer diet	M	60-190	30-60	310-500	20-90	0-4	10-30	10-20	50-80	0	0-1
	F	50-140	20-40	230-360	20-90	0-3					
Affluent diet	M	60-190	100-140	160-340	10-25	0-110	10-30	35-50	25-55	0	0-30
	F	50-140	70-100	110-250	10-25	0-80					
Healthful diet	M	60-130	30-80	310-440	35-45	0-20	10-20	10-30	50-70	0	0-5
	F	50-90	20-60	230-320	35-45	0-10					

The values given are the amounts of macronutrients considered to be adequate for a 35-55 year old man (M) of 70 kg, expending 2500 kilocalories (10400 kilojoules) per day, and for a 35-55 year old woman (F) of 58 kg, expending 1820 kilocalories (7600 kilojoules) per day. (For an explanation of these units, please see page 4.)

FIGURE 6: OUR NUTRIENT NEEDS CHANGE WITH AGE

INFANTS
- With weaning or with a change from infant formulas to cow's milk at around 6 months of age, there is a reduced intake of vitamins C and D and iron.
- Adequate exposure to sunlight usually prevents vitamin D deficiency or rickets.
- Additional sources of vitamin C and iron-containing foods are recommended at this time.
- Fluoride may be needed where water is not fluoridated.

CHILDREN
- Nutrient needs during childhood are determined both by growth and physical activity.
- A developing knowledge of and interest in food and its preparation will help children choose from a wide variety of foods.
- The principle nutritional problems of childhood in developed countries are obesity on the one hand and underweight on the other, dental caries (tooth decay) and, for a few children, food sensitivity. Food sensitivity can show up as eczema, asthma, bowel disturbances, and, possibly, behavioural problems. A lack of foods containing dietary fibre can also lead to constipation.

ADOLESCENTS
- In early adolescence or puberty there is a marked increase in rate of growth, and therefore in energy and nutrient needs. Thus foods that are energy dense (see page 17) can be tolerated at this time and nutrient-dense foods (see page 17) should be encouraged. Some foods such as nuts and meat are both energy and nutrient dense.

ADULTS
- The adult is at nutritional risk because of changing food patterns — moving from the parental home, getting a job (or not having a job), and changing patterns of physical activity. There are problems of obesity, hardening of the arteries (atherosclerosis), high blood pressure and proneness to certain cancers. To minimize these health risks the adult should maintain physical activity and control intake of energy-dense foods (especially fats) and salt.

PREGNANCY
- Energy and nutrient needs increase during pregnancy to meet the needs of the developing foetus — by about an additional 10 per cent.
- It is especially important in pregnancy to be neither overweight nor underweight. Nevertheless, pregnancy itself is not the time to be making efforts to reduce weight, because of risks to the foetus. After pregnancy, there is a greater risk of putting on excess weight and this should be guarded against.
- During pregnancy, cravings for particular foods can occur. The pregnant woman should not let these displace more important food items from her diet.
- The pregnant teenager is at extra risk because she has to meet the nutritional needs of her own growth as well as those of the foetus.
- Essential nutrients that tend to be depleted during pregnancy include protein, calcium, iron and folacin.
- Alcohol intake should be kept to a minimum because of possible harmful effects on the unborn child.

LACTATION
- Breast-feeding increases the mother's nutrient and energy needs by about 20 per cent. The more milk produced, the greater the energy and nutrient requirements.
- When a mother is breast-feeding, calcium and vitamin C are especially important, as these are present in greater concentrations in breast milk than are generally found in the diet.

ELDERLY
- When you are elderly, nutrition is an especially important factor in your diet.
- In approaching retirement, it is important to be as physically active as possible. Then you will have an appetite to eat the food you need to provide you with all the essential nutrients. Once energy intake falls below about 1200 kilocalories (5000 kilojoules), it is difficult to get all your essential nutrient needs from food.
- If you are obese, you will be less healthy and your extra weight will contribute to problems of arthritis, especially in joints such as hips and knees, which bear the weight.
- If you are well and active, your opportunities for independent shopping and food preparation are greater, and these contribute to your nutritional well-being.

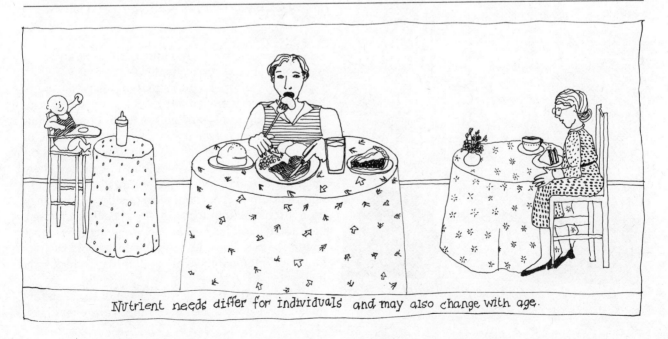

Nutrient needs differ for individuals and may also change with age.

FIGURE 7: RECOMMENDED DAILY DIETARY INTAKES FOR DIFFERENT INDIVIDUALS *

INDIVIDUAL	AGE	WEIGHT	ENERGY		PROTEIN	VITAMIN A including pro-vitamin A	VITAMIN D	VITAMIN B-1	VITAMIN B-2	NIACIN	VITAMIN B-6
	(years)	(kilograms)	(kilojoules)	(kilocalories)	(grams)	(micrograms)	(micrograms)	(milligrams)	(milligrams)	(milligrams)	(milligrams)
Men	18-35	70	11600	2800	70	750	–	1.1	1.4	18	1.3-1.9
	35-55	70	10400	2500	70	750	–	1.0	1.2	16	1.3-1.9
	55-75	70	8800	2100	70	750	–	0.8	1.0	14	1.0-1.5
Women	18-35	58	8400	2000	58	750	–	0.8	1.0	13	0.9-1.4
	35-55	58	7600	1800	58	750	–	0.7	0.9	12	0.9-1.4
	55-75	58	6400	1500	58	750	–	0.6	0.8	10	0.8-1.1
Pregnant 2nd & 3rd trimesters	18-35	68	9000	2150	66	750	–	0.9	1.1	14	1.0-1.5
	35+	68	8200	1950	66	750	–	0.8	1.0	13	1.0-1.5
Lactating	18-35	58	10800	2600	78	1200	–	1.0	1.3	17	1.6-2.2
	35+	58	10000	2400	78	1200	–	1.0	1.2	16	1.6-2.2
Infants	0-½	–	–	–	–	–	–	–	–	–	0.25
	½-1	–	460-420 (per kg)	110-100 (per kg)	2-3 (per kg)	300	10	0.4	0.5	7	0.45
Children	1-3	13	5400	1300	20-39	250	10	0.5	0.7	9	0.6-0.9
Boys	3-7	19	7200	1700	26-51	350	–	0.7	0.9	11	0.8-1.3
	7-11	28	9200	2200	37-66	500	–	0.9	1.1	15	1.1-1.6
	11-15	41	12200	2900	51-87	725	–	1.2	1.5	19	1.4-2.1
	15-18	61	12600	3000	67-90	750	–	1.2	1.5	20	1.5-2.2
Girls	3-7	18	7200	1700	25-51	350	–	0.7	0.9	11	0.8-1.3
	7-11	27	8800	2100	36-63	500	–	0.8	1.1	14	1.0-1.5
	11-15	42	10400	2500	52-75	725	–	1.0	1.3	17	1.2-1.8
	15-18	55	9200	2200	60-66	750	–	0.9	1.1	15	1.1-1.6

*These figures are for Australia but are mostly very similar to those used in other developed countries — see also Figure 8.

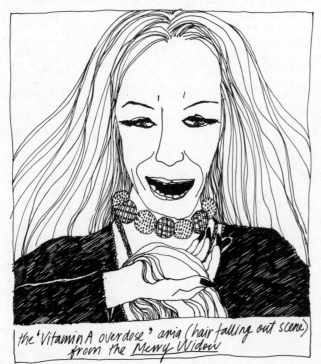

the 'Vitamin A overdose' aria (hair falling out scene) from the *Merry Widow*

HOW OUR NUTRIENT NEEDS ARE ASSESSED

How do we know the amounts of different nutrients we should eat to keep us healthy?

In many countries, committees of nutrition experts have assessed the available evidence regarding safe and adequate intakes of nutrients, and have formulated *recommended dietary intakes* (RDIs) for some of the nutrients. These recommendations are based on fairly clear evidence, and relate to the average daily amounts that are considered adequate to meet the known nutritional needs of most healthy people. They do not indicate the needs of any specific individual, but should allow for normal requirements under most circumstances. They do not allow for factors such as illness or interactions with certain drugs, which may have special needs (see Figures 19 and 20).

Where an RDI for a nutrient has not yet been formulated, a 'safe and adequate' range can generally be

INDIVIDUAL	AGE	WEIGHT	VITAMIN B-12	FOLACIN	VITAMIN C	SODIUM	POTASSIUM	CALCIUM (range)	IRON	ZINC	IODINE
	(years)	(kilograms)	(micrograms)	(micrograms)	(milligrams)	(milligrams)	(milligrams)	(milligrams)	(milligrams)	(milligrams)	(micrograms)
Men	18-35 35-55 55-75	70	2.0	200	30	920-2300	1950-5460	400-800	10	12-16	150
Women	18-35 35-55 55-75	58	2.0	200	30	920-2300	1950-5460	400-800	12	12-16	120
Pregnant 2nd & 3rd trimesters	18-35 35+	68 68	3.0	400	60	920-2300	1950-5460	900-1300	15	16-20	150
Lactating	18-35 35+	58 58	2.5	300	60	920-2300	2540-5460	900-1300	15	18-22	170
Infants	0-½ ½-1	– –	– 0.3	– 60	– 30	140-280 320-580	390-580 470-1370	– 500-700	– 4.8	3-6 4.5-6.0	50 60
Children	1-3	13	0.9	100	30	320-1150	980-2730	400-800	5	4.5-6.0	70
Boys	3-7 7-11 11-15 15-18	19 28 41 61	1.5 1.5 2.0 2.0	100 100 200 200	30 30 40 50	460-1730 600-2300 920-2300 920-2300	1560-3900 1950-5460 1950-5460 1950-5460	400-800 600-1100 600-1400 500-1400	7 10 12 12	6-9 9-14 12-18 12-18	90 120 150 150
Girls	3-7 7-11 11-15 15-18	18 27 42 55	1.5 1.5 2.0 2.0	100 100 200 200	30 30 40 50	460-1730 600-2300 920-2300 920-2300	1560-3900 1950-5460 1950-5460 1950-5460	400-800 600-1100 600-1300 500-1300	7 10 12 12	6-9 9-14 12-18 12-18	90 120 120 120

Adapted from *Dietary Allowances For Use in Australia*, Australian Government Publishing Service, Canberra, 1979.

advised. In fact, some nutritionists think that a range rather than a specific amount should be stated for all RDIs.

It is difficult to apply RDIs to an individual because what really needs to be known is that individual's particular requirements for the nutrients in question. However, if your average daily intake of any nutrient is less than two-thirds of the RDI, or is below the lower end of the 'safe and adequate' range, then you may not be getting enough of an essential nutrient. Sometimes this may be due to not eating enough food or alternatively it may be due to poor food choice.

In these few pages, you will find tables listing the general recommended dietary intakes. Differences in recommendations between countries are, by and large, of no real consequence and reflect slightly different views of scientific evidence or local differences in food supply and nutritional needs. In the latter part of this book, RDIs for individual nutrients are also shown in the Food Charts.

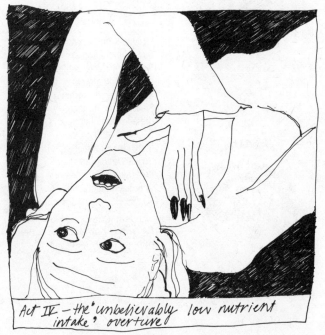

Act IV – the 'unbelievably low nutrient intake' overture

FIGURE 8: RECOMMENDED DAILY DIETARY INTAKES IN SOME DEVELOPED COUNTRIES

	AUSTRALIA		U.K.		U.S.A.	
	MEN	WOMEN	MEN	WOMEN	MEN	WOMEN
Age (years)	18-35	18-35	18-35	18-35	23-50	23-50
Weight (kilograms)	70	58	65	55	70	55
Energy (kilojoules)	11600	8400	12000	9200	11300	8400
Energy (kilocalories)	2800	2000	2900	2200	2700	2000
Protein	70	58	72	54	56	44
Vitamin A (micrograms of retinol equivalents)	750	750	750	750	1000	800
Vitamin D (micrograms)	–	–	–	–	5	5
Vitamin E (milligrams)	–	–	–	–	10	8
Vitamin B-1 (milligrams)	1.1	0.8	1.2	0.9	1.4	1.0
Vitamin B-2 (milligrams)	1.4	1.0	1.6	1.3	1.6	1.2
Niacin (milligrams of niacin equivalents)	18	13	18	15	18	13
Vitamin B-6 (milligrams)	1.3-1.9	0.9-1.4	–	–	2.2	2.0
Vitamin B-12 (micrograms)	2.0	2.0	–	–	3.0	3.0
Folacin (micrograms)	200	200	300	300	400	400
Vitamin C (milligrams)	30	30	30	30	60	60
Calcium (milligrams)	400-800	400-800	500	500	800	800
Phosphorus (milligrams)	–	–	–	–	800	800
Iron (milligrams)	10	12	10	12	10	18
Zinc (milligrams)	12-16	12-16	–	–	15	15
Magnesium (milligrams)	–	–	–	–	350	300
Iodine (micrograms)	150	120	–	–	150	150

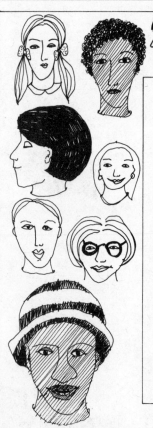

FIGURE 9: ESTIMATED SAFE AND ADEQUATE RANGE OF DAILY DIETARY INTAKES * (U.S.A.)

	MEN	WOMEN
Vitamin K (micrograms)	70-140	70-140
Biotin (micrograms)	100-200	100-200
Pantothenic acid (milligrams)	4-7	4-7
Copper (milligrams)	2-3	2-3
Manganese (milligrams)	2.5-5.0	2.5-5.0
Fluoride (milligrams)	1.5-4.0	1.5-4.0
Chromium (milligrams)	0.05-0.2	0.05-0.2
Selenium (milligrams)	0.05-0.2	0.05-0.2
Molybdenum (milligrams)	0.15-0.5	0.15-0.5
Sodium (milligrams)	1100-3300	1100-3300
Potassium (milligrams)	1875-5625	1875-5625
Chloride (milligrams)	1700-5100	1700-5100

*An 'estimated safe and adequate daily dietary intake' is given for some nutrients for which a 'recommended dietary intake' has not been established.

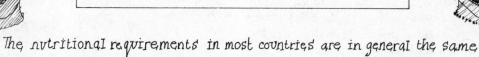

The nutritional requirements in most countries are in general the same

FIGURE 10: HOW TO CHECK YOUR INTAKE OF A PARTICULAR NUTRIENT

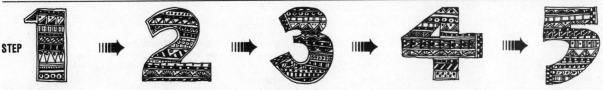

STEP

Identify foods that are good sources of the nutrient from the Food Charts in the second part of this book.	Keep a record of how often you eat those foods over one week and how much of them you eat.	Calculate the total amount of that nutrient eaten in one week and divide by 7 for the average daily intake.	Compare your average daily intake with the recommended daily intake or the safe and adequate intake.	If your intake is way below what is recommended, find, from the charts, foods that are high in that nutrient and increase them in your diet.

ENERGY BALANCE

If you eat more than your body needs to keep it working efficiently, you will get fat. Many slimming diets prefer not to emphasize this displeasing but basic fact.

When energy intake equals energy needs, our bodies are in 'energy balance'. This means that if you are fully grown, or are growing normally, and your weight is within certain limits (those that conform to longest life expectancy and least illness), you have achieved energy balance. You achieve it by balancing, on the one hand, your total energy intake, and, on the other, your level of activity. The more active you are, the more energy you need.

Energy intake, which used to be measured in Calories, is now usually measured in kilocalories or kilojoules. Nutritionists now more often use kilojoules because of newer international conventions. Remember, one kilocalorie equals one Calorie or 4.2 kilojoules.

People differ in the efficiency of their energy expenditure. This may be due to differences in efficiency of movement, or because some people are not as efficient as others in burning up their 'fuel' supplies (that is, their 'metabolic efficiency' is lower). Thus, one person may eat much more than another, with equivalent levels of activity, and yet remain similar in weight. The more 'energy-efficient' person needs to be more careful about eating too much to avoid becoming overweight. However, the same person would survive better if food supplies were short.

Energy needs vary with your age and weight, as well as with your level of activity. Figures 11 and 12 show this.

Energy is also used, with varying efficiency, to maintain body temperature, to store fuels after a meal and to form bodily wastes, as Figure 13 illustrates. So even when you are not being active your body needs energy for vital processes. This minimum level of energy expenditure is known as the 'basal metabolic rate'. It is what keeps you alive even if you are completely at rest, fasting and at a comfortable temperature.

FIGURE 11: RECOMMENDED DAILY ENERGY INTAKE VARIES WITH AGE AND WEIGHT

	BODY WEIGHT (kilograms)	RECOMMENDED ENERGY INTAKE* (kilojoules)		
		AGE		
		25 (years)	45 (years)	65 (years)
Men	55	9800	9200	7600
	60	10400	9600	8000
	65	11000	10000	8400
	70	11600	10400	8800
	75	12200	10800	9200
	80	12800	11200	9600
	85	13400	11600	10000
	90	14000	12000	10400
	95	14600	12400	10800
Women	40	7000	6200	5800
	45	7400	6600	6000
	50	7800	7000	6200
	55	8200	7400	6400
	60	8600	7800	6600
	65	9200	8200	6800
	70	9600	8600	7000
	75	10000	9000	7200

*Intake required to *maintain* weights given here. For desirable weights, see Figure 14.

FIGURE 12: ENERGY USED IN DIFFERENT PHYSICAL ACTIVITIES

PHYSICAL ACTIVITY	ENERGY EXPENDITURE (kilojoules or kilocalories per minute)			
	58-KILOGRAM WOMAN		70-KILOGRAM MAN	
	(kilojoules)	(kilocalories)	(kilojoules)	(kilocalories)
Sleeping, resting, fasting	3-5	0.5-1	4-6	1-1.5
Sitting, reading, desk work	5-7	1-1.5	6-9	1.5-2
Sitting typing, playing piano, operating controls	6-10	1.5-2.5	8-12	2-3
Light bench work, serving in shop, gardening, slow walking	9-15	2-3.5	12-18	3-4
Social sports, cycling, tennis, cricket, light factory work, light farm work	12-20	3-5	16-24	4-6
Heavy physical labour, carrying, stacking, cutting wood, jogging, competitive sports	18-30	4-7	24-36	6-8.5
Very hard physical labour, intense physical activity, heavy lifting, very vigorous sporting activity	over 40	over 10	over 50	over 12

FIGURE 13: ENERGY BALANCE

The relative amount of energy used to perform body functions varies with individuals, depending on how efficiently each function is handled.

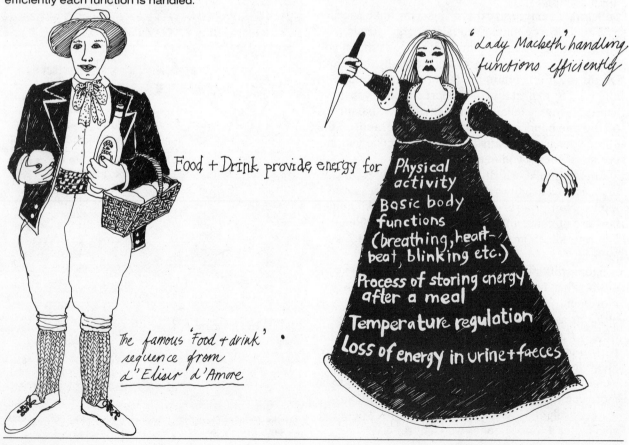

'Lady Macbeth' handling functions efficiently

Food + Drink provide energy for Physical activity
Basic body functions (breathing, heart-beat, blinking etc.)
Process of storing energy after a meal
Temperature regulation
Loss of energy in urine + faeces

The famous 'Food + drink' sequence from L'Elisir d'Amore

CONTROLLING BODY WEIGHT

When our bodies are not in energy balance, excess energy is stored as fat (in adipose tissues). Women normally have more body fat than men, and this should be taken into account when considering whether to conform to the fashion to be very slim. Desirable weights for adults of varying heights are shown in Figure 14. Those shown were obtained in 1959. Although 1979 figures are available, there is controversy about their use.

FIGURE 14: DESIRABLE WEIGHTS FOR MEN AND WOMEN (INDOOR CLOTHING)

The weight for your height in the table is the 'desirable weight' that you should maintain throughout your life. It is the weight at age 20-24 years associated with maximum life expectancy. Generally speaking, if your weight varies from the desirable weight given by up to 10 per cent (less or more), you are still within the range considered most healthy. But, depending on whether your frame is small or large, your weight may differ from the desirable weight by as much as 20 per cent without being unhealthy. Some experts believe that to weigh up to even 30 per cent more than the desirable weight is all right, depending on frame and muscularity.

MEN				WOMEN			
HEIGHT WITHOUT SHOES		WEIGHT		HEIGHT WITHOUT SHOES		WEIGHT	
(cm)	(ft in)	(kg)	(lb)	(cm)	(ft in)	(kg)	(lb)
155	5'1"	55.9	123	142	4'8"	45.9	101
158	5'2"	57.5	127	145	4'9"	47.1	104
160	5'3"	58.9	130	147	4'10"	48.4	107
163	5'4"	60.2	133	150	4'11"	49.8	110
165	5'5"	61.8	136	152	5'0"	51.2	113
168	5'6"	63.6	140	155	5'1"	52.5	116
170	5'7"	65.7	145	158	5'2"	54.1	119
173	5'8"	67.5	149	160	5'3"	55.7	123
175	5'9"	69.3	152	163	5'4"	57.5	127
178	5'10"	71.3	157	165	5'5"	59.5	131
180.5	5'11"	73.4	161	168	5'6"	61.3	135
183	6'0"	75.4	166	170	5'7"	63.1	139
185.5	6'1"	77.4	170	173	5'8"	65.0	143
187.5	6'2"	79.7	175	175	5'9"	66.8	147
190.5	6'3"	82.0	180	178	5'10"	68.6	151

Adapted from the *Statistical Bulletin*, Metropolitan Life Insurance Company, N.Y., 1959.

If you are on a weight-reduction programme, remember that body water is the main constituent lost during the first few days. It is only after 2 to 3 weeks of dieting that the loss is mainly fat. At this stage, a daily energy intake that is about 500 kilocalories (2000 kilojoules) less than the intake actually needed at a particular level of physical activity (see Figures 11 and 12) will lead to a weight loss of approximately 1 kilogram per fortnight. Remember also that not all people expend energy with the same efficiency.

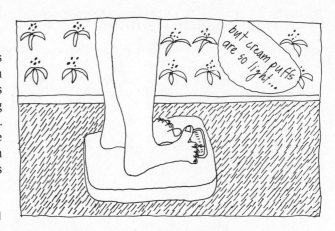

APPETITE CAN CONTROL HOW MUCH ENERGY (FOOD) WE CONSUME

Appetite has an important role in controlling energy intake. When we are physically active, appetite is more correctly related to energy need than when we are inactive. At low levels of physical activity, we are more likely to feel hungry and to eat more than we need.

Also, a diet that is low in fat and high in carbohydrate and dietary fibre seems to allow appetite to be more correctly attuned to energy need. Because fatty foods are so palatable, more of them tend to be eaten than our bodies really need. They are also more energy dense than high-carbohydrate, high-dietary-fibre foods.

ENERGY DENSITY

A high-energy-dense food has more kilocalories (or kilojoules) than the same amount of a low-energy-dense food.

The more energy dense a food is, the less of it we can eat to provide a given amount of energy. Conversely, the less energy dense a food, the more we can eat to provide us with the same amount of energy, as we can see in Figure 15.

The more water and dietary fibre, and the less fat and alcohol in a food or drink, the less energy dense it is.

NUTRIENT DENSITY

The greater the number of essential nutrients, and the larger the amount of them a food contains, the more 'nutrient dense' it is. Often foods with low energy density are quite nutrient dense, as, for example, wholegrain cereals and leguminous vegetables (like peas and beans). Some foods can be both nutrient dense and energy dense, such as a piece of steak.

FIGURE 15: ENERGY DENSITY

Some foods allow you to eat more per 25 kilocalories (100 kilojoules)

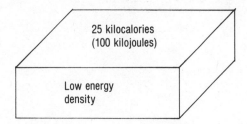

25 kilocalories
(100 kilojoules)

Low energy
density

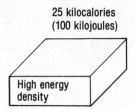

25 kilocalories
(100 kilojoules)

High energy
density

All these foods are 25 kilocalories (100 kilojoules):

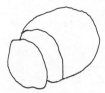 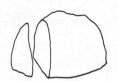 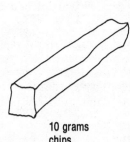 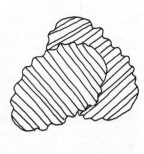

30 grams boiled potato	15 grams roast potato	10 grams chips	5 grams potato crisps
(¼ potato)	(⅛ potato)	(1 chip)	(2 crisps)

FIGURE 16: YOU CAN ASSESS YOUR NUTRITIONAL STATUS IN SEVERAL WAYS

METHOD	STEP 1	STEP 2	STEP 3	STEP 4	STEP 5
Food intake	Record food and beverage intake for one week. Compare your intake of a particular food item with the average serving size given in the Food Charts and illustrations.	From this information, convert your intake to grams of that particular item for the week. Divide by 7 to give your daily intake (grams per day).	Choose a nutrient of interest (e.g. vitamin C or energy) and, from the food charts, identify foods you have eaten that contain significant amounts of the nutrient. Calculate the amount of nutrient ingested in one day.	Find out the recommended daily intake (or safe and adequate intake) of nutrient from the Food Charts.	Calculate what percentage of the recommended amount is the amount of nutrient ingested by you. If less than 67% or greater than 200%, consider how your diet could change to give a figure nearer 100%.
Weight and height	Record your weight and height.	Read off the desirable weight for height from weight/height tables (Figure 14).	Calculate your weight as a percentage of the desirable weight.	If greater than 120% of the desirable weight, this is 'obesity'. Greater than 130% is a significant risk to health. Less than 90% of the desirable weight is also a risk to health.	
Skinfold thickness (fatty tissue under the skin)	Pinch a fold of skin on the abdomen, between thumb and forefinger.	If more than 25 millimetres thick (1 inch), this constitutes a significant risk to health.	More precise measurements of skinfold thickness can be made with calipers.	With calipers, at the rear of the mid-upper arm, measure the 'triceps skinfold' three times and average (see Figure 17).	Compare the value with those given in Figure 17 to find the percentage of fat in your body.

ASSESSING YOUR OWN NUTRITIONAL STATUS

An overall assessment of your nutritional status can be made by the methods shown in Figures 16 and 17. (You may find it helpful to refer to the introductory section of the Food Charts on page 45.)

You should be able to get an indication of whether you are consuming too much or not enough of any particular nutrient. However, this exercise is designed to help you learn about a healthy diet rather than be an exact guide. If you want to know precisely, or suspect a health problem is due to nutrient deficiency or excess, you should consult a doctor.

Figure 16 shows three ways by which you can assess your nutritional status; you can then decide from Figure 17 whether you are 'too fat'.

FIGURE 17: ARE YOU TOO FAT?

	TRICEPS SKINFOLD (millimetres)*	PER CENT DESIRABLE BODY WEIGHT	PER CENT BODY MASS AS FAT	ASSESSMENT
Men aged	6	90	15	Satisfactory
17–76 years	9	100	18.5	
	11	110	21	
	14	120	24.5	Overweight
	17	130	29.5	Significant health risk
Women aged	12	90	24	Satisfactory
17–68 years	14	100	26.5	
	17	110	29.5	
	21	120	33	Overweight
	25	130	35.5	Significant health risk

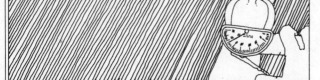

*Measured with calipers at the rear of the mid-upper arm (see skinfold thickness, Figure 16).

WATER BALANCE

Water is an essential nutrient, but the amount needed depends on climate, activity and the kinds of food we eat.

Most foods contain significant amounts of water and can contribute about half the body's daily water needs. The chemical processes within our bodies that break down food can also provide about 12 per cent of the daily water needs.

FIGURE 18: WATER INPUT AND OUTPUT

A balanced daily input and output of water, under conditions of average temperature and humidity

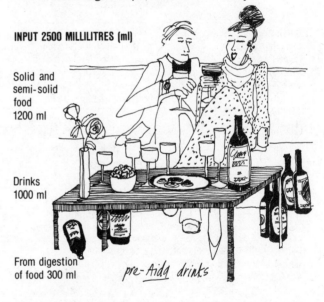

INPUT 2500 MILLILITRES (ml)

Solid and semi-solid food 1200 ml

Drinks 1000 ml

From digestion of food 300 ml

pre-Aida drinks

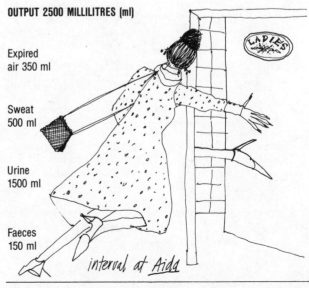

OUTPUT 2500 MILLILITRES (ml)

Expired air 350 ml

Sweat 500 ml

Urine 1500 ml

Faeces 150 ml

interval at Aida

FIGURE 19: NUTRITIONAL NEEDS OF PARTICULAR HEALTH CONDITIONS

CONDITION	NUTRITIONAL PROBLEM	REDUCED INTAKE NEEDED	INCREASED INTAKE NEEDED
Alcohol abuse	• Ethanol (alcohol) toxicity • Energy (kilocalorie or kilojoule) excess • Vitamin deficiencies: Thiamin Folacin Niacin • Element (mineral) deficiencies: Zinc Magnesium	• All alcoholic beverages	• Nutrient-dense foods (foods with a high concentration of essential nutrients)
Diabetes	• Weight control • Blood glucose (sugar) should be kept between 3.5 and 9 millimoles per litre (mmol/l). • Blood fats (cholesterol and triglycerides) should be normal (cholesterol less than 6.5 mmol/l, triglycerides less than 1.8 mmol/l).	• Energy-dense foods (foods high in calories) • Foods with little dietary fibre • Animal (saturated) fat • Large quantities of food at any one time (food intake should be spread out)	• Wholegrain cereals • Vegetables (especially legumes) • Fruits
Coronary heart disease, where blood fats are high (hyperlipidaemia) Also for other atherosclerotic vascular diseases (hardening of the arteries)	• High blood cholesterol • High blood triglycerides • Low blood level of high-density lipoprotein (HDL) • Sticky platelets (small blood cells contributing to clots and thromboses)	• Fatty foods, especially of animal origin • Cholesterol-rich foods • Foods with little dietary fibre	• Wholegrain cereals • Vegetables • Fruits • Fish
Hypertension (high blood pressure)	• Blood pressure is raised by: High sodium High potassium High ethanol High body weight Low polyunsaturated to saturated fat ratio Low dietary-fibre-rich foods	• Energy-dense foods • Alcohol • Sodium-rich foods • Animal fats	• Potassium-containing foods • Dietary-fibre-rich foods
Osteoarthritis (degeneration of weight-bearing joints such as hips and knees)	• Overweight	• Energy-dense foods (especially foods with high fat, alcohol-containing, and with low dietary fibre)	
Gout	• High uric acid level in blood and/or urine	• Alcoholic beverages • Energy-dense foods • Purine-rich foods (foods with much nucleic acid, such as organ meats and yeast)	
Coeliac disease	• Sensitivity of gut lining to gluten, resulting in poor absorption of nutrients	• Wheat flour and products containing gluten, e.g. barley, rye, buckwheat, malt, oats	• Maize, soya, rice and potato can be used safely
Cystic fibrosis (resulting in growth retardation and vitamin deficiencies)	• Inadequate digestive capacity because of reduced enzyme production by the pancreas • Altered sweat gland secretion		• Energy-dense foods according to individual tolerance • Nutrient-dense foods (some foods are both nutrient and energy dense) • Adequate salt intake

S P E C I A L
N U T R I T I O N A L
S I T U A T I O N S

As Figure 19 shows, nutritional needs can be affected by certain health conditions, and your dietary intake may need to be adjusted.

MEDICATIONS THAT ALTER NUTRITIONAL NEEDS

Some medicines may alter appetite, digestion and absorption of nutrients, and their metabolism and excretion. If you make regular or sustained use of medications, you should check with your doctor whether they affect your nutritional needs. Figure 20 illustrates how certain medications increase the need for particular nutrients.

SUGARS AND HEALTH

Sugars, and particularly sucrose, are often referred to as 'empty Calories' because they lack significant amounts of vitamins, elements (minerals) and trace elements and just provide us with energy. Some people may overeat because of their desire for sweetness. In trying to reduce weight, often the most obvious foods to exclude are sweet foods and the use of sugar. This lowers the energy intake without significantly affecting the intake of vitamins and elements. But it is not the sweet foods and sugar alone that cause people to be overweight; rather it is overeating. People who do not like or eat sweet foods can also be overweight. Indeed, obese people often eat less sucrose than others. It may be harder for these people to find a way to reduce safely their food consumption. It should also be remembered that fat and alcohol have more energy per gram than sugar and other carbohydrates. Sugar is often used to make fatty foods, for example icecream, more palatable and interesting. Obesity, resulting from excessive overeating, is associated with a number of disorders, which include high blood pressure, gallbladder disease, diabetes mellitus and heart disease.

Dietary carbohydrates and in particular sugar play an important role in tooth decay. Carbohydrates allow certain micro-organisms present in plaque (a mass of micro-organisms on the tooth surface) to produce organic acids, which demineralize teeth and cause decay. It appears that the frequency of eating and the form the sugar is in, are more important in causing decay than the actual amount consumed. Sugar in sticky foods such as caramels and toffees promotes tooth decay to a greater extent than when eaten in meals or consumed in drinks.

There are three steps that can help reduce the risk of tooth decay:

• reduce the intake of sugar and other carbohydrates particularly in sticky foods, and between meals
• increase the resistance of teeth to decay by fluoride treatment
• brush teeth after meals.

Honey is sometimes used as a substitute for sugar. Honey contains about 45 per cent fructose, 34 per cent glucose, 20 per cent water and small amounts of organic acids and other constituents. It is possible that these minor constituents in honey could have medicinal or toxic effects. Like all sugars, honey, raw sugar, brown sugar and refined sugar are not significant sources of nutrients other than carbohydrate, which only provides energy.

FIGURE 20: SOME MEDICATIONS THAT MAY INCREASE NUTRITIONAL NEEDS

MEDICATION GROUP	INCREASED REQUIREMENT *
Antibiotics	Biotin
	Vitamin K
	Iron
	Potassium
Anti-hypertensives (lower blood pressure):	
Diuretics (promote sodium and water excretion from body) e.g. chlorothiazide, frusemide	Calcium (not with chlorothiazide)
	Magnesium
	Potassium
	Zinc
Methyldopa	Folacin
	Vitamin B-12
	Iron
Hydralazine	Vitamin B-6
Heart failure treatment:	
Digoxin	General nutrient intake because of anorexia, which results if too large a dose is given
	Magnesium
	Zinc
Diuretics	(As under anti-hypertensives)
Antacids	Phosphate (phosphorus)
Analgesics (pain-killers):	
Aspirin	Vitamin C
	Iron
Indomethacin	Iron
Laxatives	Potassium
	Calcium
Oral contraceptives	Vitamin B-6
Treatment of blood clots and thromboses:	
Warfarin	Vitamin K (it can be dangerous to alter vitamin K intake during warfarin therapy)

*(under medical supervision only)

DIET AND LIFESTYLE

FIGURE 21: DIETARY INTAKE AND CULTURE OR LIFESTYLE

FOOD STYLE	CHARACTERISTIC FOODS	NUTRITIONAL ADVANTAGES	NUTRITIONAL DISADVANTAGES
Arctic (e.g. Scandinavian, Eskimo, Canadian Indian)	Fish, berries	Vitamins A and D Vitamin C Essential polyunsaturated fat (see saturated and polyunsaturated fat Chart 9)	Preservation techniques of salting and smoking may increase risk of conditions such as high blood pressure and cancer of the gut.
Mediterranean (e.g. Greek, Italian, Spanish, Yugoslavian)	Bread, olive oil, wine, vegetables	Dietary pattern protective against coronary heart disease and cancer of the large bowel	Overweight
Oriental (e.g. Chinese, Japanese)	Rice, soya sauce, monosodium glutamate (MSG), vegetables	Low fat, high carbohydrate — protective against coronary heart disease	Sometimes high in sodium (from MSG) increasing prevalence of high blood pressure
Hunter-gatherer (e.g. aboriginal Australians and Malaysians, African bushmen)	Roots, berries, nuts, leafy plants, fruit, fish	A wide variety of foods with good prospects of obtaining adequate amounts of all essential nutrients and not too much of any hazardous chemicals	
Multicultural (as in societies to which successive large migrations have occurred)	A wide range of food styles	A wide variety of foods	
Vegetarian	Cereals, vegetables, fruits } Vegan Eggs, milk and dairy products } Lacto-ovo vegetarian	Low fat, high carbohydrate, high dietary fibre — protective against coronary heart disease and large bowel cancer	May be low in some amino acids if complementary sources of protein (e.g. cereals and legumes) are not eaten
Zen macrobiotic	From 10 to 100% cereal content of diet, depending on level of adherence	At lowest level of cereal intake advantages of vegetarianism	At higher levels of cereal intake, risk of nutrient deficiency through lack of variety
Organically grown foods	Foods grown without agricultural chemicals	Possibly less pesticide residues	Inflated food prices
High fat, low carbohydrate (e.g. Dr Atkins' diet)	Dairy products, fats and oils, ruminant (beef and lamb) meats		High blood fats and increased risk of coronary heart disease Nutrient deficiency Low-dietary-fibre content leading to increased risk of disorders such as constipation and haemorrhoids Ketosis, with more acid blood
Dependence on ready-to-eat or institutionalized food sources	Fried foods, sweetened beverages, dairy products		Nutrient losses with re-heating and prolonged standing Often high in fat and sodium and low in dietary fibre
No breakfast			Mid to late morning hunger with recourse to less critical food selection of, for example, salty energy-dense snacks, sweetened beverages Fatigue or distraction due to hunger Delayed bowel movement

FOOD STYLE	CHARACTERISTIC FOODS	NUTRITIONAL ADVANTAGES	NUTRITIONAL DISADVANTAGES
Snacking	Often readily accessible foods	May avoid 'binge' eating due to hunger In those with poor appetites, or those who need to eat often (e.g. diabetics), an adequate nutrient intake may be achieved provided the snacks are nutrient dense.	More dental caries Tendency to overeat if snacks are energy dense Losing track of dietary intake
Confectionery	Sweets, chocolates		Dental caries Excessive energy intake, leading to overweight

FOOD LAW

The laws about food, food labelling and additives permitted in food vary from country to country. They are also frequently modified, added to or deleted. Doubtless there will be changes that will alter some of the statements made here about food law. Nevertheless, we feel that interested consumers should know about some of the more important current laws relating to food. People who wish to keep up to date with changes in food legislation should, in Australia, contact their State Department of Health; in the U.S.A., the Food and Drug Administration; and in the U.K., the Ministry of Agriculture, Fisheries and Food.

LABELLING AND THE LAW

The law in most Western countries requires that certain information be present on every package of food that is sold. There must be the common name of the food and the name of the manufacturer or packer. The label must not contain any statement that is false or misleading in any particular concerning the food, and must not include any statement relating to a medical condition; only claims relating to the properties of the food are allowed.

Ingredient labelling

When a statement of ingredients appears on a label, *all* the ingredients must be listed and they must be listed in descending order of their relative amounts. This is useful for giving an indication of the ingredient present in the greatest quantity. Not all foods are required to have their ingredients listed. In particular, foods that have their composition set by law do not have to list ingredients.

Nutrition labelling

Nutrition labelling is generally only required when nutrients are added to a food or a nutritional claim is made. However, many food manufacturers voluntarily include this information on their products. Nutrition information on the label must conform to a prescribed format. This makes comparison between foods much easier. In the U.S.A., this format includes the serving size, the number of servings in the container, the number of kilocalories (kilojoules), the amounts of protein, fat and carbohydrate and the amounts of vitamins and elements (minerals) in terms of the percentage of recommended daily intake per serving. In Australia, the format depends on the nutritional claim. For foods that have been supplemented or fortified with vitamins and minerals, the label must include the amount of the nutrient that is present and also the proportion of the daily allowance that a stated amount of food contains. For example, in some breakfast cereals there is 0.55 milligram of vitamin B-1 in 60 grams of the cereal. This represents 50 per cent of the daily allowance. Packaged orange juice must contain at least 80 milligrams of vitamin C per 200 millilitres, which is 270 per cent or about 2½ times the recommended daily intake in Australia. Special dietary foods in Australia have their own labelling format, which depends on the nutritive claim (see pages 25 and 26).

Date-marking of food

Many of us like to feel that the food we buy is 'fresh'. However, the term 'fresh' when applied to food has a number of meanings. How many of us realize when we see or hear the term 'farm' fresh eggs that the eggs could be up to 4 weeks old? The quality of the eggs we get on our plates depends not only on when they were laid but also on the conditions under which they were kept after laying. 'Dairy' fresh milk may be up to 11 days old before we drink it and again its quality will depend on the conditions under which it was kept. What is really meant by 'fresh fish' when it is sold far from the sea, particularly when it may have been frozen after being caught? How should the term 'fresh' be interpreted when applied to bananas or other tropical fruits that are sold in temperate regions? Would you consider bread, still steaming from the oven, 'fresh' if you knew that the flour used in its preparation was 12 months old?

It is difficult to define a meaning for 'fresh' that would be suitable for all foods. The time from the production of the food until its consumption is obviously important, but so also is the initial quality of the food or ingredients used in its preparation, and the conditions under which the item is kept until eaten. It is in the interests of both food manufacturers and consumers that food is sold in the best possible condition.

Many packaged foods have some form of date marking to indicate that if consumed within a particular time, the product should not have suffered any significant loss of 'fresh eating quality' or deteriorated to a point where it is unfit for consumption. Of course, a loss of quality is a subjective judgement, and will reflect not only the time the food has been stored prior to eating but also the temperature and moisture conditions under which the product has been kept. Temperature control is very important in maximizing the life of a food. This is obvious in the case of fruit, vegetables and frozen foods, but is also important with canned and dried foods. The rate of deterioration of canned foods greatly increases above 20°C and these foods should be stored under cool, dry conditions.

What do the different forms of date-marking mean?

In Australia, the National Health and Medical Research Council has recommended date-marking in a number of forms:

> Date of packaging or baking
> Minimum durable life
> Use-by date

Many other countries use a similar system. The 'date of packaging' or baking is of limited usefulness, as the condition or quality of the food that is purchased will depend not so much on the date of packing but on the freshness or quality of the ingredients from which it was prepared, as well as the conditions under which it was kept. The minimum durability date indicates the time up to which a food can meet consumer expectation, provided that storage instructions on the label are followed. Food can be expected to have good to fair quality for some time past this date. The use-by date refers to time after which the food should not be used, but it allows a safety margin to ensure that the food has not deteriorated to a state where it is unsafe to eat. The expected life of various foods is listed in Figures 33 to 37.

The labelling requirements of foods containing certain food additives are explained in the next section.

Special dietary foods

These are foods that meet a particular nutritive need. In Australia, the term 'special dietary food' can only be used on the labels of certain foods. The most common of these are 'low-energy' or 'low-Calorie' foods and 'carbohydrate-modified' foods. Others include low-sodium, gluten-free, and foods without added sugar. Many 'special dietary foods' other than 'low-energy' or 'low-Calorie' foods are not intended for weight control and contain as much energy as other foods.

A 'low-energy' food must meet specific energy requirements that ensure that there is significant energy reduction compared with an unmodified form of the food. For example, a 'low-energy' soft drink must contain only one-quarter of the energy (kilocalories) contained in a normal soft drink. In addition, the label must state if the drink has been sweetened with the artificial sweeteners saccharin or cyclamate and also the number of kilocalories or kilojoules in 200 millilitres of the drink. In the U.S.A., in addition to low-energy foods, there is a law that permits a label to use the term 'reduced calorie'. These foods contain more energy than 'low-energy' foods but have at least one-third lower energy than a corresponding unmodified food.

A 'special dietary food' with modified carbohydrate is *not* a low-energy food and is not useful in weight-reducing diets. These foods contain a form of carbohydrate that differs from that in the original food. As such, in limited amounts, they may be useful for diabetics. Foods that contain 'no added sugar' may not necessarily be lower in energy than the food that contains sugar because some sugar-free foods contain added sorbitol, which has the same energy content as sugar. These foods may be suitable for diabetics or useful in not promoting tooth decay. Check the label to find the energy content of the food and then compare this with the energy content of an unmodified version of the food in the energy charts.

FIGURE 22: INFORMATION ON A FOOD LABEL

Date after which the quality of the food is unlikely to meet consumer expectations. It only applies if food has been stored under recommended conditions.

Common name of the food

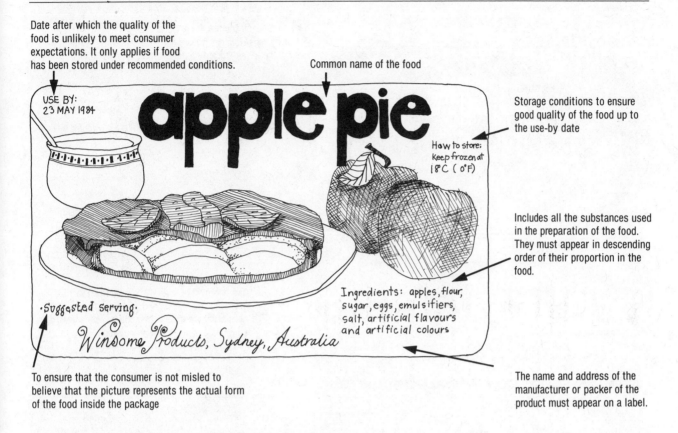

USE BY:
23 MAY 1984

apple pie

How to store:
Keep frozen at
18°C (0°F)

Ingredients: apples, flour, sugar, eggs, emulsifiers, salt, artificial flavours and artificial colours

·Suggested serving·

Winsome Products, Sydney, Australia

Storage conditions to ensure good quality of the food up to the use-by date

Includes all the substances used in the preparation of the food. They must appear in descending order of their proportion in the food.

To ensure that the consumer is not misled to believe that the picture represents the actual form of the food inside the package

The name and address of the manufacturer or packer of the product must appear on a label.

FIGURE 23: LOW-CALORIE FOODS (LOW ENERGY)

For the term 'Low Calorie' to be permitted on the label, a food must have a significant reduction in energy compared with its normal counterpart.

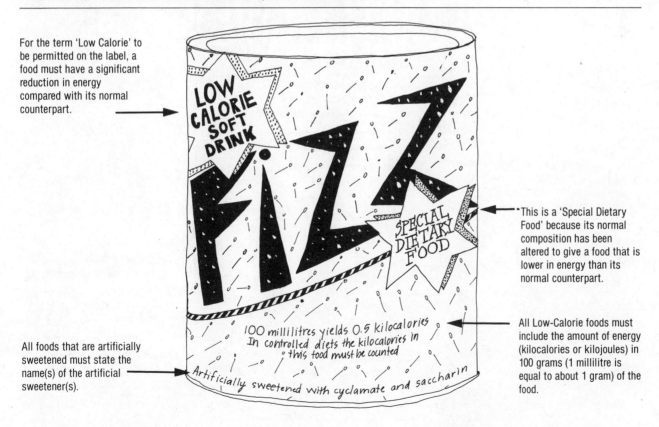

LOW CALORIE SOFT DRINK

FIZZ

SPECIAL DIETARY FOOD

100 millilitres yields 0.5 kilocalories
In controlled diets the kilocalories in
this food must be counted

Artificially sweetened with cyclamate and saccharin

This is a 'Special Dietary Food' because its normal composition has been altered to give a food that is lower in energy than its normal counterpart.

All Low-Calorie foods must include the amount of energy (kilocalories or kilojoules) in 100 grams (1 millilitre is equal to about 1 gram) of the food.

All foods that are artificially sweetened must state the name(s) of the artificial sweetener(s).

FIGURE 24: CARBOHYDRATE-MODIFIED FOODS

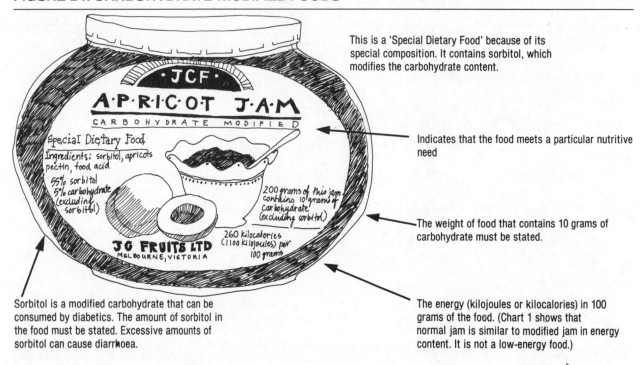

This is a 'Special Dietary Food' because of its special composition. It contains sorbitol, which modifies the carbohydrate content.

Indicates that the food meets a particular nutritive need

The weight of food that contains 10 grams of carbohydrate must be stated.

Sorbitol is a modified carbohydrate that can be consumed by diabetics. The amount of sorbitol in the food must be stated. Excessive amounts of sorbitol can cause diarrhoea.

The energy (kilojoules or kilocalories) in 100 grams of the food. (Chart 1 shows that normal jam is similar to modified jam in energy content. It is not a low-energy food.)

FIGURE 25: FOODS CONTAINING NO ADDED SUGAR

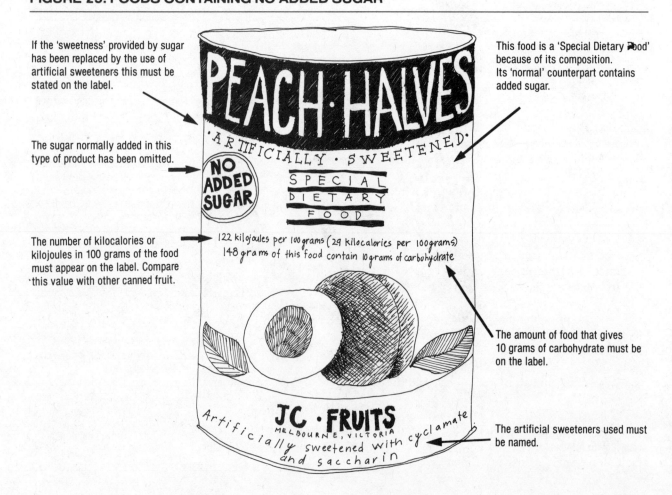

If the 'sweetness' provided by sugar has been replaced by the use of artificial sweeteners this must be stated on the label.

This food is a 'Special Dietary Food' because of its composition. Its 'normal' counterpart contains added sugar.

The sugar normally added in this type of product has been omitted.

The number of kilocalories or kilojoules in 100 grams of the food must appear on the label. Compare this value with other canned fruit.

The amount of food that gives 10 grams of carbohydrate must be on the label.

The artificial sweeteners used must be named.

F O O D
A D D I T I V E S

Food additives are substances that are intentionally added to enhance visual appearance, taste, texture, processing, or the storage life of food. In most countries the use of food additives is controlled by law. Only certain permitted additives may be used and then they are only allowed in particular foods in amounts not exceeding a stated maximum concentration. Before an additive is approved for use in a particular food it must be established that it is safe, and also that a saleable product cannot be produced without using the additive. Sometimes it is difficult to decide from laboratory tests with animals whether a substance will be harmful to people when consumed in small amounts over a long time. It is wisest to err on the side of safety. If appropriate animal tests indicate a potential hazard for people, then approval for use of the additive should not be given. As further testing and more information becomes available the list of permitted additives may need to be modified.

Many of the foods we now take for granted could not be produced without the use of food additives. We use cake mixes, requiring only addition of liquid and baking; soups and mashed potato, requiring only water and heating; the use of additives in bread maintains freshness and retards spoilage from mould and bacteria. Free-flowing salt, sausages and prepared meats, salad dressings, processed cheese, and peanut butter could not be conveniently presented without food additives.

Figure 26 gives examples of food additives, the function they perform in food and examples of foods in which they are likely to be used.

Some people would prefer to do without food additives, even if this meant limited availability, inconvenience or higher prices for food. They should have the freedom to select foods free from additives, but with the present laws governing food labelling this is not always possible. For instance, although most foods containing added colouring must declare on the label that they are artificially coloured, there are exceptions. For example, in Australia, the following foods can contain added colouring without declaration on the label: confectionery, sausage casings, cheeses, pastry mixes, custard powder, table margarine. These foods do not have to list added flavouring: chocolate, cocoa, manufactured meats, cheese, confectionery, pastry mixes, and custard powder.

FIGURE 26: THE USE OF FOOD ADDITIVES

ADDITIVE GROUP & FUNCTION	FOODS THAT MAY CONTAIN THE ADDITIVE
Anti-caking agents (e.g. sodium alumino silicate) Added to finely powdered and crystalline foods to prevent lumping	Salt, milk powder in drink-dispensing machines
Antioxidants (e.g. butylated hydroxyanisole) Preservatives to retard development of rancidity and discolouration	Edible oils and fats, margarine, 'instant' potato, dehydrated vegetables
Bleaching agents (e.g. chlorine dioxide) Added to flour to lighten its colour and improve bread-making	Flours, bread
Colours (e.g. tartrazine) To improve appearance and reinforce flavour	Pastry products, cake, cheese, confectionery, cordials, dessert mixes, flavoured milk, fruit-flavoured drinks, spreads and fillings, fruit yoghurt, ice-cream, icing mixture, jams, jellies, margarine, pickles, sauces, soft drinks
Emulsifiers, stabilizers and thickeners (e.g. glyceryl monostearate) To improve consistency, impart body and stabilize air/oil/water mixtures	Biscuits, bread, cake, canned meats, confectionery, thickened cream, 'instant' potato, dessert mixes, flavoured milk, fruit drinks, fruit yoghurt, ice cream, imitation cream, margarine, mayonnaise, peanut butter, salad dressings, soups
Flavours and flavour enhancers (e.g. vanillin) To impart taste and/or aroma to food	Pastry products, cheese, chocolate, confectionery, cordials, dessert mixes, flavoured milk, ice cream, imitation cream, jellies, manufactured meats, soft drinks, margarine, pickles. The most widely used flavour enhancer MSG (monosodium glutamate) is used in prepared meat/fish dishes, packet soups and many canned foods.
Food acids (e.g. citric acid) Give sour or tart taste, modify other flavours, aid preservation	Pastry products, cake, cheese, cider, confectionery, jellies, cordials, desserts, pickles, fruit drinks, jams, sauces, mayonnaise, salad dressings, soft drinks, soups, spreads
Humectants (e.g. glycerol) Help to retain a soft consistency during storage	Pastry products, cake, confectionery, fruit spreads and fillings, almond icing, sweetened coconut
Preservatives (e.g. benzoic acid) Prevent the growth of moulds, yeasts and bacteria	Beer, pastry products, bread, canned fruit, canned meat products, cheese, cordials, cured meat, 'instant' potato, flour, fruit drinks, fruit salad, pickles, sausages, soft drinks, tomato juice

FOOD COLOUR

From its colour, we can often tell whether food is fresh or stale, of good or poor flavour, and whether it contains particular ingredients. Because colour is important to the consumer, colours are added to food to give an attractive appearance, when it has been lost during processing or storage, or to overcome natural colour variation to ensure a consistent product.

Food colour and flavour are closely associated. When we see a food we anticipate certain flavours. We learn to reject foods that are not coloured in a familiar way. How many of us would drink black milk, even if it smelled and tasted right? We expect that a red apple will be sweet, a green plum will be sour and a brown icecream will have a chocolate flavour. Tests with testing panels showed, for example, that when children were asked to identify the flavours of red and yellow jellies, the majority identified the red jellies as strawberry flavoured and the yellow ones as lemon flavoured, regardless of the flavour actually present.

'Safe' colourings

The addition of colour to food is, for some people, an emotive issue, largely because colours are seen as cosmetic and because, from earliest times, colour was added to food sometimes to deceive the consumer as to the quality or identity of the food. Some of the colours used in food in earlier times, particularly during the nineteenth and early twentieth century, were toxic. More recently, some of the colours used are suspected of causing cancer in animals. The use of colour additives in food is controlled by law, and only those additives that are considered to be safe are permitted to be used. As more tests are performed and information becomes available the list of permitted colours may change. Some tests may cast doubt on safety and the colour should then be withdrawn from use.

Natural and synthetic colouring

Colouring that is added to food may come from natural sources or may be a synthetic product. Synthetic colours can be chemically identical to colours that occur naturally, or they may have no counterpart in nature, as with the widely used synthetic coal tar dyes. It is important to realize that there is nothing about a natural substance that makes it intrinsically more safe than a synthetic one. Figure 27 shows a list of food colourings permitted in Australia. Colours are often used in combination to produce a desired shade and this can be confusing if a person is trying to avoid a particular colouring: for example, a green cordial may be produced by using Green S or by combining tartrazine with Brilliant Blue FCF.

Eliminating a specific colouring from your diet

Tartrazine is a widely used yellow colouring, which has been associated with allergic reactions in some rare instances. Reactions have ranged from rashes and swelling to asthma and possibly even behavioural changes. If it is medically advised, diets that eliminate specific additives can be compiled. These diets should be maintained only under medical supervision, as prolonged exclusion of certain foods from the diet can lead to development of nutritional deficiencies. Although the label of most foods that have been coloured must state that colouring has been added, the name of the particular colouring(s) is usually not disclosed. This, combined with the fact that some foods are exempt from declaring the presence of added colouring on the label, make it difficult to eliminate specific colouring additives from your diet, should you need to. In the U.S.A., foods containing tartrazine (where it is known as FD&C Yellow No. 5) are required to list this colouring by name. Many drugs also contain colouring additives and this fact is sometimes overlooked when trying to avoid particular colourings.

FIGURE 27: PERMITTED COLOURING FOR FOOD*

COLOURING	SHADES
Coal tar dyes:	
Allura red	
Amaranth	
Brilliant Scarlet 4R	Reds
Carmoisine	
Sunset Yellow FCF	
Tartrazine	Yellows
Yellow 2G	
Green S	Greens
Brilliant Blue FCF	
Indigo Carmine	Blues
Chocolate Brown HT	Brown
Brilliant Black BN	Black
Others:	
Annato	
Carotenoids	
Cochineal	
Beetroot extract	
Fruit & vegetable juices/extracts	Yellows to reds
Grape skin extract	
Paprika	
Riboflavin	
Saffron	
Turmeric	
Caramel	Yellows to browns
Chlorophyll	Greens
Vegetable carbon	Black

*This list of permitted food colours is for Australia (1982). The U.K. and U.S.A. have lists that are similar but not identical.

FIGURE 28: HOW MUCH JUICE IN THE ORANGE DRINK?

Here are some useful facts about labels on orange juices, drinks and cordials.

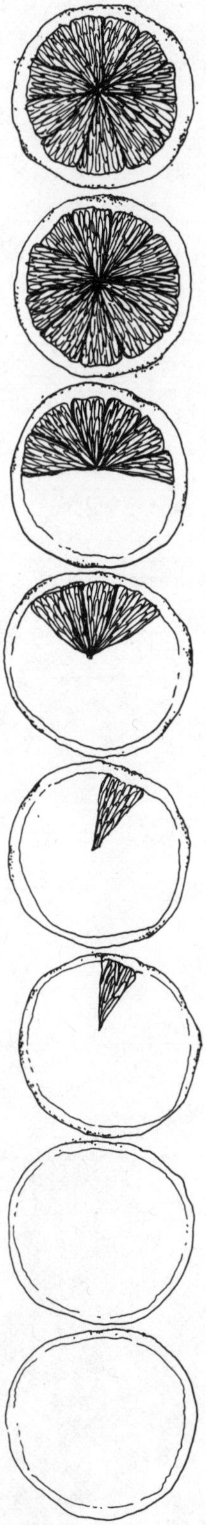

NAME ON LABEL		MINIMUM PERCENTAGE OF ORANGE JUICE ALLOWED
ORANGE JUICE		100 per cent (may contain up to 4 per cent added sugar)
SWEETENED ORANGE JUICE		100 per cent juice plus added sugar
FRESH ORANGE DRINK		50 per cent (may not contain added preservative)
ORANGE FRUIT JUICE DRINK		35 per cent
ORANGE JUICE CORDIAL		4-5 per cent when diluted
ORANGE DRINK		5 per cent
ORANGE FLAVOURED DRINK		0 per cent (flavouring extract made from fruit)
IMITATION ORANGE DRINK		0 per cent

FIGURE 29: NATURALLY OCCURRING SUBSTANCES IN FOOD THAT MAY BE HAZARDOUS TO HEALTH IN EXCESSIVE QUANTITIES

SUBSTANCE OR DISORDER	FOOD	POSSIBLE HAZARD OR POTENTIAL HAZARD
Aflatoxin	Peanuts, peanut products, corn, wheat, rice, that are grown or stored under conditions that favour mould growth	Liver damage, possibility of liver cancer
Allergens	Cereals (rice, wheat, barley, etc.), peanuts, peas, lentils, soya beans, strawberries, bananas, mangoes, pineapples, sesame, poppy and caraway seeds, tea, chocolate, coffee, yeasts, alcoholic beverages, honey and other foods likely to contain pollen	Eczema, hives, hay fever, asthma, headaches, abdominal distress, behavioural abnormalities
Caffeine	Tea, coffee, cola-type soft drinks	Increased urination, nervousness, upset stomach, tremors, irritability, possibility of birth defects, possibility of cancer of the pancreas
Cyanide	Apricot kernels, peach kernels, apple seeds, cassava, young bamboo shoots, bitter almonds, coloured varieties of lima beans	Abdominal pain, vomiting, mental confusion, sensory loss, respiratory distress, spastic weakness
Favism	Broad beans	Anaemia due to an inborn error of metabolism; the disease has an ethnic distribution around the Mediterranean and some other areas
Goitrogens	Cabbage, Brussels sprouts, broccoli, kale, turnips, swedes, mustard seeds, horseradish	Goitre, particularly in areas where the iodine content of food is low
Haemagglutinins	Uncooked legumes (castor beans, kidney beans, lima beans, soya beans, lentils, peas)	Retarded growth, diarrhoea
Lathyrogens	Chickpeas	Spastic paralysis of the legs, skeletal abnormalities
Mycotoxins: Ergotism Alimentary toxic aleukia	Mouldy rice, mouldy grain	Vomiting, damage to bone marrow, convulsions, psychotic behaviour
Oxalic acid	Spinach, rhubarb	Fatal poisoning is probably mythical; there is little danger from eating normal amounts of oxalic-acid containing plants
Nitrates and nitrites	Celery, lettuce, spinach, cabbage, cured meats	Decreased oxygen-carrying ability of blood in infants with gastro-enteritis; possible risk of gastric cancer
Pyrrolizidine alkaloids	Comfrey, some 'herbal' teas	Possibility of liver disease and liver cancer
Solanine	Sprouted and 'greening' potatoes	Vomiting, diarrhoea, abdominal pain, headache, throat irritation

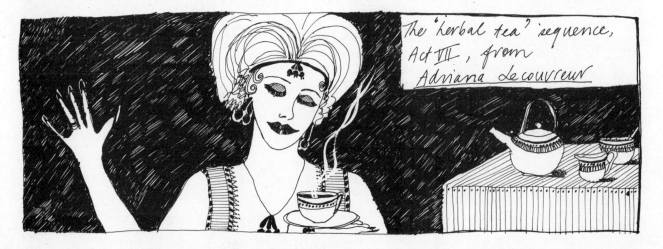

The 'herbal tea' sequence, Act III, from Adriana Lecouvreur

TOXICITY IN FOOD

IS 'NATURAL' ALWAYS GOOD?

The notion that 'natural' food *may* be harmful is not widely appreciated. The terms 'health', 'organic', 'natural', 'unprocessed', 'no added chemicals' when applied to food suggest that the food is safe or more nutritious than its conventional counterpart but this is not necessarily true. All food is made up entirely of chemicals. In addition to well-known nutrients such as carbohydrate, fat, protein and water, food contains many other substances, often in very small amounts. Any substance in food may have a degree of toxicity or 'poisonousness', whether it is natural, deliberately added, or a contaminant. There is nothing special about natural chemicals in food and no distinction should be made between natural and other substances when deciding if a food is likely to be hazardous. For example, a potato contains a number of poisonous substances such as nitrate, arsenic and solanine but in the amounts in which potatoes are normally eaten these natural substances are not hazardous. For this reason it is important not to consume large amounts of a small number of foods, as in some faddist diets, but to consume a wide variety of foods. This not only minimizes the amount of a particular potentially hazardous substance but also ensures that a range of essential nutrients are consumed.

Figure 29 lists a number of substances that occur naturally in food and have either caused illness or are suspected of being hazardous to health. Usually these effects have occurred only when *excessive* amounts of a food containing these substances have been eaten. In fact, for most of us there is little hazard from these foods. The concentration of these poisonous substances is so low in the food we eat that we would have to consume huge amounts over a long time for the toxic effect to show up. Nevertheless, it is important to realize that there are many potentially hazardous substances in our diet without any obvious effects on our health, and that this applies equally to 'natural' and processed foods. Natural foods can be harmful if they are contaminated with excessive amounts of environmental contaminants, or aflatoxin or other mycotoxins produced by some moulds.

Herbal teas

Herbal teas have become popular with an increasing number of people. Herbal and 'bush' teas contain a large number of different components, many of which have not yet been assessed for safety. Some teas can lead to disturbing effects. Tea made from the South Pacific kava plant has been associated with impaired breathing, vision and hearing, and other symptoms. Comfrey and tea made from the roots of sassafras contain substances that have caused cancer in laboratory animals. In addition, some teas can interfere with the therapeutic value of some drugs that are taken at the same time. The heavy consumption of these teas is not to be recommended. Tea, coffee and cola-type drinks contain caffeine (about 30, 40, and 10 milligrams per 100 millilitres respectively). Although individuals react differently to caffeine, the heavy consumption of these drinks can cause, in addition to stimulation, nervousness, increased urination, upset stomach and irritability (Chart 49).

ENVIRONMENTAL CONTAMINATION OF FOOD

Substances that are either real or potential risks to health may enter the food supply as a result of contamination of the environment (see Figure 30). But, in terms of the number of people affected, environmental contamination is less of a problem than illness caused by food poisoning from harmful micro-organisms in food (see page 41).

For many environmental contaminants, health authorities recommend maximum acceptable levels that are considered to be safe in food. It is illegal for foods containing higher levels to be sold although the occasional consumption of slightly higher amounts is unlikely to be harmful. Foods are monitored to check that they comply with the recommendations. Foods that contain more than the permitted amounts of the contaminants being monitored are withdrawn from sale. The effectiveness of this depends on the extent of monitoring.

In general, the level of environmental contaminants in our food complies with the limits recommended by health authorities. However, because of the uncertainty in establishing exactly what is a safe level for many of these contaminants, it is in the interests of our general health to consume as wide a variety of foods as possible. By doing this, the chances of eating large amounts of a contaminated food are minimized. Continued and extensive surveillance and control are needed.

'Heavy metals'

The common environmental contaminants of greatest concern in food are the so-called 'heavy metals', most notably cadmium, lead and mercury.

Mercury

Almost all of the mercury in food occurs in seafood. A dramatic instance of mercury poisoning occurred in the Minimata Bay area in Japan. Fish and shellfish that were heavily contaminated by industrial waste caused poisoning in many of the people who ate them, resulting in damage to the central nervous system and in some instances death. Surveys of the levels of mercury and other heavy metals in food are regularly carried out and have shown that generally the levels are below the maximum amounts permitted by health authorities. Occasionally, higher levels are detected and the food withdrawn from sale.

Lead

Lead occurs widely in the environment and it can enter our bodies through drinking water and the air we breathe, as well as through food. Children are the group at greatest risk, because even at levels below those that produce the usual signs of poisoning, lead can cause behavioural abnormalities. The levels of lead that cause these effects are uncertain so it is difficult to estimate what amount is 'safe'. In some areas, particularly where there is heavy lead pollution in the air from leaded petrol, lead levels may be hazardous for children. Legislation to limit the total environmental lead burden is being enacted in many countries.

Cadmium

Cadmium is present at very low levels in a wide variety of foods. Poisoning due to cadmium in food is rare. The upper 'acceptable' limit for cadmium in food recommended by the World Health Organisation is generally complied with. The kidneys of animals are generally higher in cadmium than are other foods. Contamination of rice, soya bean and seafood with cadmium from local industrial and mining operations has caused cadmium poisoning.

Pesticides and industrial chemicals

Two very persistent environmental contaminants are the pesticide DDT and PCBs (polychlorinated biphenyls), which have been used in electrical transformers, plastics and paints. DDT and PCBs are not easily degraded in the environment and can concentrate in the fatty tissues of many organisms as they move up the food chain. Recent surveys in Australia have not detected the presence of PCBs in food. DDT has been found in many foods but the amounts are such that the total daily intake of DDT is within the 'acceptable' upper limit recommended by the World Health Organisation.

COOKWARE AND CONTAMINATION

Cooking utensils can be made from a variety of materials: aluminium, copper, iron, steel, stainless steel, glass, earthenware. Some of these materials can find their way into food.

Usually very little aluminium migrates during cooking and at present there is no conclusive evidence that the amounts of aluminium normally consumed with our food are hazardous. Higher amounts of aluminium can transfer to food from cookware if highly acidic foods such as vinegar-containing sauces, tomatoes, and citrus fruits are left in contact with aluminium for periods longer than 5 or 6 hours. Similarly, unlined copper utensils containing acidic foods can result in migration of some copper into the food. This can cause rapid destruction of vitamin C and also possibly can lead to harmful levels of copper in food. It is better to use copper vessels that are plated with tin, stainless steel or some other material that will prevent this occurring.

Glass, enameled iron and steel and stainless steel are unlikely to cause potentially hazardous levels of material to migrate into food. Some glazes on pottery utensils that have been wrongly mixed or fired have caused potentially harmful amounts of the heavy metals lead and cadmium to migrate into acid foods that have been stored or cooked in these vessels. This is not normally a problem because modern methods of glazing produce resistant products.

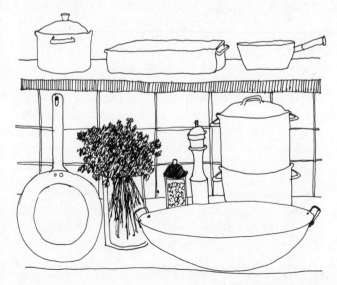

FIGURE 30: SOURCES OF ENVIRONMENTAL CONTAMINATION OF FOOD

ORIGIN	FOOD IN WHICH A CONTAMINANT IS LIKELY TO BE FOUND	POSSIBILITY OF HEALTH HAZARD FROM AMOUNTS IN FOOD, ASSUMING A NORMAL VARIED DIET
Industrial:		
Mercury	Fish	Low
Lead	All foods, water	Low
Cadmium	Fish, shellfish, kidney	Very low
Polychlorinated biphenyls	Fish, poultry, milk, eggs	Very low
Agricultural:		
Pesticides	All foods	Low
Antibiotics	Milk	Very low
Hormones	Some poultry	Very low
Food processing:		
Cleaning agents		
Lubricants		
Packing materials	Any processed food	Very low
Solvent residues		
Extraneous substances (rodent excreta, hair, insects, etc.)		

PROCESSING CAN AFFECT THE NUTRIENT CONTENT OF FOOD

There are many different forms of processing to which food may be subjected before we eat it. All of these processes have some effect on the nutrient content. Although foods are often compared before and after processing, a better comparison is at the stage when the food is eaten. For example, during the freezing of peas there is about a 10 per cent loss of vitamin C. But because they require a shorter cooking time than fresh peas, there is virtually no difference between the vitamin C content of fresh and frozen peas as they appear on our plate.

The nutritional changes that occur in the commercial preparation of food do not differ much from those in the same food prepared in the home. Both types of food preparation involve some form of processing. There may be differences in palatability and the food manufacturer may use cheaper ingredients such as emulsifiers, cereal fillers and synthetic flavours. This may be partially off-set by the fresher foods usually available to the manufacturer. The effect of the different types of processing on nutrients is discussed below.

USE OF FERTILIZERS

The use of fertilizers containing nitrogen can result in a small increase in protein content of some foods. But the amount of vitamin C is usually decreased, probably because of the increased growth of the fruit or vegetable. Since plant roots absorb nutrients in an inorganic form there is no nutritional difference between plants that have been organically fertilized and those fertilized using conventional fertilizers. The nutrients provided by both kinds of fertilizer are effectively the same.

MILLING

During the milling of cereals, part of the original grain is removed. Depending on the extent of the milling process there are large losses of fat, dietary fibre, vitamins B-1, B-2 and niacin, and elements (minerals). Foods made from wholemeal flour are better sources of these nutrients than those prepared from white flour.

CONTROLLED ATMOSPHERE (CA) STORAGE AND RIPENING, AND WAXING

This is a procedure for storing fruits and vegetables, particularly apples, under an atmosphere that differs from air. Its aim is to increase the storage life of the foods. The most important dietary component of apples is dietary fibre, which is unlikely to be changed appreciably during CA storage. Significant nutritional changes in other fruits and vegetables would not be expected. For the uniform ripening of some fruits, most notably tomatoes and bananas, brief storage under a 'ripening gas' can be used. This can initiate ripening or speed up the process. Fruit produced for market in this way is unlikely to be significantly different in nutrient composition compared with fruit that has matured normally, although it may taste differently. Without CA storage many seasonal fruits would not be available throughout the year.

Many fruits and vegetables have a natural coating of wax, which is removed when these foods are cleaned before appearing on the supermarket shelf. To make them shiny and attractive and promote their sale, some fruits and vegetables are artificially waxed. The waxes are dispersed in water and coated over the food to provide a thin film of wax, which gives a glossy appearance. Apples coated this way are likely to sell more readily. In addition to this cosmetic effect, the wax coating for a short time slows the loss of moisture, which causes weight loss and wilting. The nutritional advantage of waxing, if any, would be expected to be only very small. At present there is no reason to believe that the use of waxes approved for this purpose is hazardous to health.

CUTTING, TRIMMING AND PEELING

Trimming, peeling and cutting, used to remove inedible or undesirable portions from food, will obviously lead to nutrient loss. There is often a higher concentration of some nutrients in the outer portions of fruits and vegetables. Discarding the outer leaves of vegetables such as cabbage, spinach and lettuce and peeling fruits and vegetables such as apples, peaches, pears, potatoes and carrots, lead to a disproportionate loss of many vitamins. These foods still remain nutritious, but there would be greater benefit if they were eaten intact. It is wise to discard the outer parts only if they are inedible, limp or too difficult to clean. Removal of the stalk does not have a significant effect on nutrient content.

Trimming the fat from meat can be beneficial in reducing energy intake as well as decreasing the amount of saturated fat in the diet.

BLANCHING

Blanching is the heating of fruit or vegetables for a short time with either steam or water, and is an essential step before canning, drying or freezing of food. This heating process is not meant to cook the food but to inactivate substances that would otherwise adversely affect the nutrient content, colour, flavour or texture during subsequent processing and storage. Varying amounts of nutrients are lost in this process, in particular the water-soluble vitamins B-1, B-2, C, niacin and folacin.

COOKING

Cooking can be both detrimental and beneficial to the nutrient content of food.

Beneficial effects of cooking

Cooking is important in food processing. Although cooking results in the loss of some nutrients, it can also convert other nutrients into a form that would otherwise not be used by our bodies. Cooking also produces the desired texture, flavour and palatability we want in our food.

Starchy foods such as potatoes, corn, beans, and lentils are made more digestible by cooking. The nutritive value of the protein in legumes such as soya beans, lima beans, lentils and chick peas is also improved by cooking. Heating these foods destroys substances that would otherwise interfere with the digestibility of the protein. Adequate cooking of the foods is particularly important when they comprise the main source of protein. Other substances in soya beans, kidney beans and lentils can produce toxic effects unless cooked prior to eating. Egg whites and some fish, unless cooked, are not an effective source of the vitamins biotin and vitamin B-1 respectively. Heating flour during baking increases the amount of niacin that can be utilized by the body.

Cooking is also necessary to ensure that food is free from harmful levels of micro-organisms. As well as causing undesirable flavours and odours in food these organisms can sometimes lead to illness.

Nutrient loss during cooking

Losses of protein and carbohydrate during cooking are generally small. The amount of fat in food may be either reduced or increased depending on the method of cooking. Generally, grilling will lower the fat content and frying will increase it. The smaller the size of the pieces being fried, the greater the amount of fat that will be absorbed per 100 grams. The largest vitamin loss during cooking is usually due to destruction of vitamin C, and to a lesser extent vitamin B-1 and the other water-soluble vitamins. A few simple guidelines for maximizing vitamin retention during cooking are listed in Figure 31.

FIGURE 31: HOW TO MINIMIZE NUTRIENT LOSSES DURING COOKING

1 Choose fresh foods that are not over-ripe, bruised, cut or scraped.
2 Store foods in a cool, dark place.
3 Unless the peel or outer layer is unpalatable, damaged or contaminated, cook the food whole.
4 If it is necessary to slice the raw food, then try to keep the pieces as large as possible.
5 When boiling, add the raw food to the boiling water rather than to cold water.
6 Use the smallest amount of water possible; it is not necessary to cover the food. Steaming is a way of cooking with a minimum amount of water.
7 If possible use the cooking water for gravies, sauces or soups as it is a source of water-soluble vitamins and elements (minerals).
8 Cook for the minimum time necessary to make the food palatable and safe. Once cooked, eat as soon as possible. Do not keep the food warm for long periods.
9 Do not use baking soda to help keep the green colour of vegetables, as this increases loss of vitamin C.
10 Do not use copper utensils. (Copper helps to destroy vitamin C.)

Pressure cooking

Pressure cooking involves cooking at higher temperatures for shorter times compared with normal boiling. Because the vegetables are in contact with steam rather than boiling water, less of the water-soluble vitamins dissolve in the cooking water. Generally, pressure cooking will retain more nutrients than normal boiling. However, food steamed or boiled in a small amount of water in a tightly covered saucepan is likely to be as nutritious as food cooked in a pressure cooker.

Microwave ovens

Microwave cooking is much quicker than conventional cooking. The microwaves preferentially heat the water in food so that the cooking process is essentially similar to that of steam cooking. With meat, the differences in vitamin B-1 and vitamin B-2 retention between microwave cooking and conventional grilling or roasting are small. With vegetables, the vitamin C in microwave-cooked food is similar to that achieved by cooking with steam or using a small amount of water in a tightly covered saucepan. Generally, microwave cooking retains nutrients as well as conventional methods.

FREEZING

The major nutrient losses that occur in frozen foods are not due to freezing as such but due to the blanching that occurs before freezing, and then during subsequent thawing and cooking. In general, these losses are not greatly different from those incurred following purchase of 'market fresh' food and cooking it. The quality of some frozen fruits and vegetables is often superior to so-called 'fresh' produce, as they can be frozen very soon after being harvested.

It is important that frozen foods are stored at −18°C to prevent their rapid deterioration (see page 37). If this temperature is not maintained then some nutrient losses will occur, which are not regained by refreezing.

DEHYDRATION

Dehydration or the drying of foods is a method of preservation. With the exceptions of vitamin C and provitamin A, the nutrient losses that occur in drying are not large. Further losses can occur depending on how the dried food is further processed. If the food is eaten in the dried form, such as dried apricots, then the food is a concentrated source of many nutrients, including dietary fibre (see specific foods in the Food Charts). If the food is left in water to rehydrate, or is boiled, then there will be the additional normal cooking losses.

CANNING

Canning involves heating food in a closed container to ensure that the micro-organisms present in the raw food can no longer cause deterioration of the food or be hazardous to health. The amount of the heating depends on the type of food. Nutrient losses occur from destruction during heating and storage stages. Some nutrients, such as water-soluble vitamins and minerals, may dissolve in the water in the can, but they are lost only if this liquid is not consumed. We can reduce losses of vitamins during storage by storing the cans in a cool place.

Nutrient losses resulting from canning are generally greater than those for the same food when prepared from the fresh state in the home. However, this must be balanced against the convenience of having foods available at all times of the year no matter where we live or what the season.

PASTEURIZATION

The main pasteurized foods that contribute significant nutrients are milk and some fruit juices. Pasteurization involves heating food for a short time to kill harmful micro-organisms that are present in the food. Not all micro-organisms are destroyed, and spoilage of the food may still occur on storage, but this can be delayed by refrigeration. Nutrient losses during pasteurization of milk and fruit juices are generally small, and in the case of fruit juices they must contain not less than a specified minimum amount of vitamin C. This generally means that vitamin C is added by the processor to make up for any losses that occurred during processing. To minimize further nutrient losses, milk and fruit juices should be stored away from light and in a cool place.

TOASTING

A loss of about 10 to 30 per cent of the vitamin B-1 present in bread occurs on toasting.

SPROUTING

The consumption of seed sprouts such as beans and peas is quite widespread, particularly in China, India and Egypt. Sprouted seeds require much shorter cooking time than the dry seeds. In addition, there is an increase in the vitamin C content and also in some B-group vitamins.

STABILITY OF NUTRIENTS IN FOOD

The stability of nutrients in food depends on their environment. Nutrients can be lost to varying degrees depending on whether the food is exposed to light or air, acid or alkali, the temperature and their ability to dissolve in water. Generally the losses of carbohydrate, fat, protein, vitamin K, niacin, biotin and elements are small during processing and storage. Greatest losses are usually seen with vitamins B-1 and C, with intermediate losses shown by vitamin A, provitamin A and vitamins D, E, B-2, B-6, B-12, pantothenic acid and folacin.

Losses may be due to destruction of the nutrient or by dissolving in water that is later thrown away. The presence of acid (from other foods or addition of vinegar) or alkali (from other foods or added sodium bicarbonate (baking soda)) can cause destruction of some vitamins. The stability characteristics of nutrients are shown in Figure 32.

FIGURE 32: STABILITY OF NUTRIENTS IN FOOD

NUTRIENT	STABILITY CHARACTERISTICS
Vitamin A and provitamin A	Reasonably stable during processing. Losses occur when dehydrated foods are exposed to light and air
Vitamin D	Relatively stable but sensitive to exposure to air and light
Vitamin E	Relatively stable but foods cooked in oil can have large losses
Vitamin K	Relatively stable but sensitive to light
Vitamin B-1 (thiamin)	Large losses under neutral and alkaline conditions where baking powder is used (e.g. cakes). Dissolves in cooking water. There is reasonable retention in cooked meat
Vitamin B-2 (riboflavin)	Very sensitive to light. Relatively stable to most home cooking methods. Losses can occur in drippings from meat
Niacin	Stable to most processing. Dissolves in cooking water
Vitamin B-6	Moderate retention during most processing. In milk it is sensitive to light
Vitamin B-12	Moderate retention, but losses occur when heated under mild acid and alkaline conditions
Folacin	Relatively stable but large losses can occur on cooking. Presence of copper aids destruction
Pantothenic acid	Relatively stable during home cooking but losses occur in meat drippings and cooking water
Biotin	Good retention during most home processing
Vitamin C	Relatively unstable and losses occur from exposure to air, light, heat and copper. Dissolves in cooking water
Elements	Stable to most processing but losses can occur by dissolving in cooking water

STORAGE LIFE OF FOODS

The home storage lives of various foods are shown in Figures 33 to 37. These storage lives are only a rough approximation as the actual life of a particular food will depend on the initial quality, the type of processing, the storage temperature, the type of packaging, the moisture content of the food, the extent of contact with air and other factors. There is no precise moment at which a food suddenly becomes undesirable. There is just a gradual deterioration; the colour may darken, the texture may soften or there may be loss of flavour or development of an off-flavour. There comes a time when there is a discernible change from the initial quality. The detection of this change will vary between individuals. Changes that occur in a food when stored at temperatures higher than recommended are cumulative and cannot be reversed by returning the food to lower temperatures. The longer the storage time, the greater the deterioration in nutritional quality and palatability. In extreme cases the action of microbes can make the food unsafe to eat. Modern methods of food preservation, such as freezing, refrigeration and canning, considerably extend, above the normal, the time taken for a comparable loss of nutrients and eating quality.

Many food labels now include a date mark that gives an indication of the expected life of the food before a noticeable deterioration in quality occurs. The significance of the different forms of date marking is discussed on page 24. The 'use-by' or 'minimum durable life' date is only applicable if the food is stored under the conditions specified on the label. If no special storage conditions are required normal cupboard storage should give the stated storage life.

FROZEN FOODS

The recommended maximum storage times shown in Figure 33 for foods in the home freezer are probably conservative. If temperatures are carefully controlled at −18°C and the food was initially of high quality then longer storage times can be achieved. However, most home freezers are used for freezing as well as storage. This results in temperatures rising above −18°C, which decreases optimum storage life. Some deterioration in quality may have already taken place before the food is frozen; for instance it may have been left in a hot car while shopping. At −18°C loss in quality is very much slowed but not completely stopped. These slow changes, which limit the storage life, do not have a marked effect on nutrient content but eventually cause a noticeable change in eating quality. Frozen foods do not become unsafe to eat even if kept for many years at −18°C (see page 41 for safe handling of frozen foods).

To remain aware of storage time, each package should be marked with the date as it is placed in the freezer.

FIGURE 33: EXPECTED STORAGE LIFE FOR SOME FROZEN FOODS

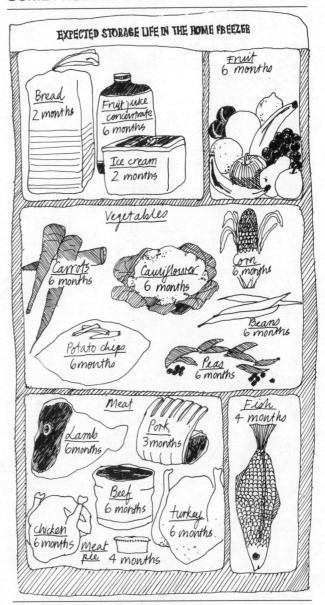

EXPECTED STORAGE LIFE IN THE HOME FREEZER

Bread 2 months
Fruit juice concentrate 6 months
Ice cream 2 months
Fruit 6 months
Vegetables
Carrots 6 months
Cauliflower 6 months
Corn 6 months
Beans 6 months
Potato chips 6 months
Peas 6 months
Meat
Lamb 6 months
Pork 3 months
Beef 6 months
Chicken 6 months
Meat pie 4 months
Turkey 6 months
Fish 4 months

Adapted from CSIRO (Australia) pamphlet: *Storage life of food.*

CANNED FOODS

The storage lives for the canned foods listed in Figure 34 are for cool, dry conditions. Some canned hams and imported fish must be refrigerated during storage. Always read labels to see if any special storage conditions are needed. Longer storage times result in a gradual decrease in quality and nutrients, but the foods are still quite safe to eat. Do not open any cans that are swollen or leaking as this indicates faulty pro-cessing; and do not buy cans that are dented or rusted. Once opened, if the contents are not eaten, they should be covered and stored in a refrigerator. Some acid and salty foods such as fruit juices, tomatoes and rhubarb should be removed from the can before refrigerating.

HOME STORAGE OF FOOD

Fruit and vegetables

The storage lives of fruit and vegetables vary enormously, being influenced by the maturity and quality of the produce at purchase and also the particular variety. Generally, the lower the storage temperature (but not below 0°C), the longer the produce can be stored. However, some fruits and vegetables, particularly bananas and most other tropical fruits, are damaged when kept in a refrigerator. Many fruits and vegetables can dry out in a refrigerator and it is a good idea, once they are chilled, to place them in the crisper or in a plastic bag with a few holes in it. If a refrigerator is not available, find a cool dry place for storage.

The storage times given in Figures 35 and 36 apply to sound, mature, ripe produce. Changes in nutritional quality and palatability are gradual and there is often no sharp cut-off point at which the food is no longer acceptable. Consequently, storage lives vary considerably, and those listed in the tables are for guidance only. Fruits and vegetables not fully ripe when purchased will have a longer storage life. Fruits ripen best at about 20°C and the unripe fruit can be removed from the refrigerator and ripened as needed. For example, unripe avocados will keep in a refrigerator for up to 3 weeks, whereas the ripe fruit will keep for a few days only. Pears bought hard and green can be kept in a refrigerator for fairly long periods; those that are bought ripe will only last a few days. Potatoes keep quite well in a cool *dark* place. You should discard any potatoes with large areas of green skin as they contain a poisonous substance called solanine (see Figure 29). Potatoes with a small area of green are safe if they are deeply peeled and the peel discarded.

FIGURE 34: EXPECTED STORAGE LIFE FOR SOME CANNED FOODS

EXPECTED STORAGE LIFE IN A COOL, DRY AREA

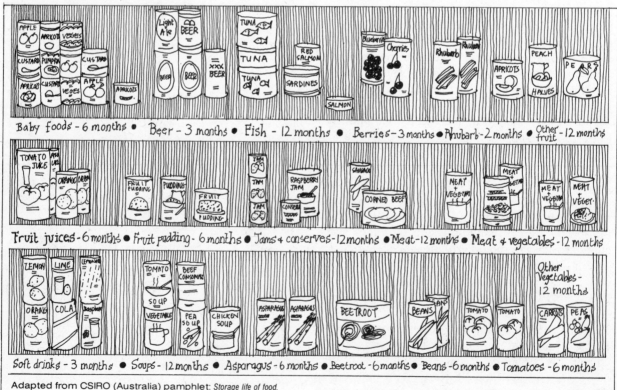

Baby foods - 6 months • Beer - 3 months • Fish - 12 months • Berries - 3 months • Rhubarb - 2 months • Other fruit - 12 months

Fruit juices - 6 months • Fruit pudding - 6 months • Jams & conserves - 12 months • Meat - 12 months • Meat & vegetables - 12 months

Soft drinks - 3 months • Soups - 12 months • Asparagus - 6 months • Beetroot - 6 months • Beans - 6 months • Tomatoes - 6 months

Adapted from CSIRO (Australia) pamphlet: *Storage life of food.*

FIGURE 35: HOME STORAGE LIFE FOR SOME RIPE FRUITS

FRUIT	CONDITIONS	APPROXIMATE STORAGE LIFE
Apples	Refrigerator	Several weeks depending on the variety
Apricots	Refrigerator	2-3 days
Avocados	Refrigerator	Several days
Bananas	Cool place	2-3 days
Cherries	Refrigerator	1-2 weeks
Grapes	Cool place	1-2 weeks
Grapefruit	Cool place	2-4 weeks
Lemons	Cool place	3-6 weeks
Pawpaw	Cool place	2-3 days
Peaches	Refrigerator	2-3 days
Pears	Refrigerator	Few days
Pineapples	Cool place	Several days
Mandarins	Cool place	2-3 weeks
Mangoes	Cool place	3-4 days
Oranges	Cool place	2-3 weeks
Passionfruit	Cool place	2 weeks
Raspberries	Refrigerator	Several days
Strawberries	Refrigerator	Several days
Watermelon	Refrigerator	1-2 weeks

Adapted from E. C. Hall, 'Handling and storing fresh fruit and vegetables in the home', *CSIRO Food Research Quarterly*, volume 39, 1979.

FIGURE 36: HOME STORAGE LIFE FOR SOME RIPE VEGETABLES

VEGETABLE	CONDITIONS	APPROXIMATE STORAGE LIFE
Asparagus	Refrigerator	2 weeks
Beetroot	Cool place	2-3 weeks
Broccoli	Refrigerator	2 weeks
Brussel sprouts	Refrigerator	2 weeks
Cabbage	Refrigerator	2-3 weeks
Capsicums	Refrigerator	1 week
Carrots	Cool place	2-3 weeks
Celery	Refrigerator	2-3 weeks
Cucumbers	Refrigerator	1 week
Lettuce	Refrigerator	7-10 days
Onions	Cool, dry place	Several weeks, depending on variety
Peas	Refrigerator	2 weeks
Parsnips	Cool place	2-3 weeks
Potatoes	Cool, dark, dry place	2-3 months
Pumpkin (whole)	Cool, dry place	2-3 months
Tomatoes	Refrigerator	7-10 days
Zucchinis	Refrigerator	1 week

Adapted from E. C. Hall, 'Handling and storing fresh fruit and vegetables in the home', *CSIRO Food Research Quarterly*, volume 39, 1979.

Other foods

The expected storage lives of foods other than fruit and vegetables are only approximate and depend very much on how the food was treated after purchase. If, for example, butter was left in a hot car for a short time, then the storage life until a deterioration in quality was noticed would be dramatically reduced. Similarly, if the packaging of breakfast cereals, for example, was damaged or opened, the storage life could not be expected to be the same as for an unopened package.

FIGURE 37: HOME STORAGE LIFE FOR SOME OTHER FOODS

FOOD	STORAGE CONDITION	EXPECTED STORAGE LIFE IN THE HOME

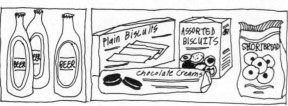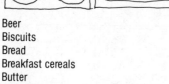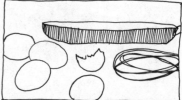

Food	Storage condition	Expected storage life
Beer	25°C or lower	3 months
Biscuits	Cool, dry place	6-10 weeks
Bread	20-25°C	1-4 days
Breakfast cereals	Cool, dry place	2-3 months
Butter	Refrigerator	6-8 weeks
Cake mixes	Cool, dry place	1-2 years

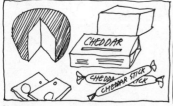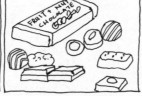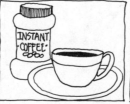

Food	Storage condition	Expected storage life
Cheese:		
Cheddar, edam, gouda	Refrigerator	3 months
Processed cheddar	25°C or lower	6-9 months
Chocolate — dark, milk	25°C or lower	3 months
Coffee — instant	25°C or lower	3 months
Eggs	25°C or lower	1-2 weeks

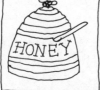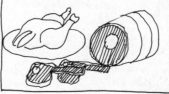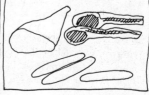

Food	Storage condition	Expected storage life
Flour	Cool, dry place	12 months
Honey	8-10°C	8 months
Margarine	Refrigerator	6-12 weeks
Meat, fresh:		
Chicken	Refrigerator	3 days
Beef, lamb, pork, veal	Refrigerator	5 days
Meat, cured — bacon, ham, frankfurters	Refrigerator	2-3 weeks

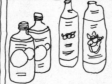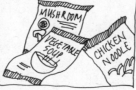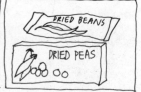

Food	Storage condition	Expected storage life
Milk	Refrigerator	5-7 days
Sauce — tomato, Worcestershire, other vinegar-based	25°C or lower	1-2 years
Soft drinks	25°C or lower	3-6 months
Soups — dried	25°C or lower	8 months
Sugar	Cool, dry place	2-3 years
Vegetables — dried	25°C or lower	6 months

Adapted from CSIRO (Australia) pamphlet: *Storage life of food.*

H E A L T H P R O B L E M S A S S O C I A T E D W I T H S O M E F O O D S

HOW TO AVOID FOOD POISONING

Micro-organisms are present almost everywhere: in the air, soil, on our hands, in our bodies and in food. Not all of these tiny organisms are harmful and some are essential for good health and the production of food and drugs. Some can cause food spoilage and illness. Most forms of food processing either destroy these micro-organisms or reduce their numbers to safe levels.

Most micro-organisms can grow and multiply at temperatures between 15°C and 63°C, with most rapid growth occurring around 37°C. It is important that food is not held in this temperature range for long periods, as the food may become contaminated with large numbers of micro-organisms and cause illness. At higher temperatures most harmful micro-organisms are destroyed, and at lower temperatures, such as in the refrigerator (1-4°C) or the deep freeze (−18°C), there is little or no growth. When cold foods are warmed, the micro-organisms will start to grow and multiply. Therefore it is important to heat food rapidly. The shorter the time spent in the temperature range where rapid growth of micro-organisms occurs, the lower the chance of food poisoning.

Some frozen foods such as vegetables, precooked foods and smaller cuts of meat can be cooked directly from the frozen state. Large cuts of meat should be thawed prior to cooking or extra cooking time should be allowed to ensure that the interior temperature reaches 71°C. Thawing is best carried out by placing the food in a refrigerator; allow at least 16 hours per kilogram. If not used after thawing it can be kept in the refrigerator chilling section for 1 to 2 days. Food that has been allowed to thaw in the kitchen should be cooked soon after thawing and not stored in a refrigerator. Packaged frozen foods have instructions on how best to prepare the food for eating. It is not advisable to re-freeze foods that have been thawed.

Because micro-organisms are very widespread, contamination of food can occur easily. Personal hygiene and a few precautions can prevent this leading to food poisoning and illness (see Figure 39).

FIGURE 38: IMPORTANT TEMPERATURES IN FOOD PREPARATION

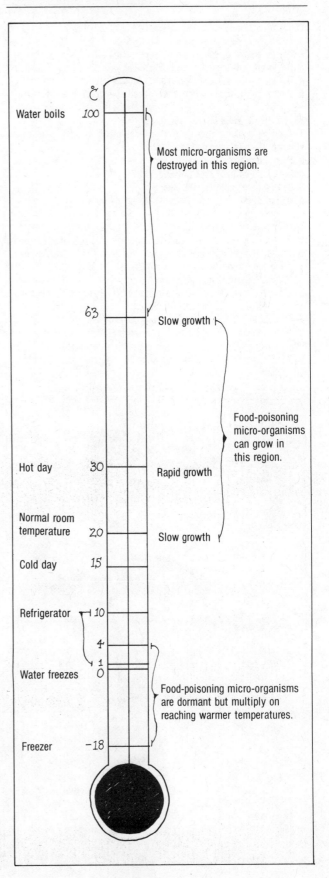

FIGURE 39: HOW TO AVOID FOOD POISONING

PERSONAL HYGIENE
1 Wash your hands before preparing food.
2 Do not smoke or comb hair when preparing food.
3 Cover any cut or pimple with dressings.
4 Do not handle pets when preparing food.
5 When tasting food do not return licked utensils to the food.

PRECAUTIONS WHEN PREPARING FOODS
1 Keep all cooking utensils and surfaces clean. Discard cracked and chipped utensils and crockery.
2 Do not use the same knives, chopping boards etc. for both raw and cooked food without first washing them.
3 Keep food as cold as possible.
4 Do not store raw food where it can contaminate cooked food. Water or blood from raw meat or fish can cause contamination by dripping onto cooked food stored below.
5 Heat food as rapidly and cook as thoroughly as possible. Remember the inside temperature can be much lower than that on the surface.
6 If the food is not to be eaten immediately after cooking, cool it as quickly as possible and keep it in the refrigerator until it is ready to be served or reheated. Large pieces of food should be sliced into smaller pieces to allow it to cool more rapidly.
7 Do not keep food warm; keep it either hot or cold.
8 When reheating food, heat quickly and thoroughly, so that even the middle of the food pieces have reached a high temperature.
9 Handle cooked food as little as possible; use serving tongs etc.
10 Discard any food that has gone 'off' (off-odour, mouldy, slimy). Storing at lower temperatures will not stop further deterioration.

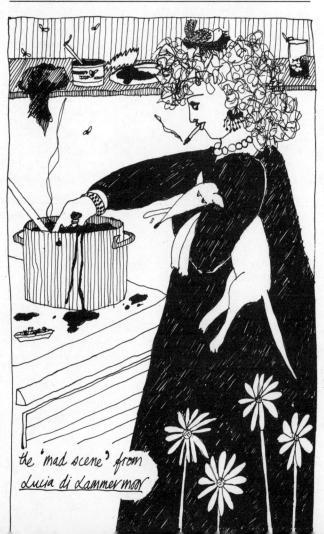

the 'mad scene' from
Lucia di Lammermoor

FOOD SENSITIVITIES

An allergic response to food can show itself in a number of ways, as indicated in Figure 40. It is important that possible causes of the disorder other than allergy be considered. A wheezing patient could have asthma due to an allergy, but the wheezing could also be due to bronchitis, infection, heart disease or cancer. Diagnosis of food allergy needs careful medical interpretation of the patient's history. This should include dietary background and the effects of 'elimination' diets, in which the suspected food(s) have first been excluded, and then reintroduced to the patient to compare the results. Although there may be improvement after the elimination diet, with a return of symptoms when the food is reintroduced, there can still be some doubt whether food allergy is the cause of the condition. There are many causes of intolerances or sensitivities to food, and not all of them are due to allergy. For example, coeliac disease (see Chart 50) can produce effects similar to cow's milk allergy.

FIGURE 40: SYMPTOMS SOMETIMES DUE TO FOOD ALLERGY

Digestive system:	Diarrhoea Vomiting Abdominal pain
Skin:	Hives Rashes Eczema Swelling or puffiness
Respiratory system:	Allergic rhinitis (hayfever, sinus trouble) Asthma Wheezy bronchitis.
Behavioural and nervous system:	Headache Irritability Fatigue Convulsive seizures Depression
Others:	Dizziness Ringing in the ears (tinnitus) Aches and pains in muscles and joints Bladder inflammation

The foods most commonly responsible for allergic reactions are listed in Figure 41. Food additives have occasionally been thought to cause allergic reactions. The additives most commonly implicated are tartrazine, a yellow dye used in many foods, beverages and pharmaceuticals; also, benzoic acid and sulphur dioxide, which are used as preservatives in some fruit drinks, cordials, soft drinks and wines.

FIGURE 41: FOODS COMMONLY RESPONSIBLE FOR ALLERGY

Dairy products:	Milk
	Cheese
Eggs	
Fish	
Shellfish	
Cereals:	Wheat
	Rice
	Corn
	Barley
	Rye
	Oats
Vegetables:	Tomatoes
	Mushrooms
Fruit:	Bananas
	Oranges
	Mangoes
	Pineapples
	Strawberries
Nuts:	Brazil
	Walnut
Seeds:	Sesame
	Poppy
	Caraway
	Fennel
	Coriander
	Anise
Meat:	Chicken
	Pork
	Veal
Chocolate	

FIGURE 42: FOODS COMMONLY REPORTED AS CAUSING MIGRAINE

Cheese
Chocolate
Alcoholic drinks
Beans
Citrus fruits
Fried, fatty food
Tomatoes
Onions
Dairy products
Pineapple

Many other foods are implicated, but less frequently. There have been conflicting results from scientific studies examining the effects of food on migraine sufferers; probably a combination of factors is involved in triggering an attack. It may be that there is a spectrum of response to dietary items, varying from very mild to very intense. With some sufferers, a particular food might always precipitate an attack, while with others, the food trigger may only be effective in combination with other factors, such as hormonal change or stress.

Diets that avoid certain foods can have serious nutritional consequences if maintained for long periods, depending on the number and type of foods avoided, and they should only be followed under the supervision of a doctor or dietitian.

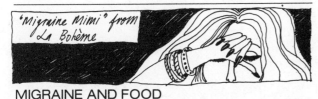

'Migraine Mimi' from La Bohème

MIGRAINE AND FOOD

A variety of factors have been reported to trigger migraine attacks. Stress is probably the most widely recognized trigger for migraine. Stress may be brought about by emotional shock, noise, glare or some other condition. Some studies on migraine have claimed that diet is a trigger factor. Between 5 and 30 per cent of migraine sufferers believe that food plays a part in their migraine. Much of the evidence linking diet and migraine is scientifically unsound. It frequently relies on the patient recognizing a link between the eating of a certain food and the attack. Such links may be difficult to establish, particularly if the food responsible is consumed up to 24 hours before the attack. The foods most commonly associated with triggering migraine are given in Figure 42.

THE FEINGOLD DIET AND HYPERKINESIS

The name hyperkinesis refers to a broad range of symptoms seen in some children. These include physical overactivity that is inappropriate for the task, short attention span and other abnormal responses. Some years ago Dr Ben Feingold, of the Allergy Department of the Kaiser-Permanente Medical Centre in San Francisco, advanced the hypothesis that salicylates (chemicals that occur naturally in some foods), food flavours and food colours were associated with hyperkinesis and learning disabilities in some children. Feingold claimed that approximately 50 per cent of children with hyperkinesis and learning difficulties improved when kept on a strict diet that excluded foods containing salicylates and artificial colours and flavours.

Many studies have been conducted to investigate this hypothesis. The results of the studies are uncertain but it is quite clear that the improvement rate is far lower than that originally claimed.

Average Serving Sizes of Sample Meals
Breakfast

Orange Juice (120g)   Toast (25g)   Eggs (2 × 60g)
Cornflakes (30g)   Butter (10g)   Bacon (40g)
Bran (8g)   Jam (30g)
Milk (115g)   Tea (230g)
Sugar (5g)

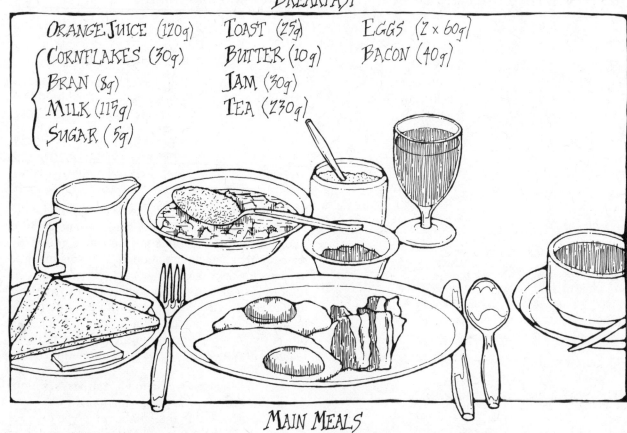

Main Meals

Tomato Soup (230g)   Tomato Juice (120g)
Chicken (130g)   Beef (120g)
Potato (120g)   Potato (120g)
Sprouts (70g)   Carrots (50g)
Cauliflower (100g)   Spinach (60g)
Peaches (120g) and Cream (30g)   Pineapple (80g) and Cream (30g)

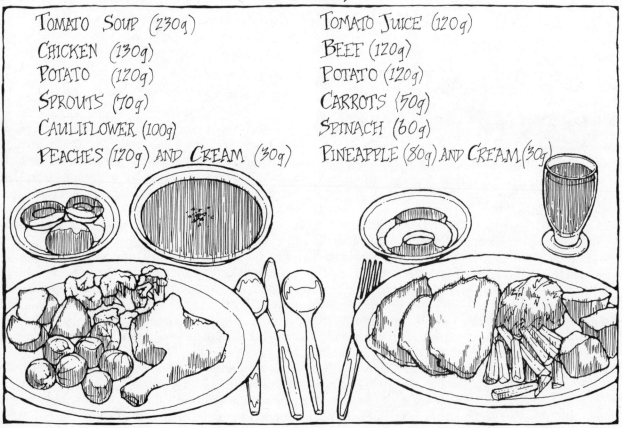

FOOD CHARTS

The food composition charts list values for all significant nutrients in many foods. Additional charts of special interest are also included. Many of the values listed are based on those in *The Composition of Foods* by A.A. Paul and D.A.T. Southgate (U.K.), and *Tables of Composition of Australian Foods* by S. Thomas and M. Corden. In addition, values from our own laboratories in the Department of Human Nutrition at Deakin University and other Australian sources are included.

Values for nutrients in food can vary widely and depend on such things as: the growing environment, the particular variety or breed, the method of processing, the storage temperature and time etc. The values given in the charts are a good indication of nutritional value. You can see at a glance which foods are rich or deficient in particular nutrients.

The charts:

• enable you to know what nutrients are present in which foods
• show which foods are particularly good or poor sources of nutrients
• give a quick comparison of the nutrient content of different foods
• allow you to estimate your own intake of a particular nutrient and compare it with that recommended (the RDI). In doing so, remember that the nutrient value given is a best estimate only, and also that recommended intakes have been developed for groups of people amongst whom there is wide individual variation.

There are 50 charts, each for one nutrient or other component of foods. Each is preceded by an introduction giving the characteristics of that particular food component. You will see that:

• the charts give nutrient values for 414 different foods. The same 414 foods are listed on most charts but there are some charts for which less information is currently available. The lists of foods in these charts is therefore shorter. In these cases, remember that if a food item is not included in the list, it does not necessarily mean that there is none of that particular component in that food.
• the foods are grouped in categories, such as Soups, Vegetables, etc. (see Figure 43B). You can find the same food in the same place in each chart. This allows a scan through each chart so that all nutrient values for a particular food can be quickly located and compared. This can be useful for assessing the nutritive value of a particular food. (For example, confectionery is very high in kilocalories and carbohydrate but a scan through other charts quickly shows it contributes insignificant amounts of other nutrients. In contrast, while a steak and kidney pie is also high in kilocalories and carbohydrate it also provides protein, several elements, vitamins B-1, B-2 and niacin.)
• each food, where practicable, is given an *average serving size* to help you work out your daily intake for a particular nutrient.

HOW TO USE THE CHARTS

The following points should help you get the best use out of the charts.

AVERAGE SERVING SIZE

Immediately after each food is a quantity given in brackets. This is the size in grams of an *average* serving. For example, 'Chicken, roast (130g)' means that the average amount of roast chicken in a single serving is 130 grams.

In the case of some food ingredients it is not possible to estimate an average serving size because this will depend on the particular food in which the ingredient is present, for example for flour; this is then indicated by a dash: '(—)'. To estimate nutrient intake from this particular ingredient you would need to know how much was present in the food you ate.

Many people eat servings that are smaller or larger than the average size. Compare your usual size with the pictures of average servings on page 44 or weigh your food before eating. You will soon be able to estimate whether your servings are average, large or small. Notice the following:

• the weight given for the average serving is for *one unit* of the food (e.g. one biscuit, one slice of melon), *unless otherwise indicated.* If an average serving usually comprises more than one unit, the average number of units is given. For example, 'Fish fingers (5 = 100g)' means 5 fish fingers comprise an average serving of 100 grams.

• the average serving size of drinks is also given in grams to make comparison of nutrients easier. Liquids are usually measured in millilitres (ml); a good approximation is that one millilitre weighs one gram.

NUTRIENT INTAKE

On the chart, the figure to the left of the food shows the amount of the nutrient that is present in 100 grams of the food. The bar which extends to the left allows comparison at a glance of the nutrient content of the food. The longer the bar, the greater the amount of nutrient in 100 grams of the food. The bar quickly allows you to identify foods that are high or low sources of a given nutrient.

When you know your serving size you can work out your nutrient intake. An average serving of boiled rice, for example, would weigh 160 grams. 100 grams of boiled rice contain 125 kilocalories of energy, so 160 grams would contain (125 ÷ 100) x 160 which is 200 kilocalories. If your serving size is very different from the average size, you will need to take this into account.

While it is interesting to calculate the values of your food intake in order to inform yourself about nutrient values, you will probably find that, as you learn, you will need to do calculations less often. You can look forward then to quick, informal scans, which just confirm what you thought — that spinach *does* contain lots of nutrients, or that 3 slices of that delicious salami *will* contain 490 kilocalories or about one-quarter of your daily energy allowance.

The amount of nutrient or food component is given as grams, milligrams, micrograms, kilocalories or kilojoules per 100 grams of food. (Some nutrients are only present in very small amounts.)

1 ounce = 28 grams
1 pound = 454 grams
1 milligram = 1/1000 gram
1 microgram = 1/1000 milligram
1 kilojoule = 1/4 kilocalorie
1 kilocalorie = 4.2 kilojoules (approximately 4)
1 millilitre (ml) approximately weighs 1 gram
1 pint = 568 millilitres

RECOMMENDED DAILY INTAKE (RDI)

The RDI for each nutrient is given, whenever available, in the introduction to each chart.

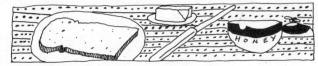

WHEN YOU CANNOT FIND THE INFORMATION

If you cannot find the information about a particular food (and have looked in the right place) it may be that the food is not listed. Obviously it is not practical to include all foods; the list would become too cumbersome. In some instances the foods may not have been analysed at all or analysed only for some nutrients and not others. This is indicated by a dash in the value column: this does not necessarily mean that there is little or none of that nutrient present.

If a food is not listed you can usually get some idea of the nutrient content by looking up similar foods (e.g. zucchini is not listed but it is very similar to marrow; the values given for marrow will be a good approximation for zucchini.) The chart of biological sources of food (Figure 3) will be helpful here.

In a similar way, you can estimate the nutrients in a particular dish by looking up values listed for the individual ingredients or food items.

SOME EXAMPLES FROM THE CHARTS

If you look up Bread on the Energy chart, you'll find: '240 Bread, brown, slice (25g)'. This means that an average slice of brown bread weighs 25 grams and that 100 grams, i.e. four slices, contain 240 kilocalories of energy. Therefore one slice will contain 240 ÷ 4 = 60 kilocalories. If you eat more than one slice you will need to count 60 kilocalories for each slice when you are working out the total amount of energy you are consuming. If you have average servings of butter and honey on each slice, you'll have to add another 73 plus 117 kilocalories for each slice.

You can see what other nutrients are in brown bread by looking this item up in each chart. For example, 100 grams contain 8 grams of protein; therefore one slice (25 grams) contains 2 grams of protein.

Similarly we can find out how much vitamin B-1 is in a slice of brown bread. A vitamin is a micronutrient, being present in minute quantities, so the value will be given in milligrams. There are 0.2 milligrams of vitamin B-1 in 100 grams of brown bread (four slices), so one slice contributes 0.05 milligrams of B-1 to a recommended daily intake of 0.8 milligrams.

Other nutrients in brown bread are present in very small or even 'trace' quantities; for example, there is only 0.4 gram of saturated fat and only a trace of vitamin E.

FIGURE 43: NOTES FOR USE OF CHARTS

(A) NUTRIENTS AND OTHER COMPONENTS LISTED IN THE CHARTS

1 Energy: kilojoules/kilocalories
2 Water
3 Dietary fibre
4 Protein
5 Phenylalanine
6 Carbohydrate
7 Fat
8 Cholesterol
9 Saturated fat and polyunsaturated fat
10 Alcohol

FAT-SOLUBLE VITAMINS

11 Vitamin A
12 Provitamin A
13 Vitamin D
14 Vitamin E
15 Vitamin K

WATER-SOLUBLE VITAMINS

16 Vitamin B-1
17 Vitamin B-2
18 Niacin
19 Vitamin B-6
20 Vitamin B-12
21 Folacin
22 Pantothenic acid
23 Biotin
24 Vitamin C

ELEMENTS

25 Sodium
26 Potassium
27 Calcium
28 Magnesium

29 Iron
30 Phosphorus
31 Sulphur
32 Chlorine
33 Copper
34 Zinc
35 Iodine
36 Fluorine
37 Chromium
38 Manganese
39 Selenium
40 Cobalt
41 Molybdenum
42 Nickel
43 Tin
44 Silicon
45 Vanadium
46 Cadmium
47 Other elements:
   Aluminium
   Antimony
   Arsenic
   Barium
   Boron
   Bromine
   Gold
   Lead
   Mercury
   Rhubidium
   Silver
   Strontium

OTHER FOOD COMPONENTS

48 Lecithin
49 Caffeine
50 Gluten

(B) FOOD CATEGORIES, AS ORDERED IN THE CHARTS

Beverages
Cereals, biscuits, cakes and desserts
Egg and cheese dishes
Fats and oils
Fish and other seafoods
Fruit
Meat and meat products
Milk and milk products
Nuts
Sauces and condiments
Soups
Sugar, jams and spreads
Sweets and confectionery
Vegetables

(C) SYMBOLS USED IN THE CHARTS

(00g) — average serving size
(—) — amount not known (the food has not yet been analysed for this nutrient)
Tr — a trace only is present; not significant
0 — none of the nutrient has been detected in the food analysed
▬▬ — bar graph representing the nutrient content (the amount of the nutrient in 100 grams of food), allowing a direct visual comparison with other foods

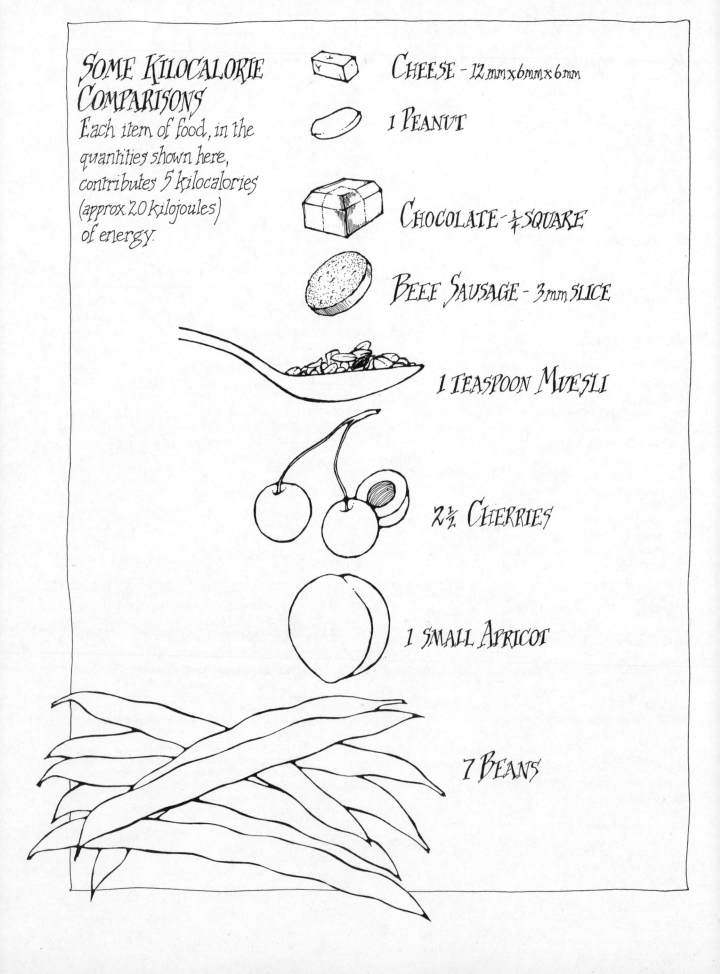

Some Kilocalorie Comparisons

Each item of food, in the quantities shown here, contributes 5 kilocalories (approx. 20 kilojoules) of energy.

Cheese - 12 mm x 6mm x 6mm

1 Peanut

Chocolate - ⅛ square

Beef Sausage - 3mm slice

1 Teaspoon Muesli

2½ Cherries

1 Small Apricot

7 Beans

1
ENERGY:
KILOCALORIES/KILOJOULES

Energy has traditionally been expressed as calories or kilocalories. More recently, the units of energy have been changed to kilojoules. There are 4.2 kilojoules in 1 kilocalorie. For convenience, both units are shown on the chart. Someone having 2000 kilocalories each day would be having 8400 kilojoules, also known as 8.4 megajoules.

The energy value of a food indicates its value to the body as a fuel. This may be less than the heat value obtained experimentally by 'burning' the food outside the body in what is called a 'bomb calorimeter'. After a food is ingested, some of its energy may be 'lost' during digestion and metabolism. Although the energy value of some foods has been found by combustion in a bomb calorimeter, more usually the amounts of the macronutrients — fat, protein, carbohydrate and alcohol (ethanol) — in a food are taken into account when assessing the total energy value of the food. The energy value for each macronutrient must be known, and an allowance made for body losses. The first system for giving energy values to the macronutrients was described by Dr W. O. Atwater in 1899. Modified, the 'Atwater factors' are:

	kilocalories per gram	kilojoules per gram
Fat	9	37
Alcohol	7	29
Protein	4	17
Carbohydrate	4	16

The energy value of a particular food is calculated from a knowledge of macronutrient composition and the modified Atwater factors for these macronutrients. The energy values shown in the chart have been obtained with this approach.

Fat is the most energy-dense macronutrient, followed by alcohol, protein and carbohydrate. For example, one double Scotch has about twice as many kilocalories as a glass of soft drink; a glass of full-cream milk has about twice the kilocalories as a glass of soft drink or of skimmed milk. Dietary fibre or roughage is not usually ascribed an energy value for humans, but it is now recognized that some dietary fibre components are used as fuels by the microflora (bacteria) of the gut, especially in the large intestine. Some of the products of dietary fibre digestion may provide energy for the gut lining and some may actually be absorbed for general bodily metabolism. Vitamins and elements have no energy value.

Energy requirement can be thought of as the amount needed to maintain the basic processes of life at rest, that is, basal metabolism, plus the amount needed for physical activity under a variety of circumstances. Body weight is an important factor in determining how much energy we need, since more energy will be needed to sustain and move a greater body mass.

You should refer to the charts of energy requirement according to age, sex and level of physical activity (Figures 11 and 12), together with the energy values of foods. However, remember that there is a great deal of individual variation in the efficiency with which ingested food energy is utilized for work by the body. If your body is relatively inefficient in its use of food energy, loss will occur in faeces and by relatively more heat production.

The word 'energy' has been used here in the nutritional sense of 'provider of fuel' and not in the sense of providing zest and vitality. High-energy foods do not necessarily affect how we feel. Food products are sometimes promoted as mood-changers on the basis of their energy value, but this is simply a reflection of the double-meaning of 'energy'.

kJ/kcal

960/230 Egg, fried (60g)
785/190 omelette (100g)
645/155 poached (55g)
610/145 raw (55g)
1020/245 scrambled (70g)
725/175 Macaroni cheese (180g)
1625/390 Quiche Lorraine (150g)

FATS AND OILS

3045/730 Butter, salted (10g)
3665/890 Dripping, beef (–)
3665/890 Lard (–)
3045/730 Margarine (10g)
3695/900 Vegetable oils (–)

FISH AND OTHER SEAFOODS

425/100 Bream, steamed (100g)
410/95 Cod, baked (100g)
835/200 fried in batter (100g)
395/95 poached (100g)
350/85 steamed (100g)
535/125 Crab, boiled (150g)
340/80 canned (90g)
785/190 Fish cakes, fried (4 = 100g)
975/235 fingers, fried (5 = 100g)
1060/250 in batter, fried (120g)
845/200 Flounder, baked (100g)
730/175 Haddock, fried (100g)
415/100 steamed (100g)
500/120 Lobster, boiled (120g)
365/85 Mussels, boiled (12 = 120g)
215/50 Oysters, raw (12 = 120g)
450/105 Prawns, boiled (6 = 120g)
845/200 Roe, cod, fried (100g)
650/155 Salmon, canned (100g)
1380/330 Sardines, canned (60g)
445/105 Scallops, steamed (10 = 100g)
1200/290 Tuna, canned in oil (120g)
800/190 Whiting, crumbed, fried (100g)
390/90 steamed (100g)

FRUIT

150/35 Apple (inc. skin, core 100g)
135/30 baked, no sugar (inc. skin 110g)
135/30 stewed, no sugar (110g)
110/25 Apricots (inc. stones 3 = 100g)

---

kJ/kcal

BEVERAGES

165/40 Beer (240g)
150/35 Cider, dry, alcoholic (180g)
175/40 sweet, alcoholic (180g)
188/45 sweet, non-alcoholic (220g)
1300/310 Cocoa powder (5g)
8/2 Coffee, percolated (230g)
170/40 Cola-type drinks (240g)
140/35 Cordil, diluted 1:4 (240g)
1555/365 Drinking chocolate (10g)
160/40 Lemonade, carbonated drinks (240g)
1785/425 Milo (10g)
1700/400 Ovaltine (10g)
655/155 Port (60g)
480/115 Sherry, dry (60g)
490/120 medium (60g)
570/130 sweet (60g)
920/220 Spirits, e.g. whisky (30g)
2/1 Tea, infusion (230g)
285/70 Wine, red (100g)
275/65 white, dry (100g)
310/70 medium (100g)
315/75 sparkling (100g)
395/95 sweet (100g)

CEREALS, BISCUITS, CAKES, DESSERTS

510/120 Barley, pearl, boiled (–)
2200/525 Biscuit, chocolate (20g)
2095/500 cream-filled (20g)
1365/320 crispbread, rye (20g)
1640/390 wheat, starch-red. (11g)
1925/455 gingernut (15g)
1925/455 semi-sweet (15g)
1965/470 short-sweet (15g)
870/205 Bran, wheat (8g)
1015/240 Bread, brown, slice (25g)
1205/285 Lebanese (pita) (¼ = 25g)
1015/240 white, slice (25g)
985/235 wholemeal, slice (25g)
1230/290 roll, brown (35g)
1630/385 starch-reduced (35g)
1230/290 white (35g)
1490/355 Cake, fruit (60g)
1650/390 plain (60g)

kJ/kcal	Food
450/105	Apricots, canned (100g)
775/180	dried (25g)
90/20	stewed, no sugar (inc. stones 110g)
920/225	Avocado pear (½=150g)
340/80	Banana (100g)
125/30	Blackberries (100g)
105/25	stewed, no sugar (100g)
65/15	Cantaloup (inc. skin 120g)
175/40	Cherries (inc. stones 20=100g)
140/35	stewed, no sugar (inc. stones 100g)
120/30	Currants, black (90g)
1040/245	dried (15g)
90/20	red (90g)
1055/250	Dates, dried (6=35g)
175/40	Figs (2=75g)
910/215	dried (2=40g)
405/95	Fruit salad, canned (120g)
215/50	Grapes, black (20=100g)
255/60	white (20=100g)
45/10	Grapefruit, whole (200g)
255/60	canned (100g)
130/30	juice, canned (120g)
260/60	Guavas, canned (100g)
65/15	Lemon, slices (2=15g)
30/7	juice (15g)
75/15	Loganberries (100g)
430/100	canned (100g)
65/15	stewed, no sugar (100g)
290/70	Lychees, canned (100g)
195/46	Mandarins (2=100g)
235/55	canned (50g)
255/60	Mango (100g)
330/75	canned (100g)
200/45	Nectarines (inc. stones 3=100g)
340/80	Olives, in brine (5=20g)
115/25	Orange, whole (130g)
160/40	juice, fresh (120g)
145/35	canned (120g)
60/15	Passionfruit, whole (30g)
170/40	Papaw (100g)
275/65	canned (100g)
135/30	Peach (inc. stones 120g)
375/85	canned (120g)
905/210	dried (25g)

kJ/kcal	Food
1940/465	Cake, sponge (60g)
1415/335	Chapati (60g)
1745/420	Cheesecake (120g)
1590/380	Cornflakes (30g)
1045/250	Crumpet (50g)
495/120	Custard (70g)
1200/285	Custard tart (120g)
1465/350	Doughnut (40g)
1570/375	Eclair (50g)
1460/350	Flour, corn- (–)
1505/360	plain (–)
1525/365	self-raising (–)
1870/445	soya, full-fat (–)
1490/350	low-fat (–)
1440/345	wholemeal (–)
1555/370	Fruit pie (150g)
1615/385	Jam tart (35g)
250/60	Jelly, made with water (100g)
1485/355	Lamington (60g)
1360/325	Lemon meringue pie (120g)
1620/380	Meringue (15g)
550/130	Milk pudding (e.g. sago) (160g)
1790/425	Muesli (30g)
625/150	Noodles (chow mein) (250g)
1285/305	Pancake (75g)
500/115	Pasta, macaroni, boiled (150g)
500/115	spaghetti, boiled (120g)
250/60	canned in tomato sauce (120g)
2355/565	Pastry, flaky (–)
2200/525	short crust (–)
980/235	Pizza, cheese and tomato (150g)
190/45	Porridge (30g)
520/125	Rice, boiled (160g)
930/220	fried (120g)
1590/380	puffed (25g)
1560/370	Scone (30g)
1445/345	Sponge pudding, steamed (100g)
675/160	Trifle (100g)
1570/375	Wheat, breakfast biscuit (35g)
715/170	Yeast, dried, baker's (–)

EGG AND CHEESE DISHES

kJ/kcal	Food
470/115	Cauliflower cheese (100g)
1030/250	Cheese soufflé (100g)
610/145	Egg, boiled (55g)

kj/kcal

kJ/kcal	Item
1175/285	cheese spread (10g)
400/95	cottage (25g)
1805/440	cream cheese (15g)
1470/355	Danish blue (25g)
1260/305	edam (25g)
1695/410	parmesan (10g)
1290/310	processed (25g)
1915/460	stilton (25g)
1585/375	Swiss (25g)
1525/365	Cream, 35% fat (30g)
950/230	sterilized, canned (15g)
705/170	Ice-cream (60g)
690/165	non-dairy (60g)
1140/265	Milk, cow's, cond. skim. sweet. (30g)
1360/320	cond. whole, sweet. (30g)
1510/355	dried, skimmed (12g)
2050/490	dried, whole (10g)
660/160	evap. whole, unsweet. (30g)
360/85	flavoured (230g)
140/35	fresh, skimmed (230g)
275/65	fresh, whole (230g)
275/65	longlife, UHT (230g)
290/70	goat's (230g)
290/70	human (100g)
510/120	Milkshake, flavoured (340g)
420/100	Yoghurt, flavoured (200g)
405/95	fruit, low-fat (200g)
215/50	natural, low-fat (200g)
325/75	plain (200g)

NUTS

kJ/kcal	Item
2335/565	Almonds (10=15g)
2545/620	Brazil nuts (5=20g)
2405/575	Cashews, roast (10=20g)
720/170	Chestnuts (4=20g)
2490/605	Coconut, desiccated (15g)
1570/380	Hazel nuts (10=15g)
2960/705	Macadamia nuts (8=20g)
2365/395	Peanuts, raw, in shells (5=25g)
1630/570	roasted, salted (30=25g)
2485/590	Pistachio nuts, shelled (25=15g)
2165/525	Walnuts (5=20g)

SAUCES & CONDIMENTS

kJ/kcal	Item
380/90	Barbecue sauce (10g)
90/20	Chilli sauce (–)

kj/kcal

kJ/kcal	Item
335/80	Peach, stewed, no sugar (120g)
125/30	Pear (inc. skin, core 120g)
325/75	canned (120g)
130/30	stewed, no sugar (120g)
195/45	Pineapple (80g)
330/75	canned (80g)
225/55	juice, canned (120g)
145/35	Plums (inc. stones 3=100g)
125/30	stewed, no sugar (inc. stones 100g)
570/135	Prunes (inc. stones 8=80g)
315/75	stewed, no sugar (inc. stones 120g)
105/25	Quince, raw (100g)
1050/245	Raisins, dried (20g)
105/25	Raspberries (100g)
370/85	canned (100g)
110/25	stewed, no sugar (100g)
25/6	Rhubarb, stewed, no sugar (120g)
110/25	Strawberries (10=100g)
345/80	canned (100g)
1065/250	Sultanas, dried (15g)
45/10	Watermelon (260g)

MEAT AND MEAT PRODUCTS

kJ/kcal	Item
1975/475	Bacon rashers, middle, fried (2=40g)
1720/415	grilled (40g)
905/215	Beef, corned, canned (90g)
835/200	fillet steak, grilled (130g)
955/230	mince, stewed (120g)
1025/245	rump steak, fried (150g)
910/220	grilled (150g)
1010/240	silverside, salted, boiled (120g)
1180/285	sirloin, roast (120g)
930/225	stewing steak, stewed (120g)
895/215	topside, roast (120g)
1100/265	Beefburger, frozen, fried (60g)
500/120	Beef stew (250g)
580/140	Bolognese sauce (100g)
765/185	Chicken, boiled (100g)
1380/330	crumbed, no bone (140g)
900/215	roast (130g)
390/90	leg quarter (inc. bone 130g)
310/75	wing quarter (inc. bone 130g)
810/195	Chicken livers, fried (130g)
1405/340	Duck, roast (100g)

660/155 Chutney, tomato (20g)
920/220 Curry powder (–)
2705/660 French dressing (15g)
1085/260 Ginger (ground) (–)
2950/720 Mayonnaise (20g)
1940/460 Mustard powder (–)
970/230 Oxo cubes (–)
1310/310 Pepper (–)
140/35 Pickles, mustard (20g)
570/135 sweet (20g)
1290/310 Salad cream (25g)
0/0 Salt, table (–)
2355/560 Sesame seeds (–)
285/70 Soy sauce (–)
2095/500 Tartare sauce (20g)
360/85 Tomato sauce (25g)
15/4 Vinegar (–)
335/80 Worcestershire sauce (–)

SOUPS (as served)
205/50 Chicken, condensed (230g)
85/20 Chicken noodle, dried (230g)
100/25 Minestrone, dried (230g)
220/55 Mushroom, canned (230g)
260/60 Tomato, condensed (230g)
130/30 Tomato, dried (230g)
160/35 Vegetable, canned (230g)

SUGARS, JAMS AND SPREADS
705/170 Fish paste (5g)
1230/390 Honey (30g)
1115/260 Jam, fruit, edible seeds (30g)
1115/260 Jam, stone fruit (30g)
1115/260 Marmalade (30g)
720/175 Meat paste (5g)
2580/625 Peanut butter (20g)
1680/395 Sugar, white (–)
1270/300 Syrup, golden (30g)
565/135 Topping, flavoured (40g)
1095/255 Treacle, black (30g)
725/174 Vegemite (3g)

SWEETS
1395/325 Boiled sweet (5g)
1760/420 Butterscotch (5g)
1710/405 Caramel (5g)

1435/340 Gelatin (–)
500/120 Ham, canned (90g)
950/225 Hamburger (170g)
1100/260 with cheese (190g)
475/115 Irish stew (250g)
525/125 Lamb, brain, boiled (150g)
1145/275 chops, loin, grilled (inc. bone 120g)
1015/245 cutlets, grilled (inc. bone 100g)
990/235 heart, roast (140g)
650/155 kidney, fried (100g)
1105/265 leg, roast (120g)
970/230 liver, fried (130g)
1310/315 shoulder, roast (120g)
1195/290 tongue, stewed (100g)
1300/315 Luncheon meat, canned (90g)
960/230 Meat pie (180g)
810/195 Moussaka (200g)
1390/330 Pastie (160g)
1075/260 Pork, chop, loin, grilled (100g)
1190/285 leg, roast (120g)
770/185 sweet and sour (250g)
1565/375 Pork pie (180g)
380/90 Rabbit, stewed (inc. bone 170g)
2030/490 Salami, slices (3=90g)
1285/310 Sausage, liver (60g)
1210/290 Sausage roll (100g)
1125/270 Sausages, beef, fried (2=120g)
1105/265 grilled (2=120g)
1135/275 frankfurter (2=100g)
1315/315 pork, fried (2=120g)
1320/320 grilled (2=120g)
1090/260 saveloy, large (2=150g)
1400/335 Spring roll, fried (200g)
1350/325 Steak and kidney pie (180g)
730/175 Stewed steak in gravy, canned (100g)
885/215 Tongue, canned (100g)
420/100 Tripe, stewed (100g)
720/170 Turkey, roast (120g)
905/215 Veal, cutlet, fried (110g)
965/230 fillet, roast (100g)
1335/320 schnitzel (140g)

MILK & MILK PRODUCTS
1245/300 Cheese, camembert (25g)
1680/405 cheddar (25g)

kJ/kcal

1775/425 Carob bar (75g)
2215/530 Chocolate square, milk (5g)
1745/415 Fruit and honey bar (50g)
1465/350 Jelly bean (5g)
1335/315 Liquorice allsort (7g)
1080/255 Pastille (5g)
1670/390 Peppermint (4g)
1605/380 Popcorn, plain unsalted (15g)
1720/410 Sesame bar (50g)
1810/430 Toffee, mixed (5g)

VEGETABLES

30/7 Artichoke, globe, boiled (100g)
40/9 Asparagus, boiled (5=100g)
105/25 Bamboo shoots (50g)
30/7 Beans, French, boiled (100g)
270/65 baked, in tomato sauce (125g)
215/50 broad, boiled (100g)
395/95 kidney (and haricot), boiled (100g)
445/105 mung, cooked dahl (100g)
545/130 soya-, boiled (100g)
190/45 Beetroot, slices, boiled (2=30g)
145/35 canned (2=30g)
80/20 Broccoli, boiled (100g)
75/20 Brussels sprouts, boiled (7=70g)
110/25 Cabbage, raw (50g)
40/9 boiled (100g)
100/25 Carrots, raw (50g)
80/20 boiled (50g)
80/20 young, canned (50g)
55/15 Cauliflower, raw (50g)
40/9 boiled (100g)
60/15 Celeriac, boiled (3=60g)
35/8 Celery, raw (50g)
20/5 boiled (50g)
610/145 Chickpeas, cooked dahl (60g)
45/10 Cucumber, slices (5=30g)
250/60 Egg plant, baked (½=100g)
50/10 Endive, raw leaves (3=15g)
105/25 Leeks, boiled (4=100g)
420/100 Lentils, split, boiled (100g)
50/10 Lettuce, raw leaves (2=20g)
30/7 Marrow, boiled (100g)
55/15 Mushrooms, raw (3=30g)
865/210 fried (6=60g)

kJ/kcal

100/25 Onions, raw (¼=20g)
55/15 boiled (100g)
1425/345 fried (70g)
150/35 spring (4=20g)
90/20 Parsley, sprigs (2=5g)
240/55 Parsnip, boiled (½=60g)
200/45 Peas, canned (60g)
340/80 canned, processed (60g)
225/50 fresh, boiled (60g)
175/40 frozen, boiled (60g)
505/120 split, boiled (60g)
65/15 Peppers, green, raw (¼=15g)
60/15 boiled (50g)
365/85 Potato, baked (inc. skin 120g)
345/80 boiled (120g)
1065/250 chips, fresh, fried (12=120g)
1215/290 chips, frozen, fried (8-14=120g)
2225/535 crisps (10=25g)
500/120 mashed (100g)
300/70 instant, cooked (100g)
325/75 new, boiled (2=100g)
225/55 new, canned (2=100g)
660/155 roast (120g)
65/15 Pumpkin (100g)
60/15 Radishes (2=20g)
130/30 Spinach, leaves, boiled (3=60g)
75/20 Swede, boiled (80g)
520/125 Sweetcorn, on cob, boiled (150g)
325/75 canned kernels (80g)
365/85 Sweet potato, boiled (100g)
60/15 Tomato, raw (120g)
50/10 canned (120g)
290/70 fried (120g)
65/15 juice, canned (120g)
60/15 Turnip, boiled (80g)
510/120 Yam, boiled (100g)

2
WATER

Water is perhaps the most essential of nutrients since we can do without it for only a short time — days at the outside. This is because, without an adequate flow of urine, waste products would build up in the body, and with the absence of moisture loss it would not be possible to regulate body temperature. However, we can obtain water from a number of sources, as can be seen by reference to Figure 18. Water may be taken as a beverage and as part of food; water is produced in our body cells following the metabolism (chemical breakdown) of fat, alcohol, protein and carbohydrate. Food usually provides more than half our daily water requirement.

The more water a food contains, the less energy dense it is, that is, water-rich foods have few kilocalories (or kilojoules) per 100 grams.

The need for water is influenced by environmental conditions. For example, in a hot climate a great deal of water can be lost not only as sweat, but also in expired air.

Making water supplies hygienic has contributed greatly to human health. More recently, the addition of fluoride to water supplies deficient in it has reduced dental decay. In Australia, nutritionists are encouraging people to drink water in preference to other beverages and to drink it in adequate amounts in dry conditions and with increased physical activity. It is sensible to have four or five glasses of 200 millilitres each day; by so doing, less energy and alcohol will be consumed. With that much water you'll be less thirsty for alcohol, coffee and other beverages and probably eat less food. Fluoride intake will be improved for many. Urine flow will increase and the risk of kidney stones decrease.

WATER INTAKE

Safe and adequate daily intake of water:

	ALL SOURCES (Millilitres)	DRINKS
Adult in a temperate climate	2500	1000 (800-1600)
Adult during exercise and thermal stress	up to 9000-10000	up to 6000-7000

Toxic level of intake

It is a most unusual event to be able to overload the body with water by drinking too much. The body compensates by increasing urine output. However, there can be an accumulation of body water in certain disease states. Occasionally, for psychological reasons, over-consumption of water does occur.

grams per 100 grams

BEVERAGES

Beer (240g)	96
Cider, dry, alcoholic (180g)	93
sweet, alcoholic (180g)	91
sweet, non-alcoholic (220g)	88
Cocoa powder (5g)	3
Coffee, percolated (230g)	100
Cola-type drinks (240g)	90
Cordial, diluted 1:4 (240g)	91
Drinking chocolate (10g)	2
Lemonade, carbonated drinks (240g)	90
Milo (10g)	3
Ovaltine (10g)	2
Port (60g)	72
Sherry, dry (60g)	82
medium (60g)	81
sweet (60g)	75
Spirits, e.g. whisky (30g)	68
Tea, infusion (230g)	100
Wine, red (100g)	88
white, dry (100g)	89
medium (100g)	86
sparkling (100g)	86
sweet (100g)	81

CEREALS, BISCUITS, CAKES, DESSERTS

Barley, pearl, boiled (–)	70
Biscuit, chocolate (20g)	2
cream-filled (20g)	3
crispbread, rye (20g)	6
wheat, starch-red. (11g)	5
gingernut (15g)	3
semi-sweet (15g)	3
short-sweet (15g)	3
Bran, wheat (8g)	8
Bread, brown, slice (25g)	39
Lebanese (pita) (¼=25g)	27
white, slice (25g)	39
wholemeal, slice (25g)	40
roll, brown (35g)	29
starch-reduced (35g)	9
white (35g)	29
Cake, fruit (60g)	20
plain (60g)	20

Egg, fried (60g)	63
omelette (100g)	69
poached (55g)	75
raw (55g)	75
scrambled (70g)	62
Macaroni cheese (180g)	67
Quiche Lorraine (150g)	35

FATS AND OILS

Butter, salted (10g)	16
Dripping, beef (–)	1
Lard (–)	1
Margarine (10g)	16
Vegetable oils (–)	Tr

FISH AND OTHER SEAFOODS

Bream, steamed (100g)	77
Cod, baked (100g)	77
fried in batter (100g)	61
poached (100g)	78
steamed (100g)	79
Crab, boiled (150g)	73
canned (90g)	79
Fish cakes, fried (4=100g)	63
fingers, fried (5=100g)	56
in batter, fried (120g)	55
Flounder, baked (100g)	60
Haddock, fried (100g)	65
steamed (100g)	75
Lobster, boiled (120g)	72
Mussels, boiled (12=120g)	79
Oysters, raw (12=120g)	86
Prawns, boiled (6=120g)	70
Roe, cod, fried (100g)	62
Salmon, canned (100g)	70
Sardines, canned (60g)	49
Scallops, steamed (10=100g)	73
Tuna, canned in oil (120g)	55
Whiting, crumbed, fried (100g)	63
steamed (100g)	77

FRUIT

Apple (inc. skin, core 100g)	65
baked, no sugar (inc. skin 110g)	68
stewed, no sugar (110g)	88
Apricots (inc. stones 3=100g)	80

Value	Food
68	Apricots, canned (100g)
15	dried (25g)
83	stewed, no sugar (inc. stones 110g)
69	Avocado pear (½ = 150g)
71	Banana (100g)
82	Blackberries (100g)
85	stewed, no sugar (100g)
57	Cantaloup (inc. skin 120g)
71	Cherries (inc. stones 20 = 100g)
73	stewed, no sugar (inc. stones 100g)
77	Currants, black (90g)
22	dried (15g)
83	red (90g)
15	Dates, dried (6 = 35g)
85	Figs (2 = 75g)
17	dried (2 = 40g)
71	Fruit salad, canned (120g)
65	Grapes, black (20 = 100g)
76	white (20 = 100g)
44	Grapefruit, whole (200g)
82	canned (100g)
90	juice, canned (120g)
78	Guavas, canned (100g)
85	Lemon, slices (2 = 15g)
91	juice (15g)
85	Loganberries (100g)
66	canned (100g)
86	stewed, no sugar (100g)
79	Lychees, canned (100g)
87	Mandarins (2 = 100g)
84	canned (50g)
83	Mango (100g)
75	canned (100g)
74	Nectarines (inc. stones 3 = 100g)
61	Olives, in brine (5 = 20g)
65	Orange, whole (130g)
88	juice, fresh (120g)
89	canned (120g)
31	Passionfruit, whole (30g)
88	Papaw (100g)
80	canned (100g)
75	Peach (inc. stones 120g)
74	canned (120g)
16	dried (25g)

Value	Food
15	Cake, sponge (60g)
29	Chapati (60g)
35	Cheesecake (120g)
3	Cornflakes (30g)
35	Crumpet (50g)
75	Custard (70g)
48	Custard tart (120g)
26	Doughnut (40g)
35	Eclair (50g)
12	Flour, corn- (–)
13	plain (–)
13	self-raising (–)
7	soya, full-fat (–)
7	low-fat (–)
14	wholemeal (–)
23	Fruit pie (150g)
19	Jam tart (35g)
84	Jelly, made with water (100g)
24	Lamington (60g)
35	Lemon meringue pie (120g)
2	Meringue (15g)
72	Milk pudding (e.g. sago) (160g)
6	Muesli (30g)
70	Noodles (chow mein) (250g)
43	Pancake (75g)
72	Pasta, macaroni, boiled (150g)
72	spaghetti, boiled (120g)
83	canned in tomato sauce (120g)
7	Pastry, flaky (–)
7	short crust (–)
51	Pizza, cheese and tomato (150g)
89	Porridge (30g)
70	Rice, boiled (160g)
50	fried (120g)
8	puffed (25g)
22	Scone (30g)
29	Sponge pudding, steamed (100g)
65	Trifle (100g)
8	Wheat, breakfast biscuit (35g)
5	Yeast, dried, baker's (–)

EGG AND CHEESE DISHES

Value	Food
78	Cauliflower cheese (100g)
57	Cheese soufflé (100g)
75	Egg, boiled (55g)

	Value
cheese spread (10g)	51
cottage (25g)	79
cream cheese (15g)	46
Danish blue (25g)	41
edam (25g)	44
parmesan (10g)	28
processed (25g)	44
stilton (25g)	28
Swiss (25g)	38
Cream, 35% fat (30g)	56
sterilized, canned (15g)	70
Ice-cream (60g)	64
non-dairy (60g)	66
Milk, cow's, cond. skim, sweet. (30g)	27
cond. whole, sweet. (30g)	26
dried, skimmed (12g)	4
dried, whole (10g)	3
evap. whole, unsweet. (30g)	69
flavoured (230g)	82
fresh, skimmed (230g)	90
fresh, whole (230g)	88
longlife, UHT (230g)	88
goat's (230g)	87
human (100g)	87
Milkshake, flavoured (340g)	75
Yoghurt, flavoured (200g)	79
fruit, low-fat (200g)	75
natural, low-fat (200g)	86
plain (200g)	84

NUTS

	Value
Almonds (10=15g)	5
Brazil nuts (5=20g)	9
Cashews, roast (10=20g)	4
Chestnuts (4=20g)	52
Coconut, desiccated (15g)	2
Hazel nuts (10=15g)	41
Macadamia nuts (8=20g)	2
Peanuts, raw, in shells (5=25g)	3
roasted, salted (30=25g)	5
Pistachio nuts, shelled (25=15g)	5
Walnuts (5=20g)	24

SAUCES & CONDIMENTS

	Value
Barbecue sauce (10g)	81
Chilli sauce (–)	94

	Value
Peach, stewed, no sugar (120g)	69
Pear (inc. skin, core 120g)	60
canned (120g)	76
stewed, no sugar (120g)	86
Pineapple (80g)	84
canned (80g)	77
juice, canned (120g)	86
Plums (inc. stones 3=100g)	70
stewed, no sugar (inc. stones 100g)	74
Prunes (inc. stones 8=80g)	19
stewed, no sugar (inc. stones 120g)	55
Quince, raw (100g)	84
Raisins, dried (20g)	22
Raspberries (100g)	83
canned (100g)	74
stewed, no sugar (100g)	82
Rhubarb, stewed, no sugar (120g)	95
Strawberries (10=100g)	89
canned (100g)	79
Sultanas, dried (15g)	18
Watermelon (260g)	47

MEAT AND MEAT PRODUCTS

	Value
Bacon rashers, middle, fried (2=40g)	29
grilled (40g)	35
Beef, corned, canned (90g)	59
fillet steak, grilled (130g)	62
mince, stewed (120g)	59
rump steak, fried (150g)	56
grilled (150g)	59
silverside, salted, boiled (120g)	55
sirloin, roast (120g)	54
stewing steak, stewed (120g)	57
topside, roast (120g)	60
Beefburger, frozen, fried (60g)	53
Beef stew (250g)	78
Bolognese sauce (100g)	75
Chicken, boiled (100g)	63
crumbed, no bone (140g)	45
roast (130g)	62
leg quarter (inc. bone 130g)	42
wing quarter (inc. bone 130g)	34
Chicken livers, fried (130g)	64
Duck, roast (100g)	50

Water	Food
13	Gelatin (–)
73	Ham, canned (90g)
51	Hamburger (170g)
48	with cheese (190g)
69	Irish stew (250g)
77	Lamb, brain, boiled (150g)
36	chops, loin, grilled (inc. bone 120g)
30	cutlets, grilled (inc. bone 100g)
57	heart, roast (140g)
67	kidney, fried (100g)
55	leg, roast (120g)
58	liver, fried (130g)
54	shoulder, roast (120g)
57	tongue, stewed (100g)
52	Luncheon meat, canned (90g)
51	Meat pie (180g)
66	Moussaka (200g)
39	Pastie (160g)
36	Pork, chop, loin, grilled (100g)
52	leg, roast (120g)
60	sweet and sour (250g)
37	Pork pie (180g)
33	Rabbit, stewed (inc. bone 170g)
28	Salami, slices (3=90g)
52	Sausage, liver (60g)
42	Sausage roll (100g)
48	Sausages, beef, fried (2=120g)
48	grilled (2=120g)
60	frankfurter (2=100g)
45	pork, fried (2=120g)
45	grilled (2=120g)
57	saveloy, large (2=150g)
40	Spring roll, fried (200g)
43	Steak and kidney pie (180g)
70	Stewed steak in gravy, canned (100g)
64	Tongue, canned (100g)
79	Tripe, stewed (100g)
65	Turkey, roast (120g)
55	Veal, cutlet, fried (110g)
55	fillet, roast (100g)
49	schnitzel (140g)

MILK & MILK PRODUCTS

Water	Food
48	Cheese, camembert (25g)
37	cheddar (25g)

Water	Food
58	Chutney, tomato (20g)
–	Curry powder (–)
24	French dressing (15g)
–	Ginger (ground) (–)
28	Mayonnaise (20g)
–	Mustard powder (–)
9	Oxo cubes (–)
Tr	Pepper (–)
86	Pickles, mustard (20g)
59	sweet (20g)
53	Salad cream (25g)
Tr	Salt, table (–)
5	Sesame seeds (–)
63	Soy sauce (–)
34	Tartare sauce (20g)
82	Tomato sauce (25g)
95	Vinegar (–)
80	Worcestershire sauce (–)

SOUPS (as served)

Water	Food
91	Chicken, condensed (230g)
94	Chicken noodle, dried (230g)
93	Minestrone, dried (230g)
89	Mushroom, canned (230g)
85	Tomato, condensed (230g)
91	Tomato, dried (230g)
86	Vegetable, canned (230g)

SUGARS, JAMS AND SPREADS

Water	Food
67	Fish paste (5g)
23	Honey (30g)
30	Jam, fruit, edible seeds (30g)
30	Jam, stone fruit (30g)
28	Marmalade (30g)
67	Meat paste (5g)
1	Peanut butter (20g)
Tr	Sugar, white (–)
20	Syrup, golden (30g)
66	Topping, flavoured (40g)
29	Treacle, black (30g)
37	Vegemite (3g)

SWEETS

Water	Food
Tr	Boiled sweet (5g)
2	Butterscotch (5g)
7	Caramel (5g)

	Water
Onions, raw (¼=20g)	93
boiled (100g)	97
fried (70g)	42
spring (4=20g)	87
Parsley, sprigs (2=5g)	79
Parsnip, boiled (½=60g)	83
Peas, canned (60g)	82
canned, processed (60g)	72
fresh, boiled (60g)	80
frozen, boiled (60g)	81
split, boiled (60g)	67
Peppers, green, raw (¼=15g)	94
boiled (50g)	94
Potato, baked (inc. skin 120g)	58
boiled (120g)	81
chips, fresh, fried (12=120g)	47
chips, frozen, fried (8-14=120g)	48
crisps (10=25g)	3
mashed (100g)	77
instant, cooked (100g)	79
new, boiled (2=100g)	79
new, canned (2=100g)	84
roast (120g)	64
Pumpkin (100g)	95
Radishes (2=20g)	93
Spinach, leaves, boiled (3=60g)	85
Swede, boiled (80g)	92
Sweetcorn, on cob, boiled (150g)	65
canned kernels (80g)	73
Sweet potato, boiled (100g)	72
Tomato, raw (120g)	94
canned (120g)	94
fried (120g)	87
juice, canned (120g)	93
Turnip, boiled (80g)	95
Yam, boiled (100g)	66

	Water
Carob bar (75g)	4
Chocolate square, milk (5g)	2
Fruit and honey bar (50g)	11
Jelly bean (5g)	9
Liquorice allsort (7g)	7
Pastille (5g)	10
Peppermint (4g)	Tr
Popcorn, plain unsalted (15g)	4
Sesame bar (50g)	11
Toffee, mixed (5g)	5

VEGETABLES

	Water
Artichoke, globe, boiled (100g)	36
Asparagus, boiled (5=100g)	46
Bamboo shoots (50g)	91
Beans, French, boiled (100g)	96
baked, in tomato sauce (125g)	74
broad, boiled (100g)	84
kidney (and haricot), boiled (100g)	70
mung, cooked dahl (100g)	73
soya-, boiled (100g)	70
Beetroot, slices, boiled (2=30g)	83
canned (2=30g)	90
Broccoli, boiled (100g)	90
Brussels sprouts, boiled (7=70g)	92
Cabbage, raw (50g)	90
boiled (100g)	96
Carrots, raw (50g)	90
boiled (50g)	92
young, canned (50g)	91
Cauliflower, raw (50g)	93
boiled (100g)	95
Celeriac, boiled (3=60g)	90
Celery, raw (50g)	94
boiled (50g)	96
Chickpeas, cooked dahl (60g)	66
Cucumber, slices (5=30g)	96
Egg plant, baked (½=100g)	89
Endive, raw leaves (13=15g)	94
Leeks, boiled (4=100g)	91
Lentils, split, boiled (100g)	72
Lettuce, raw leaves (2=20g)	96
Marrow, boiled (100g)	98
Mushrooms, raw (3=30g)	92
fried (6=60g)	64

3

D I E T A R Y   F I B R E

Dietary fibre is a term that refers to a group of food components that pass through the stomach and small intestine undigested and reach the large intestine virtually unchanged. Most other nutrients are digested and are being used in other parts of the body by this stage. During its passage through the *large* intestine some components of dietary fibre are broken down to varying degrees and absorbed by the body; the remaining components are excreted in the faeces. Diets that are high in dietary fibre produce a slower rate of stomach emptying and bulky faeces, which pass more quickly through the large intestine.

The current attention being given to the role of dietary fibre in prevention of certain diseases is largely due to the observation that patterns of disease observed in Africa and Asia were different from those in Western countries. It was suggested that the dietary fibre content was associated with this difference. Although it is not yet proven, there is evidence to suggest that a diet high in dietary fibre can be of value for treating or preventing such disorders as constipation, irritable bowel syndrome, diverticular disease, hiatus hernia and haemorrhoids. Some components of dietary fibre may also be of value in reducing the level of cholesterol in blood and thereby decreasing a risk factor for coronary heart disease and the development of gallstones. Dietary fibre is beneficial in the treatment of some diabetics.

The actual role of dietary fibre in many of these disorders is not known. It may be that dietary fibre as such is not the major factor. When high dietary fibre foods are eaten, other foods, which may be responsible for the disease, are either reduced in quantity or completely excluded. For example, diets that are high in fibre tend to be low in energy and these diets can be useful in weight control. People who are grossly overweight (more than 130 per cent of ideal weight) are more prone to heart disease and diabetes.

The analysis of dietary fibre in food is very complex and only a limited number of foods have been examined. Dietary fibre from different foods, and even different samples of the same food, contain varying quantities of the components that collectively make up dietary fibre. Each of these components has different biological properties and it is frequently not clear which of these is most beneficial. The different components of dietary fibre and their sources are shown in Figure 44. Foods of animal origin do not contain dietary fibre.

FIGURE 44: COMPONENTS OF DIETARY FIBRE

COMPONENT	SOURCE
Cellulose	All food plants
Hemicellulose	All food plants, especially cereal bran
Pectin	Mainly fruit
Lignin	Mainly cereals and 'woody' vegetables
Gums and some food thickeners	Food additives in processed foods

INTAKE OF DIETARY FIBRE

There is no recommended dietary intake (RDI) for fibre as such in Australia. However, the Australian Department of Health has among its dietary goals for Australians an increased intake of fruit, vegetables, bread and cereals, all of which are sources of dietary fibre. The greatest amount of dietary fibre in wheat is in the outer layer, or bran, of the wheat grain. When white flour is produced, the bran layer is removed and the dietary-fibre content of the flour is greatly reduced. Flour made from whole grains contains about three times as much dietary fibre as white flour.

grams per 100 grams

BEVERAGES

–	Beer (240g)
–	Cider, dry, alcoholic (180g)
–	sweet, alcoholic (180g)
–	sweet, non-alcoholic (220g)
–	Cocoa powder (5g)
–	Coffee, percolated (230g)
0	Cola-type drinks (240g)
–	Cordial, diluted 1:4 (240g)
–	Drinking chocolate (10g)
0	Lemonade, carbonated drinks (240g)
–	Milo (10g)
–	Ovaltine (10g)
–	Port (60g)
–	Sherry, dry (60g)
–	medium (60g)
–	sweet (60g)
–	Spirits, e.g. whisky (30g)
–	Tea, infusion (230g)
–	Wine, red (100g)
–	white, dry (100g)
–	medium (100g)
–	sparkling (100g)
–	sweet (100g)

CEREALS, BISCUITS, CAKES, DESSERTS

2	Barley, pearl, boiled (–)
3	Biscuit, chocolate (20g)
–	cream-filled (20g)
12	crispbread, rye (20g)
5	wheat, starch-red. (11g)
2	gingernut (15g)
2.5	semi-sweet (15g)
1.5	short-sweet (15g)
44	Bran, wheat (8g)
5	Bread, brown, slice (25g)
–	Lebanese (pita) (¼=25g)
3	white, slice (25g)
7	wholemeal, slice (25g)
7	roll, brown (35g)
2	starch-reduced (35g)
3	white (35g)
3	Cake, fruit (60g)
1.5	plain (60g)

(Eggs)

–	Egg, fried (60g)
–	omelette (100g)
–	poached (55g)
–	raw (55g)
–	scrambled (70g)
.6	Macaroni cheese (180g)
.8	Quiche Lorraine (150g)

FATS AND OILS

–	Butter, salted (10g)
–	Dripping, beef (–)
–	Lard (–)
–	Margarine (10g)
–	Vegetable oils (–)

FISH AND OTHER SEAFOODS

–	Bream, steamed (100g)
–	Cod, baked (100g)
.3	fried in batter (100g)
–	poached (100g)
–	steamed (100g)
–	Crab, boiled (150g)
–	canned (90g)
.7	Fish cakes, fried (4=100g)
.7	fingers, fried (5=100g)
–	in batter, fried (120g)
–	Flounder, baked (100g)
–	Haddock, fried (100g)
–	steamed (100g)
–	Lobster, boiled (120g)
–	Mussels, boiled (12=120g)
–	Oysters, raw (12=120g)
–	Prawns, boiled (6=120g)
–	Roe, cod, fried (100g)
–	Salmon, canned (100g)
–	Sardines, canned (60g)
–	Scallops, steamed (10=100g)
–	Tuna, canned in oil (120g)
–	Whiting, crumbed, fried (100g)
–	steamed (100g)

FRUIT

1.5	Apple (inc. skin, core 100g)
2	baked, no sugar (inc. skin 110g)
2	stewed, no sugar (110g)
2	Apricots (inc. stones 3=100g)

	Fibre (g)	Food
	1.5	Apricots, canned (100g)
	24	dried (25g)
	1.5	stewed, no sugar (inc. stones 110g)
	2	Avocado pear (½=150g)
	1.3	Banana (100g)
	7.5	Blackberries (100g)
	6.5	stewed, no sugar (100g)
	.5	Cantaloup (inc. skin 120g)
	1.5	Cherries (inc. stones 20=100g)
	1	stewed, no sugar (inc. stones 100g)
	8.5	Currants, black (90g)
	6.5	dried (15g)
	8	red (90g)
	8.5	Dates, dried (6=35g)
	2.5	Figs (2=75g)
	18.5	dried (2=40g)
	1	Fruit salad, canned (120g)
	.5	Grapes, black (20=100g)
	1	white (20=100g)
	.5	Grapefruit, whole (200g)
	.5	canned (100g)
	–	juice, canned (120g)
	3.5	Guavas, canned (100g)
	5	Lemon, slices (2=15g)
	–	juice (15g)
	6	Loganberries (100g)
	3.5	canned (100g)
	5.5	stewed, no sugar (100g)
	.5	Lychees, canned (100g)
	–	Mandarins (2=100g)
	.5	canned (50g)
	1.5	Mango (100g)
	1	canned (100g)
	2	Nectarines (inc. stones 3=100g)
	3.5	Olives, in brine (5=20g)
	1.5	Orange, whole (130g)
	–	juice, fresh (120g)
	–	canned (120g)
	6.5	Passionfruit, whole (30g)
	–	Papaw (100g)
	.5	canned (100g)
	1	Peach (inc. stones 120g)
	1	canned (120g)
	14.5	dried (25g)

	Fibre (g)	Food
	1	Cake, sponge (60g)
	3.5	Chapati (60g)
	1	Cheesecake (120g)
	–	Cornflakes (30g)
	–	Crumpet (50g)
	–	Custard (70g)
	1	Custard tart (120g)
	–	Doughnut (40g)
	–	Eclair (50g)
	–	Flour, corn– (–)
	3.5	plain (–)
	3.5	self-raising (–)
	12	soya, full-fat (–)
	14.5	low-fat (–)
	9.5	wholemeal (–)
	2.5	Fruit pie (150g)
	1.5	Jam tart (35g)
	1.5	Jelly, made with water (100g)
	–	Lamington (60g)
	.5	Lemon meringue pie (120g)
	–	Meringue (15g)
	–	Milk pudding (e.g. sago) (160g)
	–	Muesli (30g)
	–	Noodles (chow mein) (250g)
	–	Pancake (75g)
	.5	Pasta, macaroni, boiled (150g)
	–	spaghetti, boiled (120g)
	–	canned in tomato sauce (120g)
	2	Pastry, flaky (–)
	2	short crust (–)
	1.8	Pizza, cheese and tomato (150g)
	1	Porridge (30g)
	1	Rice, boiled (160g)
	–	fried (120g)
	–	puffed (25g)
	2	Scone (30g)
	1	Sponge pudding, steamed (100g)
	–	Trifle (100g)
	–	Wheat, breakfast biscuit (35g)
	22	Yeast, dried, baker's (–)

EGG AND CHEESE DISHES

	Fibre (g)	Food
	1.2	Cauliflower cheese (100g)
	.3	Cheese soufflé (100g)
	–	Egg, boiled (55g)

Value	Food
5.5	Peach, stewed, no sugar (120g)
1.5	Pear (inc. skin, core 120g)
1.5	canned (120g)
2.5	stewed, no sugar (120g)
1	Pineapple (80g)
1	canned (80g)
0	juice, canned (120g)
4	Plums (inc. stones 3 = 100g)
3	stewed, no sugar (inc. stones 100g)
13.5	Prunes (inc. stones 8 = 80g)
7.5	stewed, no sugar (inc. stones 120g)
6.5	Quince, raw (100g)
7	Raisins, dried (20g)
7.5	Raspberries (100g)
5	canned (100g)
7.8	stewed, no sugar (100g)
2.5	Rhubarb, stewed, no sugar (120g)
2	Strawberries (10 = 100g)
1	canned (100g)
7	Sultanas, dried (15g)
–	Watermelon (260g)

MEAT AND MEAT PRODUCTS

Value	Food
–	Bacon rashers, middle, fried (2 = 40g)
–	grilled (40g)
–	Beef, corned, canned (90g)
–	fillet steak, grilled (130g)
–	mince, stewed (120g)
–	rump steak, fried (150g)
–	grilled (150g)
–	silverside, salted, boiled (120g)
–	sirloin, roast (120g)
–	stewing steak, stewed (120g)
.3	topside, roast (120g)
.3	Beefburger, frozen, fried (60g)
.7	Beef stew (250g)
.2	Bolognese sauce (100g)
–	Chicken, boiled (100g)
–	crumbed, no bone (140g)
–	roast (130g)
–	leg quarter (inc. bone 130g)
–	wing quarter (inc. bone 130g)
–	Chicken livers, fried (130g)
–	Duck, roast (100g)

Value	Food
–	cheese spread (10g)
–	cottage (25g)
–	cream cheese (15g)
–	Danish blue (25g)
–	edam (25g)
–	parmesan (10g)
–	processed (25g)
–	stilton (25g)
–	Swiss (25g)
–	Cream, 35% fat (30g)
–	sterilized, canned (15g)
–	Ice-cream (60g)
–	non-dairy (60g)
–	Milk, cow's, cond. skim, sweet. (30g)
–	cond. whole, sweet. (30g)
–	dried, skimmed (12g)
–	dried, whole (10g)
–	evap. whole, unsweet. (30g)
–	flavoured (230g)
–	fresh, skimmed (230g)
–	fresh, whole (230g)
–	longlife, UHT (230g)
–	goat's (230g)
–	human (100g)
–	Milkshake, flavoured (340g)
–	Yoghurt, flavoured (200g)
–	fruit, low-fat (200g)
–	natural, low-fat (200g)
–	plain (200g)

NUTS

Value	Food
14.5	Almonds (10 = 15g)
9	Brazil nuts (5 = 20g)
–	Cashews, roast (10 = 20g)
7	Chestnuts (4 = 20g)
23.5	Coconut, desiccated (15g)
6	Hazel nuts (10 = 15g)
–	Macadamia nuts (8 = 20g)
5.5	Peanuts, raw, in shells (5 = 25g)
8.1	roasted, salted (30 = 25g)
–	Pistachio nuts, shelled (25 = 15g)
5	Walnuts (5 = 20g)

SAUCES & CONDIMENTS

Value	Food
–	Barbecue sauce (10g)
–	Chilli sauce (–)

Food	Fibre (g)
Gelatin (–)	–
Ham, canned (90g)	–
Hamburger (170g)	–
with cheese (190g)	–
Irish stew (250g)	1.2
Lamb, brain, boiled (150g)	–
chops, loin, grilled (inc. bone 120g)	–
cutlets, grilled (inc. bone 100g)	–
heart, roast (140g)	–
kidney, fried (100g)	–
leg, roast (120g)	–
liver, fried (130g)	–
shoulder, roast (120g)	–
tongue, stewed (100g)	–
Luncheon meat, canned (90g)	.2
Meat pie (180g)	–
Moussaka (200g)	.9
Pastie (160g)	1.3
Pork, chop, loin, grilled (100g)	–
leg, roast (120g)	–
sweet and sour (250g)	–
Pork pie (180g)	1
Rabbit, stewed (inc. bone 170g)	–
Salami, slices (3=90g)	.1
Sausage, liver (60g)	.2
Sausage roll (100g)	1.3
Sausages, beef, fried (2=120g)	.6
grilled (2=120g)	.6
frankfurter (2=100g)	.1
pork, fried (2=120g)	.5
grilled (2=120g)	.5
saveloy, large (2=150g)	.4
Spring roll, fried (200g)	–
Steak and kidney pie (180g)	.7
Stewed steak in gravy, canned (100g)	–
Tongue, canned (100g)	–
Tripe, stewed (100g)	–
Turkey, roast (120g)	–
Veal, cutlet, fried (110g)	–
fillet, roast (100g)	–
schnitzel (140g)	–
MILK & MILK PRODUCTS	
Cheese, camembert (25g)	–
cheddar (25g)	–

Food	Fibre (g)
Chutney, tomato (20g)	2
Curry powder (–)	–
French dressing (15g)	0
Ginger (ground) (–)	–
Mayonnaise (20g)	0
Mustard powder (–)	–
Oxo cubes (–)	0
Pepper (–)	–
Pickles, mustard (20g)	2
sweet (20g)	1.5
Salad cream (25g)	–
Salt, table (–)	0
Sesame seeds (–)	–
Soy sauce (–)	–
Tartare sauce (20g)	–
Tomato sauce (25g)	2
Vinegar (–)	0
Worcestershire sauce (–)	–
SOUPS (as served)	
Chicken, condensed (230g)	–
Chicken noodle, dried (230g)	–
Minestrone, dried (230g)	.5
Mushroom, canned (230g)	–
Tomato, condensed (230g)	–
Tomato, dried (230g)	.5
Vegetable, canned (230g)	–
SUGARS, JAMS AND SPREADS	
Fish paste (5g)	–
Honey (30g)	–
Jam, fruit, edible seeds (30g)	1
Jam, stone fruit (30g)	1
Marmalade (30g)	.5
Meat paste (5g)	.1
Peanut butter (20g)	7.5
Sugar, white (–)	0
Syrup, golden (30g)	0
Topping, flavoured (40g)	–
Treacle, black (30g)	0
Vegemite (3g)	–
SWEETS	
Boiled sweet (5g)	0
Butterscotch (5g)	–
Caramel (5g)	–

Food	Fibre (g)
Carob bar (75g)	–
Chocolate square, milk (5g)	–
Fruit and honey bar (50g)	–
Jelly bean (5g)	–
Liquorice allsort (7g)	–
Pastille (5g)	–
Peppermint (4g)	0
Popcorn, plain unsalted (15g)	–
Sesame bar (50g)	–
Toffee, mixed (5g)	–

VEGETABLES

Food	Fibre (g)
Artichoke, globe, boiled (100g)	–
Asparagus, boiled (5=100g)	1
Bamboo shoots (50g)	–
Beans, French, boiled (100g)	3
baked, in tomato sauce (125g)	7.3
broad, boiled (100g)	4
kidney (and haricot), boiled (100g)	7.5
mung, cooked dahl (100g)	6.5
soya-, boiled (100g)	–
Beetroot, slices, boiled (2=30g)	2.5
canned (2=30g)	2.8
Broccoli, boiled (100g)	4
Brussels sprouts, boiled (7=70g)	3
Cabbage, raw (50g)	3
boiled (100g)	2.5
Carrots, raw (50g)	3
boiled (50g)	3
young, canned (50g)	3.5
Cauliflower, raw (50g)	2
boiled (100g)	2
Celeriac, boiled (3=60g)	5
Celery, raw (50g)	2
boiled (50g)	2
Chickpeas, cooked dahl (60g)	6
Cucumber, slices (5=30g)	.5
Egg plant, baked (½=100g)	–
Endive, raw leaves (3=15g)	2
Leeks, boiled (4=100g)	4
Lentils, split, boiled (100g)	4
Lettuce, raw leaves (2=20g)	.8
Marrow, boiled (100g)	.5
Mushrooms, raw (3=30g)	2.5
fried (6=60g)	4
Onions, raw (¼=20g)	1.5
boiled (100g)	1.5
fried (70g)	4.5
spring (4=20g)	3
Parsley, sprigs (2=5g)	9
Parsnip, boiled (½=60g)	2.5
Peas, canned (60g)	6.5
canned, processed (60g)	8
fresh, boiled (60g)	5
frozen, boiled (60g)	12
split, boiled (60g)	5
Peppers, green, raw (¼=15g)	1
boiled (50g)	1
Potato, baked (inc. skin 120g)	2
boiled (120g)	1
chips, fresh, fried (12=120g)	–
chips, frozen, fried (8-14=120g)	3
crisps (10=25g)	3.8
mashed (100g)	1
instant, cooked (100g)	3.5
new, boiled (2=100g)	2
new, canned (2=100g)	2.5
roast (120g)	–
Pumpkin (100g)	2.2
Radishes (2=20g)	1
Spinach, leaves, boiled (3=60g)	6.5
Swede, boiled (80g)	3
Sweetcorn, on cob, boiled (150g)	1.7
canned kernels (80g)	5.5
Sweet potato, boiled (100g)	2.5
Tomato, raw (120g)	1.5
canned (120g)	1
fried (120g)	3
juice, canned (120g)	–
Turnip, boiled (80g)	2
Yam, boiled (100g)	4

4

PROTEIN

Protein is an essential part of the diet. It is made up of various combinations of small organic chemicals called amino acids. When we eat food containing protein it is broken down during digestion into its constituent amino acids. These amino acids are absorbed by our bodies and are used to produce new proteins and other necessary substances. Our bodies can make some of the amino acids needed to manufacture proteins, but others must be obtained from the diet; these are the eight so-called 'essential' amino acids. In addition, one other amino acid is needed by infants during early growth and development.

Proteins form part of the structure of the body, so that a continual supply of amino acids is needed. Our bodies are able to put these basic amino acid units together, using different arrangements of amino acids, to produce specific proteins, which can only be produced if all the necessary amino acids are available.

The nutritional value of a protein food can be judged by its ability to provide both the quantity and number of essential amino acids needed by the body. Different food sources contain different groups of proteins, which are made up of different arrangements and amounts of amino acids. In general, proteins from animal sources are of greater nutritional value because they usually contain all the essential amino acids. Proteins from plant sources, such as cereals and vegetables, may be deficient in one or other of the essential amino acids. For example, the proteins obtained from wheat lack adequate quantities of one essential amino acid, and those from beans are deficient in another.

Because the deficiency is different in each food, when they are eaten together they complement each other and the mixture is of higher nutritional value than the separate foods, and is as good as animal protein. It is important, particularly for strict vegetarians who do not consume dairy or egg products (see Figure 21), that a variety of different types of protein foods are eaten.

Cooking can alter the amino-acid composition of protein and this usually results in desirable flavour and browning development. Very little nutritional value is lost.

RECOMMENDED DAILY DIETARY INTAKE OF PROTEIN IN AUSTRALIA

The recommended dietary intake (RDI) in Australia is one gram per kilogram of body weight per day. The protein intake for a 70-kilogram man is 70 grams and for a 58-kilogram woman, 58 grams per day. Growing children and pregnant and lactating women have a greater requirement for protein because of the additional needs of these conditions (see Figure 6). People who have had severe infections or surgery may require additional protein. Because of the margin of safety in the RDI for protein it is usually not necessary to increase protein intake for additional muscular activity such as required for heavy work or training.

A deficiency of protein in the diet can lead to muscle wasting, oedema, anaemia and, in children, a slowing or stopping of growth. These conditions are usually seen as a result of chronic protein malnutrition. Having an adequate energy intake (see Figures 11 and 12) will almost always ensure an adequate protein intake.

Higher levels of protein consumption appear to be neither beneficial nor harmful. However, it is possible that additional calcium may be required to counterbalance an excessive protein intake. Also there is a higher load of protein breakdown products, which must be excreted by the kidneys.

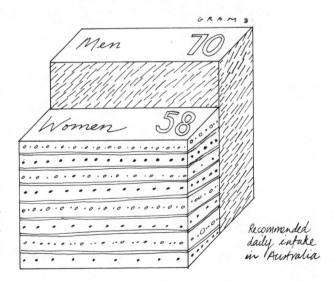

Recommended daily intake in Australia

grams per 100 grams

BEVERAGES

Beer (240g)	.3
Cider, dry, alcoholic (180g)	Tr
sweet, alcoholic (180g)	Tr
sweet, non-alcoholic (220g)	.1
Cocoa powder (5g)	19
Coffee, percolated (230g)	.2
Cola-type drinks (240g)	Tr
Cordial, diluted 1:4 (240g)	Tr
Drinking chocolate (10g)	6
Lemonade, carbonated drinks (240g)	Tr
Milo (10g)	13
Ovaltine (10g)	13
Port (60g)	.1
Sherry, dry (60g)	.2
medium (60g)	.1
sweet (60g)	.3
Spirits, e.g. whisky (30g)	Tr
Tea, infusion (230g)	.1
Wine, red (100g)	.2
white, dry (100g)	.1
medium (100g)	.1
sparkling (100g)	.3
sweet (100g)	.2

CEREALS, BISCUITS, CAKES, DESSERTS

Barley, pearl, boiled (–)	3
Biscuit, chocolate (20g)	6
cream-filled (20g)	5
crispbread, rye (20g)	9
wheat, starch-red. (11g)	45
gingernut (15g)	6
semi-sweet (15g)	7
short-sweet (15g)	6
Bran, wheat (8g)	14
Bread, brown, slice (25g)	8
Lebanese (pita) (¼=25g)	10
white, slice (25g)	8
wholemeal, slice (25g)	9
roll, brown (35g)	12
starch-reduced (35g)	44
white (35g)	12
Cake, fruit (60g)	5
plain (60g)	5

Egg, fried (60g)	14
omelette (100g)	11
poached (55g)	12
raw (55g)	12
scrambled (70g)	11
Macaroni cheese (180g)	7
Quiche Lorraine (150g)	15

FATS AND OILS

Butter, salted (10g)	.4
Dripping, beef (–)	Tr
Lard (–)	Tr
Margarine (10g)	.4
Vegetable oils (–)	Tr

FISH AND OTHER SEAFOODS

Bream, steamed (100g)	18
Cod, baked (100g)	21
fried in batter (100g)	20
poached (100g)	21
steamed (100g)	19
Crab, boiled (150g)	20
canned (90g)	18
Fish cakes, fried (4=100g)	9
fingers, fried (5=100g)	14
in batter, fried (120g)	14
Flounder, baked (100g)	25
Haddock, fried (100g)	21
steamed (100g)	23
Lobster, boiled (120g)	22
Mussels, boiled (12=120g)	17
Oysters, raw (12=120g)	11
Prawns, boiled (6=120g)	23
Roe, cod, fried (100g)	21
Salmon, canned (100g)	20
Sardines, canned (60g)	20
Scallops, steamed (10=100g)	23
Tuna, canned in oil (120g)	23
Whiting, crumbed, fried (100g)	18
steamed (100g)	21

FRUIT

Apple (inc. skin, core 100g)	.2
baked, no sugar (inc. skin 110g)	.3
stewed, no sugar (110g)	.3
Apricots (inc. stones 3=100g)	.5

Protein (g)	Food
6	Cake, sponge (60g)
8	Chapati (60g)
4	Cheesecake (120g)
7	Cornflakes (30g)
8	Crumpet (50g)
4	Custard (70g)
6	Custard tart (120g)
6	Doughnut (40g)
4	Eclair (50g)
.4	Flour, corn- (–)
11	plain (–)
11	self-raising (–)
37	soya, full-fat (–)
45	low-fat (–)
12	wholemeal (–)
4	Fruit pie (150g)
4	Jam tart (35g)
1	Jelly, made with water (100g)
6	Lamington (60g)
6	Lemon meringue pie (120g)
5	Meringue (15g)
4	Milk pudding (e.g. sago) (160g)
9	Muesli (30g)
8	Noodles (chow mein) (250g)
6	Pancake (75g)
4	Pasta, macaroni, boiled (150g)
4	spaghetti, boiled (120g)
2	canned in tomato sauce (120g)
7	Pastry, flaky (–)
7	short crust (–)
9	Pizza, cheese and tomato (150g)
1	Porridge (30g)
2	Rice, boiled (160g)
6	fried (120g)
6	puffed (25g)
8	Scone (30g)
7	Sponge pudding, steamed (100g)
4	Trifle (100g)
10	Wheat, breakfast biscuit (35g)
36	Yeast, dried, baker's (–)

EGG AND CHEESE DISHES

Protein (g)	Food
6	Cauliflower cheese (100g)
12	Cheese soufflé (100g)
12	Egg, boiled (55g)

Protein (g)	Food
.5	Apricots, canned (100g)
5	dried (25g)
.4	stewed, no sugar (inc. stones 110g)
4	Avocado pear (½ = 150g)
1	Banana (100g)
1	Blackberries (100g)
1	stewed, no sugar (100g)
.6	Cantaloup (inc. skin 120g)
.5	Cherries (inc. stones 20 = 100g)
.4	stewed, no sugar (inc. stones 100g)
.9	Currants, black (90g)
2	dried (15g)
1	red (90g)
2	Dates, dried (6 = 35g)
1	Figs (2 = 75g)
4	dried (2 = 40g)
.3	Fruit salad, canned (120g)
.6	Grapes, black (20 = 100g)
.6	white (20 = 100g)
.3	Grapefruit, whole (200g)
.5	canned (100g)
.3	juice, canned (120g)
.4	Guavas, canned (100g)
.8	Lemon, slices (2 = 15g)
.3	juice (15g)
1	Loganberries (100g)
.6	canned (100g)
1	stewed, no sugar (100g)
.4	Lychees, canned (100g)
.8	Mandarins (2 = 100g)
.6	canned (50g)
.5	Mango (100g)
.3	canned (100g)
.9	Nectarines (inc. stones 3 = 100g)
.7	Olives, in brine (5 = 20g)
.6	Orange, whole (130g)
.6	juice, fresh (120g)
.4	canned (120g)
1	Passionfruit, whole (30g)
.6	Papaw (100g)
.2	Peach (inc. stones 120g)
.6	canned (120g)
.4	dried (120g)
3	dried (25g)

Food	Protein
cheese spread (10g)	18
cottage (25g)	14
cream cheese (15g)	8
Danish blue (25g)	23
edam (25g)	24
parmesan (10g)	35
processed (25g)	22
stilton (25g)	26
Swiss (25g)	29
Cream, 35% fat (30g)	2
sterilized, canned (15g)	3
Ice-cream (60g)	4
non-dairy (60g)	3
Milk, cow's, cond. skim, sweet. (30g)	10
cond. whole, sweet. (30g)	8
dried, skimmed (12g)	36
dried, whole (10g)	26
evap. whole, unsweet. (30g)	9
flavoured (230g)	3
fresh, skimmed (230g)	3
fresh, whole (230g)	3
longlife, UHT (230g)	3
goat's (230g)	3
human (100g)	1
Milkshake, flavoured (340g)	3
Yoghurt, flavoured (200g)	4
fruit, low-fat (200g)	5
natural, low-fat (200g)	5
plain (200g)	4

NUTS

Food	Protein
Almonds (10=15g)	17
Brazil nuts (5=20g)	12
Cashews, roast (10=20g)	18
Chestnuts (4=20g)	2
Coconut, desiccated (15g)	6
Hazel nuts (10=15g)	8
Macadamia nuts (8=20g)	8
Peanuts, raw, in shells (5=25g)	24
roasted, salted (30=25g)	17
Pistachio nuts, shelled (25=15g)	19
Walnuts (5=20g)	11

SAUCES & CONDIMENTS

Food	Protein
Barbecue sauce (10g)	2
Chilli sauce (–)	1

Food	Protein
Peach, stewed, no sugar (120g)	.1
Pear (inc. skin, core 120g)	.2
canned (120g)	.4
stewed, no sugar (120g)	.3
Pineapple (80g)	.5
canned (80g)	.3
juice, canned (120g)	.4
Plums (inc. stones 3=100g)	.5
stewed, no sugar (inc. stones 100g)	.4
Prunes (inc. stones 8=80g)	2
stewed, no sugar (inc. stones 120g)	1
Quince, raw (100g)	.3
Raisins, dried (20g)	1
Raspberries (100g)	.9
canned (100g)	.6
stewed, no sugar (100g)	.9
Rhubarb, stewed, no sugar (120g)	.6
Strawberries (10=100g)	.6
canned (100g)	.4
Sultanas, dried (15g)	2
Watermelon (260g)	.2

MEAT AND MEAT PRODUCTS

Food	Protein
Bacon rashers, middle, fried (2=40g)	24
grilled (40g)	25
Beef, corned, canned (90g)	27
fillet steak, grilled (130g)	28
mince, stewed (120g)	23
rump steak, fried (150g)	29
grilled (150g)	27
silverside, salted, boiled (120g)	29
sirloin, roast (120g)	24
stewing steak, stewed (120g)	31
topside, roast (120g)	27
Beefburger, frozen, fried (60g)	20
Beef stew (250g)	10
Bolognese sauce (100g)	8
Chicken, boiled (100g)	29
crumbed, no bone (140g)	24
roast (130g)	23
leg quarter (inc. bone 130g)	15
wing quarter (inc. bone 130g)	12
Chicken livers, fried (130g)	21
Duck, roast (100g)	20

Value	Food
84	Gelatin (–)
27	Ham, canned (90g)
14	Hamburger (170g)
11	with cheese (190g)
5	Irish stew (250g)
12	Lamb, brain, boiled (150g)
18	chops, loin, grilled (inc. bone 120g)
15	cutlets, grilled (inc. bone 100g)
26	heart, roast (140g)
25	kidney, fried (100g)
26	leg, roast (120g)
23	liver, fried (130g)
20	shoulder, roast (120g)
18	tongue, stewed (100g)
13	Luncheon meat, canned (90g)
8	Meat pie (180g)
9	Moussaka (200g)
8	Pastie (160g)
22	Pork, chop, loin, grilled (100g)
27	leg, roast (120g)
7	sweet and sour (250g)
10	Pork pie (180g)
14	Rabbit, stewed (inc. bone 170g)
19	Salami, slices (3=90g)
13	Sausage, liver (60g)
8	Sausage roll (100g)
13	Sausages, beef, fried (2=120g)
13	grilled (2=120g)
10	frankfurter (2=100g)
14	pork, fried (2=120g)
13	grilled (2=120g)
10	saveloy, large (2=150g)
5	Spring roll, fried (200g)
9	Steak and kidney pie (180g)
15	Stewed steak in gravy, canned (100g)
16	Tongue, canned (100g)
15	Tripe, stewed (100g)
28	Turkey, roast (120g)
31	Veal, cutlet, fried (110g)
32	fillet, roast (100g)
21	schnitzel (140g)

MILK & MILK PRODUCTS

Value	Food
23	Cheese, camembert (25g)
26	Cheddar (25g)

Value	Food
1	Chutney, tomato (20g)
10	Curry powder (–)
.1	French dressing (15g)
7	Ginger (ground) (–)
2	Mayonnaise (20g)
29	Mustard powder (–)
38	Oxo cubes (–)
9	Pepper (–)
1	Pickles, mustard (20g)
.6	sweet (20g)
2	Salad cream (25g)
0	Salt, table (–)
19	Sesame seeds (–)
6	Soy sauce (–)
1	Tartare sauce (20g)
2	Tomato sauce (25g)
.4	Vinegar (–)
1	Worcestershire sauce (–)

SOUPS (as served)

Value	Food
1	Chicken, condensed (230g)
.8	Chicken noodle, dried (230g)
.8	Minestrone, dried (230g)
1	Mushroom, canned (230g)
.9	Tomato, condensed (230g)
.6	Tomato, dried (230g)
2	Vegetable, canned (230g)

SUGARS, JAMS AND SPREADS

Value	Food
15	Fish paste (5g)
.4	Honey (30g)
.6	Jam, fruit, edible seeds (30g)
.4	Jam, stone fruit (30g)
.1	Marmalade (30g)
15	Meat paste (5g)
23	Peanut butter (20g)
Tr	Sugar, white (–)
.3	Syrup, golden (30g)
.1	Topping, flavoured (40g)
1	Treacle, black (30g)
30	Vegemite (3g)

SWEETS

Value	Food
Tr	Boiled sweet (5g)
Tr	Butterscotch (5g)
4	Caramel (5g)

9	Carob bar (75g)
8	Chocolate square, milk (5g)
11	Fruit and honey bar (50g)
.1	Jelly bean (5g)
4	Liquorice allsort (7g)
5	Pastille (5g)
.5	Peppermint (4g)
6	Popcorn, plain unsalted (15g)
11	Sesame bar (50g)
2	Toffee, mixed (5g)

VEGETABLES

.5	Artichoke, globe, boiled (100g)
2	Asparagus, boiled (5=100g)
3	Bamboo shoots (50g)
.8	Beans, French, boiled (100g)
5	baked, in tomato sauce (125g)
4	broad, boiled (100g)
7	kidney (and haricot), boiled (100g)
6	mung, cooked dahl (100g)
11	soya-, boiled (100g)
2	Beetroot, slices, boiled (2=30g)
1	canned (2=30g)
3	Broccoli, boiled (100g)
3	Brussels sprouts, boiled (7=70g)
3	Cabbage, raw (50g)
1	boiled (100g)
.7	Carrots, raw (50g)
.6	boiled (50g)
.7	young, canned (50g)
2	Cauliflower, raw (50g)
2	boiled (100g)
2	Celeriac, boiled (3=60g)
.9	Celery, raw (50g)
.6	boiled (50g)
8	Chickpeas, cooked dahl (60g)
.6	Cucumber, slices (5=30g)
1	Egg plant, baked (½=100g)
2	Endive, raw leaves (13=15g)
2	Leeks, boiled (4=100g)
8	Lentils, split, boiled (100g)
1	Lettuce, raw leaves (2=20g)
.5	Marrow, boiled (100g)
2	Mushrooms, raw (3=30g)
2	fried (6=60g)

.9	Onions, raw (¼=20g)
.6	boiled (100g)
2	fried (70g)
.9	spring (4=20g)
5	Parsley, sprigs (2=5g)
1	Parsnip, boiled (½=60g)
5	Peas, canned (60g)
6	canned, processed (60g)
5	fresh, boiled (60g)
5	frozen, boiled (60g)
8	split, boiled (60g)
.9	Peppers, green, raw (¼=15g)
.9	boiled (50g)
2	Potato, baked (inc. skin 120g)
1	boiled (120g)
4	chips, fresh, fried (12=120g)
3	chips, frozen, fried (8-14=120g)
6	crisps (10=25g)
2	mashed (100g)
2	instant, cooked (100g)
2	new, boiled (2=100g)
1	new, canned (2=100g)
3	roast (120g)
.6	Pumpkin (100g)
1	Radishes (2=20g)
5	Spinach, leaves, boiled (3=60g)
.9	Swede, boiled (80g)
4	Sweetcorn, on cob, boiled (150g)
3	canned kernels (80g)
1	Sweet potato, boiled (100g)
.9	Tomato, raw (120g)
1	canned (120g)
1	fried (120g)
1	juice, canned (120g)
.7	Turnip, boiled (80g)
2	Yam, boiled (100g)

5
PHENYLALANINE

Phenylalanine is a small organic chemical belonging to a group of substances called amino acids. Amino acids are combined in nature to form proteins. When we eat foods containing proteins, the proteins are broken down during digestion into their constituent amino acids. Our bodies use some of these to make new proteins and other substances that are essential for life. Phenylalanine is one of the so-called 'essential' amino acids and must be obtained by the body from food. You can obtain all the essential amino acids by consuming a mixed diet containing the recommended intake of protein (see Chart 4).

However, there are some disorders in which the normal metabolism of amino acids is defective. These are genetically determined and can usually be detected soon after birth. *Phenylketonuria* (PKU) is an inherited defect in which phenylalanine is incompletely and abnormally metabolized. Unless detected and treated early this can lead to mental retardation. Tests to detect this disorder are routinely carried out on all new babies born in a hospital.

Treatment for PKU consists in strictly limiting the amount of phenylalanine in the diet. Because phenylalanine is an essential amino acid, its complete absence will retard growth and development. Therefore diets for PKU children restrict the amount of phenylalanine to a level that will allow both normal growth and normal intelligence. They must be planned in consultation with a doctor and a dietitian. A woman who was a PKU child and who subsequently becomes pregnant must restrict her phenylalanine intake during the pregnancy to avoid the possibility of damage to the baby.

PHENYLALANINE INTAKE

Only children who have phenylketonuria (PKU) must strictly control the foods they eat to ensure that they do not have an excessive intake of phenylalanine. This must be under the supervision of a dietitian or doctor. The chart gives the approximate amount of phenylalanine in a variety of foods.

milligrams per 100 grams

BEVERAGES

10	Beer (240g)
–	Cider, dry, alcoholic (180g)
–	sweet, alcoholic (180g)
–	sweet, non-alcoholic (220g)
780	Cocoa powder (5g)
10	Coffee, percolated (230g)
–	Cola-type drinks (240g)
–	Cordial, diluted 1:4 (240g)
220	Drinking chocolate (10g)
–	Lemonade, carbonated drinks (240g)
–	Milo (10g)
–	Ovaltine (10g)
–	Port (60g)
–	Sherry, dry (60g)
–	medium (60g)
–	sweet (60g)
–	Spirits, e.g. whisky (30g)
–	Tea, infusion (230g)
–	Wine, red (100g)
–	white, dry (100g)
–	medium (100g)
–	sparkling (100g)
–	sweet (100g)

CEREALS, BISCUITS, CAKES, DESSERTS

150	Barley, pearl, boiled (–)
300	Biscuit, chocolate (20g)
–	cream-filled (20g)
450	crispbread, rye (20g)
2380	wheat, starch-red. (11g)
290	gingernut (15g)
350	semi-sweet (15g)
320	short-sweet (15g)
580	Bran, wheat (8g)
440	Bread, brown, slice (25g)
–	Lebanese (pita) (¼=25g)
420	white, slice (25g)
420	wholemeal, slice (25g)
570	roll, brown (35g)
2320	starch-reduced (35g)
610	white (35g)
170	Cake, fruit (60g)
300	plain (60g)

720	Egg, fried (60g)
530	omelette (100g)
640	poached (55g)
630	raw (55g)
540	scrambled (70g)
390	Macaroni cheese (180g)
740	Quiche Lorraine (150g)

FATS AND OILS

20	Butter, salted (10g)
–	Dripping, beef (–)
–	Lard (–)
10	Margarine (10g)
–	Vegetable oils (–)

FISH AND OTHER SEAFOODS

–	Bream, steamed (100g)
890	Cod, baked (100g)
820	fried in batter (100g)
870	poached (100g)
780	steamed (100g)
800	Crab, boiled (150g)
730	canned (90g)
–	Fish cakes, fried (4=100g)
580	fingers, fried (5=100g)
–	in batter, fried (120g)
–	Flounder, baked (100g)
890	Haddock, fried (100g)
950	steamed (100g)
890	Lobster, boiled (120g)
720	Mussels, boiled (12=120g)
450	Oysters, raw (12=120g)
910	Prawns, boiled (6=120g)
–	Roe, cod, fried (100g)
840	Salmon, canned (100g)
820	Sardines, canned (60g)
970	Scallops, steamed (10=100g)
950	Tuna, canned in oil (120g)
750	Whiting, crumbed, fried (100g)
870	steamed (100g)

FRUIT

2	Apple (inc. skin, core 100g)
10	baked, no sugar (inc. skin 110g)
10	stewed, no sugar (110g)
10	Apricots (inc. stones 3=100g)

Food	mg	Food	mg
Cake, sponge (60g)	330	Apricots, canned (100g)	10
Chapati (60g)	400	dried (25g)	80
Cheesecake (120g)	220	stewed, no sugar (inc. stones 110g)	10
Cornflakes (30g)	430	Avocado pear (½=150g)	150
Crumpet (50g)	–	Banana (100g)	50
Custard (70g)	300	Blackberries (100g)	–
Custard tart (120g)	310	stewed, no sugar (100g)	–
Doughnut (40g)	310	Cantaloup (inc. skin 120g)	30
Eclair (50g)	230	Cherries (inc. stones 20=100g)	–
Flour, corn- (–)	–	stewed, no sugar (inc. stones 100g)	–
plain (–)	520	Currants, black (90g)	–
self-raising (–)	490	dried (15g)	40
soya, full-fat (–)	2000	red (90g)	–
low-fat (–)	2460	Dates, dried (6=35g)	60
wholemeal (–)	630	Figs (2=75g)	30
Fruit pie (150g)	90	dried (2=40g)	90
Jam tart (35g)	170	Fruit salad, canned (120g)	–
Jelly, made with water (100g)	30	Grapes, black (20=100g)	10
Lamington (60g)	–	white (20=100g)	10
Lemon meringue pie (120g)	230	Grapefruit, whole (200g)	10
Meringue (15g)	310	canned (100g)	20
Milk pudding (e.g. sago) (160g)	220	juice, canned (120g)	10
Muesli (30g)	690	Guavas, canned (100g)	10
Noodles (chow mein) (250g)	–	Lemon, slices (2=15g)	30
Pancake (75g)	320	juice (15g)	–
Pasta, macaroni, boiled (150g)	230	Loganberries (100g)	–
spaghetti, boiled (120g)	220	canned (100g)	–
canned in tomato sauce (120g)	90	stewed, no sugar (100g)	–
Pastry, flaky (–)	310	Lychees, canned (100g)	–
short crust (–)	360	Mandarins (2=100g)	–
Pizza, cheese and tomato (150g)	490	canned (50g)	20
Porridge (30g)	70	Mango (100g)	–
Rice, boiled (160g)	110	canned (100g)	–
fried (120g)	–	Nectarines (inc. stones 3=100g)	20
puffed (25g)	–	Olives, in brine (5=20g)	–
Scone (30g)	400	Orange, whole (130g)	20
Sponge pudding, steamed (100g)	310	juice, fresh (120g)	20
Trifle (100g)	180	canned (120g)	20
Wheat, breakfast biscuit (35g)	550	Passionfruit, whole (30g)	–
Yeast, dried, baker's (–)	1710	Papaw (100g)	–
EGG AND CHEESE DISHES		canned (100g)	–
Cauliflower cheese (100g)	280	Peach (inc. stones 120g)	10
Cheese soufflé (100g)	590	canned (120g)	10
Egg, boiled (55g)	630	dried (25g)	80

Food	Phenylalanine
cheese spread (10g)	980
cottage (25g)	730
cream cheese (15g)	170
Danish blue (25g)	1230
edam (25g)	1300
parmesan (10g)	1870
processed (25g)	1150
stilton (25g)	1370
Swiss (25g)	–
Cream, 35% fat (30g)	100
sterilized, canned (15g)	140
Ice-cream (60g)	200
non-dairy (60g)	180
Milk, cow's, cond. skim, sweet. (30g)	530
cond. whole, sweet. (30g)	440
dried, skimmed (12g)	1940
dried, whole (10g)	1400
evap. whole, unsweet. (30g)	460
flavoured (230g)	–
fresh, skimmed (230g)	180
fresh, whole (230g)	180
longlife, UHT (230g)	180
goat's (230g)	–
human (100g)	50
Milkshake, flavoured (340g)	–
Yoghurt, flavoured (200g)	–
fruit, low-fat (200g)	280
natural, low-fat (200g)	290
plain (200g)	–

NUTS

Food	Phenylalanine
Almonds (10=15g)	980
Brazil nuts (5=20g)	530
Cashews, roast (10=20g)	–
Chestnuts (4=20g)	–
Coconut, desiccated (15g)	290
Hazel nuts (10=15g)	330
Macadamia nuts (8=20g)	–
Peanuts, raw, in shells (5=25g)	960
roasted, salted (30=25g)	1400
Pistachio nuts, shelled (25=15g)	–
Walnuts (5=20g)	540

SAUCES & CONDIMENTS

Food	Phenylalanine
Barbecue sauce (10g)	–
Chilli sauce (–)	–

Food	Phenylalanine
Peach, stewed, no sugar (120g)	30
Pear (inc. skin, core 120g)	5
canned (120g)	10
stewed, no sugar (120g)	5
Pineapple (80g)	10
canned (80g)	10
juice, canned (120g)	10
Plums (inc. stones 3 = 100g)	–
stewed, no sugar (inc. stones 100g)	–
Prunes (inc. stones 8 = 80g)	–
stewed, no sugar (inc. stones 120g)	–
Quince, raw (100g)	–
Raisins, dried (20g)	20
Raspberries (100g)	–
canned (100g)	–
stewed, no sugar (100g)	–
Rhubarb, stewed, no sugar (120g)	–
Strawberries (10 = 100g)	20
canned (100g)	10
Sultanas, dried (15g)	40
Watermelon (260g)	–

MEAT AND MEAT PRODUCTS

Food	Phenylalanine
Bacon rashers, middle, fried (2=40g)	1040
grilled (40g)	1080
Beef, corned, canned (90g)	1120
fillet steak, grilled (130g)	–
mince, stewed (120g)	1030
rump steak, fried (150g)	1280
grilled (150g)	1220
silverside, salted, boiled (120g)	1280
sirloin, roast (120g)	1060
stewing steak, stewed (120g)	1380
topside, roast (120g)	1190
Beefburger, frozen, fried (60g)	880
Beef stew (250g)	430
Bolognese sauce (100g)	330
Chicken, boiled (100g)	1310
crumbed, no bone (140g)	–
roast (130g)	1110
leg quarter (inc. bone 130g)	690
wing quarter (inc. bone 130g)	560
Chicken livers, fried (130g)	1030
Duck, roast (100g)	1130

1980	Gelatin (–)
740	Ham, canned (90g)
–	Hamburger (170g)
–	with cheese (190g)
190	Irish stew (250g)
600	Lamb, brain, boiled (150g)
700	chops, loin, grilled (inc. bone 120g)
580	cutlets, grilled (inc. bone 100g)
1210	heart, roast (140g)
1220	kidney, fried (100g)
1000	leg, roast (120g)
1140	liver, fried (130g)
760	shoulder, roast (120g)
640	tongue, stewed (100g)
490	Luncheon meat, canned (90g)
–	Meat pie (180g)
430	Moussaka (200g)
370	Pastie (160g)
850	Pork, chop, loin, grilled (100g)
1030	leg, roast (120g)
–	sweet and sour (250g)
480	Pork pie (180g)
650	Rabbit, stewed (inc. bone 170g)
800	Salami, slices (3=90g)
560	Sausage, liver (60g)
340	Sausage roll (100g)
540	Sausages, beef, fried (2=120g)
540	grilled (2=120g)
410	frankfurter (2=100g)
550	pork, fried (2=120g)
530	grilled (2=120g)
330	saveloy, large (2=150g)
–	Spring roll, fried (200g)
720	Steak and kidney pie (180g)
590	Stewed steak in gravy, canned (100g)
770	Tongue, canned (100g)
570	Tripe, stewed (100g)
1290	Turkey, roast (120g)
1410	Veal, cutlet, fried (110g)
1410	fillet, roast (100g)
–	schnitzel (140g)

MILK & MILK PRODUCTS

1220	Cheese, camembert (25g)
1390	cheddar (25g)

20	Chutney, tomato (20g)
–	Curry powder (–)
–	French dressing (15g)
–	Ginger (ground) (–)
90	Mayonnaise (20g)
–	Mustard powder (–)
–	Oxo cubes (–)
–	Pepper (–)
–	Pickles, mustard (20g)
–	sweet (20g)
–	Salad cream (25g)
–	Salt, table (–)
–	Sesame seeds (–)
–	Soy sauce (–)
–	Tartare sauce (25g)
70	Tomato sauce (25g)
–	Vinegar (–)
–	Worcestershire sauce (–)

SOUPS (as served)

–	Chicken, condensed (230g)
–	Chicken noodle, dried (230g)
–	Minestrone, dried (230g)
–	Mushroom, canned (230g)
–	Tomato, condensed (230g)
–	Tomato, dried (230g)
–	Vegetable, canned (230g)

SUGARS, JAMS AND SPREADS

–	Fish paste (5g)
–	Honey (30g)
–	Jam, fruit, edible seeds (30g)
–	Jam, stone fruit (30g)
2	Marmalade (30g)
580	Meat paste (5g)
1290	Peanut butter (20g)
–	Sugar, white (–)
–	Syrup, golden (30g)
–	Topping, flavoured (40g)
–	Treacle, black (30g)
–	Vegemite (3g)

SWEETS

–	Boiled sweet (5g)
–	Butterscotch (5g)
–	Caramel (5g)

Food	Phe
Carob bar (75g)	–
Chocolate square, milk (5g)	550
Fruit and honey bar (50g)	–
Jelly bean (5g)	–
Liquorice allsort (7g)	–
Pastille (5g)	–
Peppermint (4g)	–
Popcorn, plain unsalted (15g)	–
Sesame bar (50g)	–
Toffee, mixed (5g)	–

VEGETABLES

Food	Phe
Artichoke, globe, boiled (100g)	–
Asparagus, boiled (5 = 100g)	40
Bamboo shoots (50g)	–
Beans, French, boiled (100g)	30
baked, in tomato sauce (125g)	270
broad, boiled (100g)	180
kidney (and haricot), boiled (100g)	350
mung, cooked dahl (100g)	–
soya-, boiled (100g)	
Beetroot, slices, boiled (2 = 30g)	60
canned (2 = 30g)	–
Broccoli, boiled (100g)	110
Brussels sprouts, boiled (7 = 70g)	100
Cabbage, raw (50g)	100
boiled (100g)	40
Carrots, raw (50g)	20
boiled (50g)	20
young, canned (50g)	20
Cauliflower, raw (50g)	60
boiled (100g)	60
Celeriac, boiled (3 = 60g)	–
Celery, raw (50g)	40
boiled (50g)	30
Chickpeas, cooked dahl (60g)	460
Cucumber, slices (5 = 30g)	10
Egg plant, baked (½ = 100g)	–
Endive, raw leaves (3 = 15g)	–
Leeks, boiled (4 = 100g)	–
Lentils, split, boiled (100g)	400
Lettuce, raw leaves (2 = 20g)	50
Marrow, boiled (100g)	–
Mushrooms, raw (3 = 30g)	80
fried (6 = 60g)	120
Onions, raw (¼ = 20g)	30
boiled (100g)	20
fried (70g)	50
spring (4 = 20g)	30
Parsley, sprigs (2 = 5g)	–
Parsnip, boiled (½ = 60g)	–
Peas, canned (60g)	220
canned, processed (60g)	290
fresh, boiled (60g)	230
frozen, boiled (60g)	250
split, boiled (60g)	390
Peppers, green, raw (¼ = 15g)	–
boiled (50g)	–
Potato, baked (inc. skin 120g)	90
boiled (120g)	60
chips, fresh, fried (12 = 120g)	170
chips, frozen, fried (8-14 = 120g)	130
crisps (10 = 25g)	270
mashed (100g)	130
instant, cooked (100g)	90
new, boiled (2 = 100g)	70
new, canned (2 = 100g)	50
roast (120g)	120
Pumpkin (100g)	–
Radishes (2 = 20g)	–
Spinach, leaves, boiled (3 = 60g)	310
Swede, boiled (80g)	–
Sweetcorn, on cob, boiled (150g)	200
canned kernels (80g)	150
Sweet potato, boiled (100g)	40
Tomato, raw (120g)	20
canned (120g)	20
fried (120g)	20
juice, canned (120g)	10
Turnip, boiled (80g)	10
Yam, boiled (100g)	70

6

CARBOHYDRATE

Carbohydrates can be divided into three main groups:

- sugars
- starches
- cellulose and other complex substances that are not digested by humans.

Sugars and starches in food are sources of energy. Australians obtain 20 to 60 per cent of their total dietary energy from carbohydrate. Cellulose and some related substances are not used by our bodies as a significant source of energy. Nevertheless, these components are very important as, together with other indigestible substances, they constitute dietary fibre. The role of dietary fibre is discussed on page 61.

SUGARS

The main sugars in food are sucrose, glucose, fructose, maltose and lactose. Sucrose is obtained from sugar cane and is usually called 'sugar'. In addition, sucrose (as well as glucose and fructose) is found in fruit, fruit juices and honey. Besides providing energy, sugars also produce the sensation of sweetness. Each sugar contributes the same amount of energy (kilocalories) to our diet regardless of its sweetness. Different sugars are not equally sweet and the degree of sweetness of a food is often not a good indication of the amount of sugars present. For example, as shown in Figure 45, maltose is only half as sweet as sucrose.

FIGURE 45: SWEETNESS OF SUGARS RELATIVE TO SUCROSE

SUGAR	RELATIVE SWEETNESS	OTHER NAME
Sucrose	1	Sugar
Glucose	0.7	Grape sugar
Fructose	1.1	Fruit sugar
Lactose	0.4	Milk sugar
Maltose	0.5	Malt sugar
Sorbitol	0.5	—

Sugars are widely distributed in foods, particularly processed foods where their sweetness may sometimes be masked or hidden by other ingredients.

Often the list of ingredients on the label will give an indication of the relative amount of sugar present. For a fuller discussion on sugars, see page 21.

The use of non-nutritive or artificial sweeteners can be used to make food and drink sweet without contributing significant amounts of energy. Although there is controversy about their safety, the most widely used artificial sweeteners are saccharin and cyclamate. The label of any food or drink containing these sweeteners must indicate that they are present. An artificial sweetener recently approved by some health authorities is aspartame. It has about the same energy value as sugar but because it is 180 times sweeter, very little needs to be used. The amount of aspartame providing sweetness equivalent to one teaspoon of sugar will only provide one-tenth of a kilocalorie.

STARCH

Starch is the main form of carbohydrate in our food. It is present in a variety of cereals, vegetables and fruit, with major contributions from flour, potatoes and legumes (beans, peas). Starchy foods are usually cooked to improve digestibility and give a more desirable texture and flavour. During the ripening of fruit, starch is changed into sugars, which give sweetness to ripe fruits. In contrast to sugars, starch is often accompanied by significant amounts of other nutrients including dietary fibre. Starch has the same energy value as sugars. Health authorities are in agreement that we should increase our consumption of foods containing starch, such as wholegrain bread, cereals, fruits, vegetables and nuts.

CARBOHYDRATE INTAKE

There is no specific dietary requirement for carbohydrate because energy can also be derived from protein, fat and alcohol. However, a diet that does not contain carbohydrate can lead to muscle breakdown, ketosis and dehydration. This can be prevented by 50 to 100 grams of carbohydrate per day, but levels above this are desirable. Sources of complex carbohydrates, such as starch, are recommended as these often also provide necessary vitamins, elements (minerals) and dietary fibre.

grams per 100 grams

BEVERAGES

2	Beer (240g)
3	Cider, dry, alcoholic (180g)
4	sweet, alcoholic (180g)
12	sweet, non-alcoholic (220g)
12	Cocoa powder (5g)
0	Coffee, percolated (230g)
11	Cola-type drinks (240g)
9	Cordial, diluted 1:4 (240g)
77	Drinking chocolate (10g)
10	Lemonade, carbonated drinks (240g)
68	Milo (10g)
79	Ovaltine (10g)
12	Port (60g)
1	Sherry, dry (60g)
4	medium (60g)
7	sweet (60g)
Tr	Spirits, e.g. whisky (30g)
Tr	Tea, infusion (230g)
Tr	Wine, red (100g)
1	white, dry (100g)
3	medium (100g)
1	sparkling (100g)
6	sweet (100g)

CEREALS, BISCUITS, CAKES, DESSERTS

28	Barley, pearl, boiled (–)
67	Biscuit, chocolate (20g)
67	cream-filled (20g)
70	crispbread, rye (20g)
37	wheat, starch-red. (11g)
79	gingernut (15g)
75	semi-sweet (15g)
62	short-sweet (15g)
27	Bran, wheat (8g)
48	Bread, brown, slice (25g)
53	Lebanese (pita) (¼=25g)
49	white, slice (25g)
47	wholemeal, slice (25g)
57	roll, brown (35g)
46	starch-reduced (35g)
57	white (35g)
58	Cake, fruit (60g)
58	plain (60g)

Tr	Egg, fried (60g)
Tr	omelette (100g)
Tr	poached (55g)
Tr	raw (55g)
Tr	scrambled (70g)
15	Macaroni cheese (180g)
21	Quiche Lorraine (150g)

FATS AND OILS

Tr	Butter, salted (10g)
0	Dripping, beef (–)
0	Lard (–)
Tr	Margarine (10g)
0	Vegetable oils (–)

FISH AND OTHER SEAFOODS

0	Bream, steamed (100g)
0	Cod, baked (100g)
8	fried in batter (100g)
0	poached (100g)
0	steamed (100g)
0	Crab, boiled (150g)
0	canned (90g)
15	Fish cakes, fried (4=100g)
17	fingers, fried (5=100g)
14	in batter, fried (120g)
0	Flounder, baked (100g)
4	Haddock, fried (100g)
0	steamed (100g)
0	Lobster, boiled (120g)
Tr	Mussels, boiled (12=120g)
Tr	Oysters, raw (12=120g)
0	Prawns, boiled (6=120g)
3	Roe, cod, fried (100g)
0	Salmon, canned (100g)
0	Sardines, canned (60g)
Tr	Scallops, steamed (10=100g)
0	Tuna, canned in oil (120g)
7	Whiting, crumbed, fried (100g)
0	steamed (100g)

FRUIT

9	Apple (inc. skin, core 100g)
8	baked, no sugar (inc. skin 110g)
8	stewed, no sugar (110g)
6	Apricots (inc. stones 3=100g)

Value	Food
28	Apricots, canned (100g)
43	dried (25g)
5	stewed, no sugar (inc. stones 110g)
2	Avocado pear (½=150g)
19	Banana (100g)
6	Blackberries (100g)
6	stewed, no sugar (100g)
3	Cantaloup (inc. skin 120g)
10	Cherries (inc. stones 20=100g)
8	stewed, no sugar (inc. stones 100g)
7	Currants, black (90g)
63	dried (15g)
4	red (90g)
64	Dates, dried (6=35g)
10	Figs (2=75g)
53	dried (2=40g)
25	Fruit salad, canned (120g)
13	Grapes, black (20=100g)
15	white (20=100g)
3	Grapefruit, whole (200g)
16	canned (100g)
8	juice, canned (120g)
16	Guavas, canned (100g)
3	Lemon, slices (2=15g)
2	juice (15g)
3	Loganberries (100g)
26	canned (100g)
3	stewed, no sugar (100g)
18	Lychees, canned (100g)
11	Mandarins (2=100g)
14	canned (50g)
15	Mango (100g)
20	canned (100g)
11	Nectarines (inc. stones 3=100g)
Tr	Olives, in brine (5=20g)
6	Orange, whole (130g)
9	juice, fresh (120g)
9	canned (120g)
3	Passionfruit, whole (30g)
11	Papaw (100g)
17	canned (100g)
8	Peach (inc. stones 120g)
23	canned (120g)
53	dried (25g)

Value	Food
53	Cake, sponge (60g)
50	Chapati (60g)
35	Cheesecake (120g)
87	Cornflakes (30g)
52	Crumpet (50g)
4	Custard (70g)
17	Custard tart (120g)
49	Doughnut (40g)
38	Eclair (50g)
87	Flour, corn- (–)
75	plain (–)
74	self-raising (–)
24	soya, full-fat (–)
28	low-fat (–)
72	wholemeal (–)
57	Fruit pie (150g)
63	Jam tart (35g)
14	Jelly, made with water (100g)
56	Lamington (60g)
46	Lemon meringue pie (120g)
96	Meringue (15g)
20	Milk pudding (e.g. sago) (160g)
56	Muesli (30g)
8	Noodles (chow mein) (250g)
36	Pancake (75g)
25	Pasta, macaroni, boiled (150g)
26	spaghetti, boiled (120g)
12	canned in tomato sauce (120g)
41	Pastry, flaky (–)
32	short crust (–)
25	Pizza, cheese and tomato (150g)
8	Porridge (30g)
30	Rice, boiled (160g)
30	fried (120g)
88	puffed (25g)
56	Scone (30g)
46	Sponge pudding, steamed (100g)
24	Trifle (100g)
75	Wheat, breakfast biscuit (35g)
4	Yeast, dried, baker's (–)

EGG AND CHEESE DISHES

Value	Food
5	Cauliflower cheese (100g)
9	Cheese soufflé (100g)
Tr	Egg, boiled (55g)

Food	Carbohydrate (g)
cheese spread (10g)	Tr
cottage (25g)	1
cream cheese (15g)	Tr
Danish blue (25g)	Tr
edam (25g)	Tr
parmesan (10g)	Tr
processed (25g)	Tr
stilton (25g)	Tr
Swiss (25g)	Tr
Cream, 35% fat (30g)	3
sterilized, canned (15g)	3
Ice-cream (60g)	25
non-dairy (60g)	21
Milk, cow's, cond. skim, sweet. (30g)	60
cond. whole, sweet. (30g)	56
dried, skimmed (12g)	53
dried, whole (10g)	39
evap. whole, unsweet. (30g)	11
flavoured (230g)	10
fresh, skimmed (230g)	5
fresh, whole (230g)	5
longlife, UHT (230g)	5
goat's (230g)	5
human (100g)	7
Milkshake, flavoured (340g)	17
Yoghurt, flavoured (200g)	11
fruit, low-fat (200g)	18
natural, low-fat (200g)	6
plain (200g)	6

NUTS

Food	Carbohydrate (g)
Almonds (10=15g)	4
Brazil nuts (5=20g)	4
Cashews, roast (10=20g)	28
Chestnuts (4=20g)	37
Coconut, desiccated (15g)	6
Hazel nuts (10=15g)	7
Macadamia nuts (8=20g)	14
Peanuts, raw, in shells (5=25g)	6
roasted, salted (30=25g)	9
Pistachio nuts, shelled (25=15g)	19
Walnuts (5=20g)	5

SAUCES & CONDIMENTS

Food	Carbohydrate (g)
Barbecue sauce (10g)	8
Chilli sauce (–)	4

Food	Carbohydrate (g)
Peach, stewed, no sugar (120g)	20
Pear (inc. skin, core 120g)	8
canned (120g)	20
stewed, no sugar (120g)	8
Pineapple (80g)	12
canned (80g)	20
juice, canned (120g)	13
Plums (inc. stones 3=100g)	9
stewed, no sugar (inc. stones 100g)	7
Prunes (inc. stones 8=80g)	34
stewed, no sugar (inc. stones 120g)	19
Quince, raw (100g)	6
Raisins, dried (20g)	64
Raspberries (100g)	6
canned (100g)	23
stewed, no sugar (100g)	6
Rhubarb, stewed, no sugar (120g)	1
Strawberries (10=100g)	6
canned (100g)	21
Sultanas, dried (15g)	65
Watermelon (260g)	3

MEAT AND MEAT PRODUCTS

Food	Carbohydrate (g)
Bacon rashers, middle, fried (2=40g)	0
grilled (40g)	0
Beef, corned, canned (90g)	0
fillet steak, grilled (130g)	0
mince, stewed (120g)	0
rump steak, fried (150g)	0
grilled (150g)	0
silverside, salted, boiled (120g)	0
sirloin, roast (120g)	0
stewing steak, stewed (120g)	0
topside, roast (120g)	0
Beefburger, frozen, fried (60g)	7
Beef stew (250g)	4
Bolognese sauce (100g)	3
Chicken, boiled (100g)	0
crumbed, no bone (140g)	10
roast (130g)	0
leg quarter (inc. bone 130g)	0
wing quarter (inc. bone 130g)	0
Chicken livers, fried (130g)	3
Duck, roast (100g)	0

Food	Carbohydrate
Gelatin (–)	0
Ham, canned (90g)	0
Hamburger (170g)	22
with cheese (190g)	21
Irish stew (250g)	9
Lamb, brain, boiled (150g)	0
chops, loin, grilled (inc. bone 120g)	0
cutlets, grilled (inc. bone 100g)	0
heart, roast (140g)	0
kidney, fried (100g)	0
leg, roast (120g)	0
liver, fried (130g)	4
shoulder, roast (120g)	0
tongue, stewed (100g)	0
Luncheon meat, canned (90g)	6
Meat pie (180g)	18
Moussaka (200g)	10
Pastie (160g)	31
Pork, chop, loin, grilled (100g)	0
leg, roast (120g)	0
sweet and sour (250g)	18
Pork pie (180g)	25
Rabbit, stewed (inc. bone 170g)	0
Salami, slices (3 = 90g)	2
Sausage, liver (60g)	4
Sausage roll (100g)	24
Sausages, beef, fried (2 = 120g)	15
grilled (2 = 120g)	15
frankfurter (2 = 100g)	3
pork, fried (2 = 120g)	11
grilled (2 = 120g)	12
saveloy, large (2 = 150g)	10
Spring roll, fried (200g)	29
Steak and kidney pie (180g)	26
Stewed steak in gravy, canned (100g)	1
Tongue, canned (100g)	0
Tripe, stewed (100g)	Tr
Turkey, roast (120g)	0
Veal, cutlet, fried (110g)	4
fillet, roast (100g)	0
schnitzel (140g)	10

MILK & MILK PRODUCTS

Food	Carbohydrate
Cheese, camembert (25g)	Tr
cheddar (25g)	Tr

Food	Carbohydrate
Chutney, tomato (20g)	40
Curry powder (–)	26
French dressing (15g)	Tr
Ginger (ground) (–)	60
Mayonnaise (20g)	Tr
Mustard powder (–)	21
Oxo cubes (–)	12
Pepper (–)	68
Pickles, mustard (20g)	6
sweet (20g)	34
Salad cream (25g)	15
Salt, table (–)	0
Sesame seeds (–)	22
Soy sauce (–)	10
Tartare sauce (20g)	6
Tomato sauce (25g)	8
Vinegar (–)	1
Worcestershire sauce (–)	18

SOUPS (as served)

Food	Carbohydrate
Chicken, condensed (230g)	3
Chicken noodle, dried (230g)	4
Minestrone, dried (230g)	4
Mushroom, canned (230g)	4
Tomato, canned (230g)	7
Tomato, dried (230g)	6
Vegetable, canned (230g)	7

SUGARS, JAMS AND SPREADS

Food	Carbohydrate
Fish paste (5g)	4
Honey (30g)	76
Jam, fruit, edible seeds (30g)	69
Jam, stone fruit (30g)	69
Marmalade (30g)	70
Meat paste (5g)	3
Peanut butter (20g)	13
Sugar, white (–)	100
Syrup, golden (30g)	79
Topping, flavoured (40g)	34
Treacle, black (30g)	67
Vegemite (3g)	13

CONFECTIONERY

Food	Carbohydrate
Boiled sweet (5g)	87
Butterscotch (5g)	90
Caramel (5g)	77

37	Carob bar (75g)
59	Chocolate square, milk (5g)
25	Fruit and honey bar (50g)
90	Jelly bean (5g)
74	Liquorice allsort (7g)
62	Pastille (5g)
100	Peppermint (4g)
85	Popcorn, plain unsalted (15g)
23	Sesame bar (50g)
71	Toffee, mixed (5g)

VEGETABLES

1	Artichoke, globe, boiled (100g)
1	Asparagus, boiled (5=100g)
5	Bamboo shoots (50g)
1	Beans, French, boiled (100g)
10	baked, in tomato sauce (125g)
7	broad, boiled (100g)
17	kidney (and haricot), boiled (100g)
11	mung, cooked dahl (100g)
11	soya-, boiled (100g)
10	Beetroot, slices, boiled (2=30g)
8	canned (2=30g)
2	Broccoli, boiled (100g)
2	Brussels sprouts, boiled (7=70g)
3	Cabbage, raw (50g)
1	boiled (100g)
5	Carrots, raw (50g)
4	boiled (50g)
5	young, canned (50g)
2	Cauliflower, raw (50g)
1	boiled (100g)
2	Celeriac, boiled (3=60g)
1	Celery, raw (50g)
1	boiled (50g)
22	Chickpeas, cooked dahl (60g)
2	Cucumber, slices (5=30g)
4	Egg plant, baked (½=100g)
1	Endive, raw leaves (3=15g)
5	Leeks, boiled (4=100g)
17	Lentils, split, boiled (100g)
1	Lettuce, raw leaves (2=20g)
1	Marrow, boiled (100g)
0	Mushrooms, raw (3=30g)
0	fried (6=60g)

5	Onions, raw (¼=20g)
3	boiled (100g)
10	fried (70g)
9	spring (4=20g)
Tr	Parsley, sprigs (2=5g)
14	Parsnip, boiled (½=60g)
7	Peas, canned (60g)
14	canned, processed (60g)
8	fresh, boiled (60g)
4	frozen, boiled (60g)
22	split, boiled (60g)
2	Peppers, green, raw (¼=15g)
2	boiled (50g)
20	Potato, baked (inc. skin 120g)
20	boiled (120g)
37	chips, fresh, fried (12=120g)
29	chips, frozen, fried (8-14=120g)
49	crisps (10=25g)
18	mashed (100g)
16	instant, cooked (100g)
18	new, boiled (2=100g)
13	new, canned (2=100g)
27	roast (120g)
3	Pumpkin (100g)
3	Radishes (2=20g)
1	Spinach, leaves, boiled (3=60g)
4	Swede, boiled (80g)
23	Sweetcorn, on cob, boiled (150g)
16	canned kernels (80g)
20	Sweet potato, boiled (100g)
3	Tomato, raw (120g)
2	canned (120g)
3	fried (120g)
3	juice, canned (120g)
2	Turnip, boiled (80g)
30	Yam, boiled (100g)

7

F A T

Fat is also known as lipid and is mainly present in food in a form called 'triglycerides'. Butter and margarine, for example, are almost entirely made up of triglycerides. Triglycerides consist of glycerol and three ('tri') fatty acids. The fatty acids can be mainly 'saturated' as in butter or mainly 'polyunsaturated' as in some margarines (see Figure 47). There are also monounsaturated fatty acids, which occur in quantity in the triglyceride of olive oil and peanut oil.

Food may contain other fats, such as cholesterol and phospholipids, in addition to triglycerides. Lecithin is a phospholipid, made up of glycerol, choline and fatty acids, which again may be mainly saturated or polyunsaturated (see Chart 48 on lecithin).

Fat is energy dense, having an Atwater factor of 9 kilocalories, or 37 kilojoules, per gram. Also, it does not mix with water, so that the food in which it is found tends to be more energy dense because of the relative lack of water. If it is a fat of plant origin, it may be associated with dietary fibre, giving bulk and reducing energy density, as, for example, with the cereal oats that are relatively high in fat for a cereal, but also relatively high in dietary fibre. If the fat is from animal sources, the energy density will be rather high, not only because of the fat and the low amount of water, but also because there is no dietary fibre.

If we are very physically active and in need of energy then fat can be a useful source of the energy. Conversely, if we are physically inactive, too much fat in our diet can lead to overweight.

It is possible to eat very little fat and maintain good health. There are traditional dietary patterns in which the contribution of fat to energy intake is as low as 10 per cent. However, in the 'affluent' diet, it may contribute up to 50 per cent of energy intake (see Figure 5).

Fat also confers texture and flavour on food, enhancing its palatability. Many flavours are fat soluble; unfortunately it is these desirable properties that encourage over-eating.

FAT INTAKE

The acceptable range for fat intake:

About 10-30 per cent of energy intake, which for a 35-55 year old man would be 30-80 grams of fat per day, and for a 35-55 year old woman would be 20-60 grams of fat per day.

grams per 100 grams

BEVERAGES

Food	Fat (g/100g)
Beer (240g)	Tr
Cider, dry, alcoholic (180g)	0
sweet, alcoholic (180g)	0
sweet, non-alcoholic (220g)	Tr
Cocoa powder (5g)	22
Coffee, percolated (230g)	Tr
Cola-type drinks (240g)	0
Cordial, diluted 1:4 (240g)	–
Drinking chocolate (10g)	6
Lemonade, carbonated drinks (240g)	0
Milo (10g)	10
Ovaltine (10g)	3
Port (60g)	0
Sherry, dry (60g)	0
medium (60g)	0
sweet (60g)	0
Spirits, e.g. whisky (30g)	0
Tea, infusion (230g)	Tr
Wine, red (100g)	0
white, dry (100g)	0
medium (100g)	0
sparkling (100g)	0
sweet (100g)	0

CEREALS, BISCUITS, CAKES, DESSERTS

Food	Fat (g/100g)
Barley, pearl, boiled (–)	1
Biscuit, chocolate (20g)	28
cream-filled (20g)	25
crispbread, rye (20g)	2
wheat, starch-red. (11g)	8
gingernut (15g)	15
semi-sweet (15g)	17
short-sweet (15g)	23
Bran, wheat (8g)	6
Bread, brown, slice (25g)	2
Lebanese (pita) (¼=25g)	2
white, slice (25g)	2
wholemeal, slice (25g)	2
roll, brown (35g)	3
starch-reduced (35g)	4
white (35g)	3
Cake, fruit (60g)	13
plain (60g)	17

Food	Fat (g/100g)
Egg, fried (60g)	20
omelette (100g)	16
poached (55g)	12
raw (55g)	11
scrambled (70g)	23
Macaroni cheese (180g)	10
Quiche Lorraine (150g)	28

FATS AND OILS

Food	Fat (g/100g)
Butter, salted (10g)	81
Dripping, beef (–)	100
Lard (–)	100
Margarine (10g)	80
Vegetable oils (–)	100

FISH AND OTHER SEAFOODS

Food	Fat (g/100g)
Bream, steamed (100g)	3
Cod, baked (100g)	1
fried in batter (100g)	10
poached (100g)	1
steamed (100g)	1
Crab, boiled (150g)	5
canned (90g)	1
Fish cakes, fried (4=100g)	11
fingers, fried (5=100g)	13
in batter, fried (120g)	16
Flounder, baked (100g)	11
Haddock, fried (100g)	8
steamed (100g)	1
Lobster, boiled (120g)	3
Mussels, boiled (12=120g)	2
Oysters, raw (12=120g)	1
Prawns, boiled (6=120g)	2
Roe, cod, fried (100g)	12
Salmon, canned (100g)	8
Sardines, canned (60g)	28
Scallops, steamed (10=100g)	1
Tuna, canned in oil (120g)	22
Whiting, crumbed, fried (100g)	10
steamed (100g)	1

FRUIT

Food	Fat (g/100g)
Apple (inc. skin, core 100g)	Tr
baked, no sugar (inc. skin 110g)	Tr
stewed, no sugar (110g)	Tr
Apricots (inc. stones 3 = 100g)	Tr

Fat (g)	Food
27	Cake, sponge (60g)
13	Chapati (60g)
35	Cheesecake (120g)
Tr	Cornflakes (30g)
1	Crumpet (50g)
4	Custard (70g)
17	Custard tart (120g)
16	Doughnut (40g)
24	Eclair (50g)
Tr	Flour, corn- (–)
2	plain (–)
2	self-raising (–)
24	soya, full-fat (–)
7	low-fat (–)
3	wholemeal (–)
16	Fruit pie (150g)
15	Jam tart (35g)
0	Jelly, made with water (100g)
13	Lamington (60g)
15	Lemon meringue pie (120g)
0	Meringue (15g)
4	Milk pudding (e.g. sago) (160g)
20	Muesli (30g)
10	Noodles (chow mein) (250g)
16	Pancake (75g)
1	Pasta, macaroni, boiled (150g)
Tr	spaghetti, boiled (120g)
1	canned in tomato sauce (120g)
41	Pastry, flaky (–)
32	short crust (–)
12	Pizza, cheese and tomato (150g)
1	Porridge (30g)
Tr	Rice, boiled (160g)
9	fried (120g)
Tr	puffed (25g)
15	Scone (30g)
16	Sponge pudding, steamed (100g)
6	Trifle (100g)
1	Wheat, breakfast biscuit (35g)
2	Yeast, dried, baker's (–)

EGG AND CHEESE DISHES

Fat (g)	Food
8	Cauliflower cheese (100g)
19	Cheese soufflé (100g)
11	Egg, boiled (55g)

Fat (g)	Food
Tr	Apricots, canned (100g)
Tr	dried (25g)
Tr	stewed, no sugar (inc. stones 110g)
22	Avocado pear (½=150g)
Tr	Banana (100g)
Tr	Blackberries (100g)
Tr	stewed, no sugar (100g)
Tr	Cantaloup (inc. skin 120g)
Tr	Cherries (inc. stones 20=100g)
Tr	stewed, no sugar (inc. stones 100g)
Tr	Currants, black (90g)
Tr	dried (90g)
Tr	red (15g)
Tr	Dates, dried (6=35g)
Tr	Figs (2=75g)
Tr	dried (2=40g)
Tr	Fruit salad, canned (120g)
Tr	Grapes, black (20=100g)
Tr	white (20=100g)
Tr	Grapefruit, whole (200g)
Tr	canned (100g)
Tr	juice, canned (120g)
Tr	Guavas, canned (100g)
Tr	Lemon, slices (2=15g)
Tr	juice (15g)
Tr	Loganberries (100g)
Tr	canned (100g)
Tr	stewed, no sugar (100g)
Tr	Lychees, canned (100g)
Tr	Mandarins (2=100g)
Tr	canned (50g)
Tr	Mango (100g)
Tr	canned (100g)
Tr	Nectarines (inc. stones 3=100g)
9	Olives, in brine (5=20g)
Tr	Orange, whole (130g)
Tr	juice, fresh (120g)
Tr	canned (120g)
Tr	Passionfruit, whole (30g)
Tr	Papaw (100g)
Tr	canned (100g)
Tr	Peach (inc. stones 120g)
Tr	canned (120g)
Tr	dried (25g)

Food	Fat
cheese spread (10g)	23
cottage (25g)	4
cream cheese (15g)	47
Danish blue (25g)	29
edam (25g)	23
parmesan (10g)	30
processed (25g)	25
stilton (25g)	40
Swiss (25g)	29
Cream, 35% fat (30g)	38
sterilized, canned (15g)	23
Ice-cream (60g)	7
non-dairy (60g)	8
Milk, cow's, cond. skim. sweet. (30g)	Tr
cond. whole, sweet. (30g)	9
dried, skimmed (12g)	1
dried, whole (10g)	26
evap. whole, unsweet. (30g)	9
flavoured (230g)	4
fresh, skimmed (230g)	Tr
fresh, whole (230g)	4
longlife, UHT (230g)	4
goat's (230g)	5
human (100g)	4
Milkshake, flavoured (340g)	5
Yoghurt, flavoured (200g)	4
fruit, low-fat (200g)	1
natural, low-fat (200g)	1
plain (200g)	4

NUTS

Food	Fat
Almonds (10=15g)	54
Brazil nuts (5=20g)	62
Cashews, roast (10=20g)	47
Chestnuts (4=20g)	3
Coconut, desiccated (15g)	62
Hazel nuts (10=15g)	36
Macadamia nuts (8=20g)	74
Peanuts, raw, in shells (5=25g)	34
roasted, salted (30=25g)	49
Pistachio nuts, shelled (25=15g)	54
Walnuts (5=20g)	52

SAUCES & CONDIMENTS

Food	Fat
Barbecue sauce (10g)	7
Chilli sauce (–)	.6

Food	Fat
Peach, stewed, no sugar (120g)	Tr
Pear (inc. skin, core 120g)	Tr
canned (120g)	Tr
stewed, no sugar (120g)	Tr
Pineapple (80g)	Tr
canned (80g)	Tr
juice, canned (120g)	Tr
Plums (inc. stones 3=100g)	Tr
stewed, no sugar (inc. stones 100g)	Tr
Prunes (inc. stones 8=80g)	Tr
stewed, no sugar (inc. stones 120g)	Tr
Quince, raw (100g)	Tr
Raisins, dried (20g)	Tr
Raspberries (100g)	Tr
canned (100g)	Tr
stewed, no sugar (100g)	Tr
Rhubarb, stewed, no sugar (120g)	Tr
Strawberries (10=100g)	Tr
canned (100g)	Tr
Sultanas, dried (15g)	Tr
Watermelon (260g)	Tr

MEAT AND MEAT PRODUCTS

Food	Fat
Bacon rashers, middle, fried (2=40g)	42
grilled (40g)	35
Beef, corned, canned (90g)	12
fillet steak, grilled (130g)	9
mince, stewed (120g)	23
rump steak, fried (150g)	29
grilled (150g)	27
silverside, salted, boiled (120g)	29
sirloin, roast (120g)	24
stewing steak, stewed (120g)	31
topside, roast (120g)	27
Beefburger, frozen, fried (60g)	17
Beef stew (250g)	8
Bolognese sauce (100g)	11
Chicken, boiled (100g)	7
crumbed, no bone (140g)	22
roast (130g)	14
leg quarter (inc. bone 130g)	3
wing quarter (inc. bone 130g)	3
Chicken livers, fried (130g)	11
Duck, roast (100g)	29

Tr	Gelatin (–)
5	Ham, canned (90g)
10	Hamburger (170g)
13	with cheese (190g)
7	Irish stew (250g)
9	Lamb, brain, boiled (150g)
18	chops, loin, grilled (inc. bone 120g)
15	cutlets, grilled (inc. bone 100g)
15	heart, roast (140g)
6	kidney, fried (100g)
26	leg, roast (120g)
14	liver, fried (130g)
26	shoulder, roast (120g)
24	tongue, stewed (100g)
27	Luncheon meat, canned (90g)
14	Meat pie (180g)
13	Moussaka (200g)
20	Pastie (160g)
19	Pork, chop, loin, grilled (100g)
20	leg, roast (120g)
9	sweet and sour (250g)
27	Pork pie (180g)
4	Rabbit, stewed (inc. bone 170g)
45	Salami, slices (3=90g)
27	Sausage, liver (60g)
18	Sausage roll (100g)
18	Sausages, beef, fried (2=120g)
17	grilled (2=120g)
25	frankfurter (2=100g)
25	pork, fried (2=120g)
25	grilled (2=120g)
21	saveloy, large (2=150g)
22	Spring roll, fried (200g)
21	Steak and kidney pie (180g)
13	Stewed steak in gravy, canned (100g)
17	Tongue, canned (100g)
5	Tripe, stewed (100g)
7	Turkey, roast (120g)
8	Veal, cutlet, fried (110g)
12	fillet, roast (100g)
21	schnitzel (140g)

MILK & MILK PRODUCTS

23	Cheese, camembert (25g)
34	cheddar (25g)

Tr	Chutney, tomato (20g)
10	Curry powder (–)
73	French dressing (15g)
3	Ginger (ground) (–)
79	Mayonnaise (20g)
29	Mustard powder (–)
3	Oxo cubes (–)
7	Pepper (–)
1	Pickles, mustard (20g)
Tr	sweet (20g)
27	Salad cream (25g)
0	Salt, table (–)
49	Sesame seeds (–)
1	Soy sauce (–)
54	Tartare sauce (20g)
5	Tomato sauce (25g)
0	Vinegar (–)
0	Worcestershire sauce (–)

SOUPS (as served)

4	Chicken, condensed (230g)
Tr	Chicken noodle, dried (230g)
1	Minestrone, dried (230g)
4	Mushroom, canned (230g)
3	Tomato, condensed (230g)
1	Tomato, dried (230g)
1	Vegetable, canned (230g)

SUGARS, JAMS AND SPREADS

10	Fish paste (5g)
Tr	Honey (30g)
0	Jam, fruit, edible seeds (30g)
0	Jam, stone fruit (30g)
0	Marmalade (30g)
11	Meat paste (5g)
54	Peanut butter (20g)
0	Sugar, white (–)
0	Syrup, golden (30g)
Tr	Topping, flavoured (40g)
0	Treacle, black (30g)
0	Vegemite (3g)

SWEETS

Tr	Boiled sweet (5g)
8	Butterscotch (5g)
11	Caramel (5g)

	Food	Fat (g)
27	Carob bar (75g)	
30	Chocolate square, milk (5g)	
31	Fruit and honey bar (50g)	
Tr	Jelly bean (5g)	
2	Liquorice allsort (7g)	
0	Pastille (5g)	
1	Peppermint (4g)	
4	Popcorn, plain unsalted (15g)	
31	Sesame bar (50g)	
17	Toffee, mixed (5g)	

VEGETABLES

	Food	Fat (g)
Tr	Artichoke, globe, boiled (100g)	
Tr	Asparagus, boiled (5=100g)	
Tr	Bamboo shoots (50g)	
Tr	Beans, French, boiled (100g)	
1	baked, in tomato sauce (125g)	
1	broad, boiled (100g)	
1	kidney (and haricot), boiled (100g)	
4	mung, cooked dahl (100g)	
6	soya-, boiled (100g)	
Tr	Beetroot, slices, boiled (2=30g)	
Tr	canned (2=30g)	
Tr	Broccoli, boiled (100g)	
Tr	Brussels sprouts, boiled (7=70g)	
Tr	Cabbage, raw (50g)	
Tr	boiled (100g)	
Tr	Carrots, raw (50g)	
Tr	boiled (50g)	
Tr	young, canned (50g)	
Tr	Cauliflower, raw (50g)	
Tr	boiled (100g)	
Tr	Celeriac, boiled (3=60g)	
Tr	Celery, raw (50g)	
Tr	boiled (50g)	
3	Chickpeas, cooked dahl (60g)	
Tr	Cucumber, slices (5=30g)	
5	Egg plant, baked (½=100g)	
Tr	Endive, raw leaves (3=15g)	
Tr	Leeks, boiled (4=100g)	
1	Lentils, split, boiled (100g)	
Tr	Lettuce, raw leaves (2=20g)	
Tr	Marrow, boiled (100g)	
1	Mushrooms, raw (3=30g)	
22	fried (6=60g)	
Tr	Onions, raw (¼=20g)	
Tr	boiled (100g)	
33	fried (70g)	
Tr	spring (4=20g)	
Tr	Parsley, sprigs (2=5g)	
Tr	Parsnip, boiled (½=60g)	
Tr	Peas, canned (60g)	
Tr	canned, processed (60g)	
Tr	fresh, boiled (60g)	
Tr	frozen, boiled (60g)	
Tr	split, boiled (60g)	
Tr	Peppers, green, raw (¼=15g)	
Tr	boiled (50g)	
Tr	Potato, baked (inc. skin 120g)	
Tr	boiled (120g)	
11	chips, fresh, fried (12=120g)	
19	chips, frozen, fried (8-14=120g)	
36	crisps (10=25g)	
5	mashed (100g)	
Tr	instant, cooked (100g)	
Tr	new, boiled (2=100g)	
Tr	new, canned (2=100g)	
5	roast (120g)	
Tr	Pumpkin (100g)	
Tr	Radishes (2=20g)	
1	Spinach, leaves, boiled (3=60g)	
Tr	Swede, boiled (80g)	
2	Sweetcorn, on cob, boiled (150g)	
1	canned kernels (80g)	
1	Sweet potato, boiled (100g)	
Tr	Tomato, raw (120g)	
Tr	canned (120g)	
6	fried (120g)	
Tr	juice, canned (120g)	
Tr	Turnip, boiled (80g)	
Tr	Yam, boiled (100g)	

8

CHOLESTEROL

There is another type of fat, called sterols. Cholesterol is the sterol found in all animal tissues; in plants, the sterols are of a different kind.

Cholesterol forms a part of all animal cell walls (membranes). It is also used to make hormones like cortisol and to make bile acids.

Unfortunately, it can also accumulate in the inner parts of arteries, leading to progressive reduction in the diameter of blood vessels and in blood flow. This in turn leads to heart attacks, angina, abnormal heart rhythms and heart failure when the vessels affected are the coronary arteries supplying the heart. Arteries supplying blood to the brain, the legs, the kidneys and the gut can also be affected.

The extent to which cholesterol accumulates in arteries depends in part on the level of cholesterol in the blood. When high, this is called hypercholesterolaemia. Not only dietary cholesterol, but also dietary saturated fat, elevate the blood cholesterol level. Polyunsaturated fat and certain kinds of dietary fibre lower the blood cholesterol level.

It is worth remembering that the body can make its own cholesterol so that dietary cholesterol is not an essential nutrient.

Note: In seafood, some of the sterols that were once believed to be cholesterol are actually a different kind, so the values shown in Figure 46 for seafood may be less than in some other references.

CHOLESTEROL INTAKE

The safe range of cholesterol intake is 200-400 milligrams per day.

FIGURE 46: THE CHOLESTEROL CONTENT OF FOOD

FOOD*	CHOLESTEROL (milligrams per 100 grams of food)	

CEREALS, BISCUITS, CAKES AND DESSERTS:

Bread	1	(25g) †
Cake, sponge	130	(60g)
Cornflakes	0	(30g)
Custard (no egg)	15	(70g)
Custard tart	60	(120g)
Eclairs	90	(50g)
Jelly, made with water	0	(100g)
Lemon meringue pie	90	(120g)
Meringues	0	(15g)
Milk pudding	15	(160g)
Pancakes	65	(75g)
Pizza, cheese and tomato	20	(150g)
Rice, boiled	0	(160g)
Rice, puffed	0	(25g)
Scones	5	(30g)
Sponge pudding, steamed	80	(100g)
Trifle	50	(100g)
Wheat flakes	0	(35g)

EGG AND CHEESE DISHES:

Cauliflower cheese	17	(100g)
Eggs, boiled	450	(55g)
Eggs, fried	480	(60g)
Egg omelette	410	(100g)
Eggs, poached	480	(55g)
Eggs, scrambled	410	(70g)
Macaroni cheese	17	(180g)
Quiche lorraine	130	(150g)

FATS AND OILS:

Butter, salted	260	(10g)
Dripping, beef	95	(—)
Lard	95	(—)
Margarine (all vegetable)	0-5	(10g)

FISH AND OTHER SEAFOODS:

Bream	130	(100g)
Cod, steamed	40	(100g)
Crab	65	(150g)
Flathead	60	(100g)
Fish fingers, fried	50	(5 = 100g)
Haddock, steamed	75	(100g)
Lobster	70	(120g)
Mussels	55	(12 = 120g)
Oysters, raw	40	(12 = 120g)
Prawns, boiled	170	(6 = 120g)
Roe, cod, fried	500	(100g)
Salmon, canned	90	(100g)
Sardines, canned	80	(60g)
Scallops, steamed	30	(10 = 100g)
Tuna, canned in oil	90	(120g)
Whiting, steamed	110	(100g)

MEAT AND MEAT PRODUCTS:

Bacon, rashers, fried	80	(2 = 40g)
Bacon, rashers, grilled	75	(40g)
Beef, corned, canned	85	(90g)
Beef, cooked	80	(120g)
Beefburgers, frozen, fried	70	(60g)
Beef stew	30	(250g)
Bolognese sauce	25	(100g)
Chicken, boiled	90	(100g)
Chicken, roast	100	(130g)
Duck, roast	160	(100g)
Ham, canned	35	(90g)
Hamburger, cheese	34	(190g)
Hamburger, plain	20	(170g)
Irish stew	35	(250g)
Lamb, brain, boiled	2200	(150g)
Lamb, cooked	110	(120g)
Lamb, kidney, fried	610	(100g)
Lamb, tongue, stewed	270	(100g)
Luncheon meat, canned	55	(90g)
Meat paste	70	(5g)
Meat pie	20	(180g)
Moussaka	40	(200g)
Pastie	50	(160g)
Pork, cooked	110	(120g)
Pork, pie	50	(180g)
Salami, slices	80	(3 = 90g)
Sausage roll	20	(100g)
Sausage, liver	120	(60g)
Sausages, beef, fried	40	(2 = 120g)
Sausages, beef, grilled	40	(2 = 120g)
Sausages, pork, fried	55	(2 = 120g)
Sausages, pork, grilled	55	(2 = 120g)
Sausages, saveloy	45	(2 = 150g)
Steak and kidney pie	125	(180g)
Tongue, canned	110	(100g)
Tripe, stewed	160	(100g)
Turkey, roast	80	(120g)

MILK AND MILK PRODUCTS:

Cheese, camembert type	70	(25g)
Cheese, cheddar type	70	(25g)
Cheese, cottage	15	(25g)
Cheese, cream	95	(15g)
Cheese, danish blue type	90	(25g)
Cheese, edam type	70	(25g)
Cheese, parmesan	90	(10g)
Cheese, processed	90	(25g)
Cheese, spread	70	(10g)
Cream	100	(30g)
Cream, sterilized, canned	75	(15g)
Ice cream	45	(60g)
Milk, cow's, condensed, skimmed, sweetened	3	(30g)
Milk, cow's, condensed, whole, sweetened	35	(30g)
Milk, cow's, dried, skimmed	20	(12g)
Milk, cow's, dried, whole	120	(10g)
Milk, cow's, evaporated, whole, unsweetened	35	(30g)
Milk, cow's, fresh, skimmed	2	(230g)
Milk, cow's, fresh, whole	10	(230g)
Milk, cow's, longlife (UHT treated)	10	(230g)
Milk, human	15	(100g)
Yoghurt, low fat, fruit	5	(200g)
Yoghurt, low fat, plain	5	(200g)

SUGAR, JAMS AND SPREADS:

Honey	0	(30g)
Jam	0	(30g)
Sugar	0	(—)
Syrup, golden	0	(30g)
Treacle, black	0	(30g)
Vegemite	0	(3g)

SWEETS AND CONFECTIONERY:

Boiled sweets	0	(5g)
Chocolate, milk	90	(5g)

*Cholesterol is not found in plant foods — cereals, fruit, nuts and vegetables. The amount of cholesterol in food depends on the amount of animal produce used.

†Values in parentheses are average serving sizes.

9

SATURATED AND POLY-
UNSATURATED FAT

There are several types of fats, the chief ones being called triglycerides, cholesterol esters, and phospholipids. They contain fatty acids, which may be saturated, monounsaturated or polyunsaturated.

Some polyunsaturated fatty acids are essential for humans because they cannot be made in our bodies. One group of essential fatty acids comes from plant sources; these fatty acids are found in considerable quantity in polyunsaturated margarine and in vegetable oils. We need about 1 to 2 per cent of our energy to come from this type of fatty acid, although a higher intake, up to about 10 per cent of energy, may be protective against coronary heart disease. The requirements of another type of essential fatty acid have not been worked out, but they are obtained mainly from seafood and, in a different way, seem protective against coronary heart disease — they reduce the 'stickiness' of the blood. Both kinds of essential fatty acids can lower high levels of blood fats.

Saturated fatty acids come chiefly from ruminant animals, such as sheep and cattle, and from milk and dairy products of these animals. In the stomachs of ruminants the polyunsaturated fatty acids that are present in fodder are broken down to a large extent to saturated fatty acids so that the fatty tissues of animals such as cattle are mostly saturated. On the other hand, animals with a single stomach (monogastric) absorb the range of fatty acids, saturated and polyunsaturated, present in the diet. Pigs and humans are similar in this respect. Furthermore, domesticated animals have more carcass fat than wild animals so that the advent of animal production for human consumption has led to a great increase in the consumption of saturated fat.

Saturated fat increases the amount of cholesterol in blood. Monounsaturated fat does not change the blood cholesterol level (olive oil and peanut oil provide monounsaturated fat), while polyunsaturated fat decreases it. Traditional cultures that use olive oil in food preparation or a lot of groundnuts (peanuts) have little coronary heart disease. Cholesterol in food increases the level of cholesterol in blood.

Saturated fat also increases the amount of triglyceride in the blood. Both blood cholesterol and blood triglyceride, when elevated, increase the risk of hardening of the arteries (atherosclerosis), with consequent coronary heart disease.

The desirable ratio of polyunsaturated to saturated fat in the diet is 1 : 1 (i.e. 50 : 50).

SPECIAL POLYUNSATURATED PRODUCTS

Some novel food products have been developed to decrease the saturated and increase the polyunsaturated fat of the total diet. Foods traditionally high in saturated fat, such as icecream made with milkfat, are now available made from polyunsaturated vegetable oils.

Dairy and beef cattle have been fed polyunsaturated fat protected from digestive breakdown so that the dairy and beef products are more polyunsaturated. Eggs have also had the yolk, rich in cholesterol, removed and replaced with a polyunsaturated oil substitute — hence 'polyunsaturated egg mix', with the main advantage being a low cholesterol content.

SATURATED AND POLYUNSATURATED FAT IN MARGARINE AND VEGETABLE OILS

Approximate amounts of saturated and polyunsaturated fat in different types of margarine are shown in Figure 47, and the amounts in different vegetable oils are shown in Figure 48.

FIGURE 47: APPROXIMATE AMOUNTS OF SATURATED AND POLYUNSATURATED FAT IN MARGARINES

TYPE OF MARGARINE	SATURATED FAT	POLYUNSATURATED FAT
	(grams per 100 grams of margarine)	
Hard (animal and vegetable oils)	30	14
Hard (vegetable oils only)	30	10
Soft (animal and vegetable oils)	25	16
Soft (vegetable oils only)	26	18
Polyunsaturated	19	60

FIGURE 48: APPROXIMATE AMOUNTS OF SATURATED AND POLYUNSATURATED FAT IN DIFFERENT VEGETABLE OILS

TYPE OF OIL	SATURATED FAT	POLYUNSATURATED FAT
	(grams per 100 grams of oil)	
Coconut oil	85	2
Maize oil	16	49
Olive oil	14	11
Palm oil	45	8
Peanut oil	19	29
Safflower oil	10	72
Soya bean oil	14	57
Sunflower oil	13	50

	Polyunsaturated Fats grams per 100 grams	Saturated Fats grams per 100 grams
BEVERAGES		
Beer (240g)	–	–
Cider, dry, alcoholic (180g)	–	–
sweet, alcoholic (180g)	–	–
sweet, non-alcoholic (220g)	–	–
Cocoa powder (5g)	.6	13
Coffee, percolated (230g)	–	–
Cola-type drinks (240g)	–	–
Cordial, diluted 1:4 (240g)	–	–
Drinking chocolate (10g)	.2	4
Lemonade, carbonated drinks (240g)	–	–
Milo (10g)	–	–
Ovaltine (10g)	–	–
Port (60g)	–	–
Sherry, dry (60g)	–	–
medium (60g)	–	–
sweet (60g)	–	–
Spirits, e.g. whisky (30g)	–	–
Tea, infusion (230g)	–	–
Wine, red (100g)	–	–
white, dry (100g)	–	–
medium (100g)	–	–
sparkling (100g)	–	–
sweet (100g)	–	–
CEREALS, BISCUITS, CAKES, DESSERTS		
Barley, pearl, boiled (–)	.3	.1
Biscuit, chocolate (20g)	1	17
cream-filled (20g)	–	–
crispbread, rye (20g)	1	.3
wheat, starch-red. (11g)	1	3
gingernut (15g)	1	7
semi-sweet (15g)	2	8
short-sweet (15g)	2	12
Bran, wheat (8g)	3	.9
Bread, brown, slice (25g)	.9	.4
Lebanese (pita) (¼=25g)	–	–
white, slice (25g)	.7	.4
wholemeal, slice (25g)	1	.5
roll, brown (35g)	1	.6
starch-reduced (35g)	2	.6
white (35g)	1	.8
Cake, fruit (60g)	2	4

Food	Left	Right
plain (60g)	1	6
Cake, sponge (60g)	4	10
Chapati (60g)	–	–
Cheesecake (120g)	2	19
Cornflakes (30g)	.8	.3
Crumpet (50g)	–	–
Custard (70g)	.3	3
Custard tart (120g)	2	7
Doughnut (40g)	–	–
Eclair (50g)	2	12
Flour, corn- (–)	–	–
plain (–)	.5	.2
self-raising (–)	.5	.2
soya, full-fat (–)	13	3
low-fat (–)	4	1
wholemeal (–)	.9	.3
Fruit pie (150g)	–	–
Jam tart (35g)	2	6
Jelly, made with water (100g)	–	–
Lamington (60g)	–	–
Lemon meringue pie (120g)	2	6
Meringue (15g)	–	–
Milk pudding (e.g. sago) (160g)	.1	3
Muesli (30g)	3	1
Noodles (chow mein) (250g)	–	–
Pancake (75g)	1	7
Pasta, macaroni, boiled (150g)	.3	.1
spaghetti, boiled (120g)	.1	.04
canned in tomato sauce (120g)	–	–
Pastry, flaky (–)	5	16
short crust (–)	4	13
Pizza, cheese and tomato (150g)	.7	5
Porridge (30g)	.4	.1
Rice, boiled (160g)	.1	.1
fried (120g)	–	–
puffed (25g)	–	–
Scone (30g)	2	6
Sponge pudding, steamed (100g)	3	6
Trifle (100g)	.4	3
Wheat, breakfast biscuit (35g)	–	–
Yeast, dried, baker's (–)	–	–

EGG AND CHEESE DISHES

Food	Left	Right
Cauliflower cheese (100g)	.6	4
Cheese soufflé (100g)	2	8

Food	Polyunsaturated Fats	Saturated Fats
Egg, boiled (55g)	1	3
Egg, fried (60g)	–	–
omelette (100g)	1	5
poached (55g)	1	4
raw (55g)	1	3
scrambled (70g)	1	11
Macaroni cheese (180g)	.7	5
Quiche Lorraine (150g)	2	13
FATS AND OILS		
Butter, salted (10g)	2	49
Dripping, beef (–)	4	43
Lard (–)	9	42
Margarine (10g)	–	–
Vegetable oils (–)	–	–
FISH AND OTHER SEAFOODS		
Bream, steamed (100g)	–	–
Cod, baked (100g)	.1	.5
fried in batter (100g)	–	–
poached (100g)	.1	.4
steamed (100g)	.1	.3
Crab, boiled (150g)	1	2
canned (90g)	.1	.3
Fish cakes, fried (4=100g)	–	–
fingers, fried (5=100g)	–	–
in batter, fried (120g)	–	–
Flounder, baked (100g)	–	–
Haddock, fried (100g)	–	–
steamed (100g)	.1	.3
Lobster, boiled (120g)	.7	1
Mussels, boiled (12=120g)	.4	.6
Oysters, raw (12=120g)	.1	.3
Prawns, boiled (6=120g)	.3	.7
Roe, cod, fried (100g)	–	–
Salmon, canned (100g)	3	2
Sardines, canned (60g)	7	6
Scallops, steamed (10=100g)	.1	.3
Tuna, canned in oil (120g)	9	8
Whiting, crumbed fried (100g)	–	–
steamed (100g)	.3	.2
FRUIT		
Apple (inc. skin, core 100g)	–	–
baked, no sugar (inc. skin 110g)	–	–

stewed, no sugar (110g)	—	—
Apricots (inc. stones 3=100g)	—	—
Apricots, canned (100g)	—	—
dried (25g)	—	—
stewed, no sugar (inc. stones 110g)	—	—
Avocado pear (½=150g)	2	3
Banana (100g)	.1	.1
Blackberries (100g)	—	—
stewed, no sugar (100g)	—	—
Cantaloup (inc. skin 120g)	—	—
Cherries (inc. stones 20=100g)	—	—
stewed, no sugar (inc. stones 100g)	—	—
Currants, black (90g)	—	—
dried (15g)	—	—
red (90g)	—	—
Dates, dried (6=35g)	—	—
Figs (2=75g)	—	—
dried (2=40g)	—	—
Fruit salad, canned (120g)	—	—
Grapes, black (20=100g)	—	—
white (20=100g)	—	—
Grapefruit, whole (200g)	—	—
canned (100g)	—	—
juice, canned (120g)	—	—
Guavas, canned (100g)	—	—
Lemon, slices (2=15g)	—	—
juice (15g)	—	—
Loganberries (100g)	—	—
canned (100g)	—	—
stewed, no sugar (100g)	—	—
Lychees, canned (100g)	—	—
Mandarins (2=100g)	—	—
canned (50g)	—	—
Mango (100g)	—	—
canned (100g)	—	—
Nectarines (inc. stones 3=100g)	—	—
Olives, in brine (5=20g)	1	1
Orange, whole (130g)	—	—
juice, fresh (120g)	—	—
canned (120g)	—	—
Passionfruit, whole (30g)	—	—
Papaw (100g)	—	—
canned (100g)	—	—
Peach (inc. stones 120g)	—	—

Food	Polyunsaturated Fats	Saturated Fats
canned (120g)	–	–
dried (25g)	–	–
Peach, stewed, no sugar (120g)	–	–
Pear (inc. skin, core 120g)	–	–
canned (120g)	–	–
stewed, no sugar (120g)	–	–
Pineapple (80g)	–	–
canned (80g)	–	–
juice, canned (120g)	–	–
Plums (inc. stones 3=100g)	–	–
stewed, no sugar (inc. stones 100g)	–	–
Prunes (inc. stones 8=80g)	–	–
stewed, no sugar (inc. stones 120g)	–	–
Quince, raw (100g)	–	–
Raisins, dried (20g)	–	–
Raspberries (100g)	–	–
canned (100g)	–	–
stewed, no sugar (100g)	–	–
Rhubarb, stewed, no sugar (120g)	–	–
Strawberries (10=100g)	–	–
canned (100g)	–	–
Sultanas, dried (15g)	–	–
Watermelon (260g)	–	–
MEAT AND MEAT PRODUCTS		
Bacon rashers, middle, fried (2=40g)	3	17
grilled (40g)	3	14
Beef, corned, canned (90g)	.5	5
fillet steak, grilled (130g)	–	–
mince, stewed (120g)	.6	6
rump steak, fried (150g)	.6	6
grilled (150g)	.5	5
silverside, salted, boiled (120g)	.6	6
sirloin, roast (120g)	.9	9
stewing steak, stewed (120g)	.4	5
topside, roast (120g)	.5	5
Beefburger, frozen, fried (60g)	.7	7
Beef stew (250g)	.4	3
Bolognese sauce (100g)	3	3
Chicken, boiled (100g)	1	2
crumbed, no bone (140g)	–	–
roast (130g)	.8	2
leg quarter (inc. bone 130g)	.5	1

Food	Poly-unsaturated	Saturated
wing quarter (inc. bone 130g)	.9	.4
Chicken livers, fried (130g)	-	-
Duck, roast (100g)	3	1
Gelatin (-)	-	-
Ham, canned (90g)	2	.5
Hamburger (170g)	-	-
with cheese (190g)	-	-
Irish stew (250g)	3	.3
Lamb, brain, boiled (150g)	2	1
chops, loin, grilled (inc. bone 120g)	11	1
cutlets, grilled (inc. bone 100g)	10	1
heart, roast (140g)	6	1
kidney, fried (100g)	-	-
leg, roast (120g)	9	.8
liver, fried (130g)	-	-
shoulder, roast (120g)	13	1
tongue, stewed (100g)	8	1
Luncheon meat, canned (90g)	10	2
Meat pie (180g)	-	-
Moussaka (200g)	5	3
Pastie (160g)	-	-
Pork, chop, loin, grilled (100g)	7	1
leg, roast (120g)	8	2
sweet and sour (250g)	-	-
Pork pie (180g)	-	1
Rabbit, stewed (inc. bone 170g)	2	1
Salami, slices (3=90g)	18	4
Sausage, liver (60g)	8	2
Sausage roll (100g)	14	4
Sausages, beef, fried (2=120g)	-	-
grilled (2=120g)	-	.8
frankfurter (2=100g)	10	2
pork, fried (2=120g)	-	-
grilled (2=120g)	10	2
saveloy, large (2=150g)	-	-
Spring roll, fried (200g)	-	2
Steak and kidney pie (180g)	7	2
Stewed steak in gravy, canned (100g)	5	.5
Tongue, canned (100g)	-	-
Tripe, stewed (100g)	2	.1
Turkey, roast (120g)	.9	.9
Veal, cutlet, fried (110g)	3	.3
fillet, roast (100g)	5	.5
schnitzel (140g)	-	-

Saturated Fats / **Polyunsaturated Fats**

Food	Saturated Fats	Polyunsaturated Fats
MILK & MILK PRODUCTS		
Cheese, camembert (25g)	14	.6
cheddar (25g)	20	1
cheese spread (10g)	14	.6
cottage (25g)	2	.1
cream cheese (15g)	28	1
Danish blue (25g)	17	.8
edam (25g)	14	.6
parmesan (10g)	18	.8
processed (25g)	15	.7
stilton (25g)	24	1
Swiss (25g)	–	–
Cream, 35% fat (30g)	21	1
sterilized, canned (15g)	14	.6
Ice-cream (60g)	4	.2
non-dairy (60g)	4	.6
Milk, cow's, cond. skim, sweet. (30g)	.1	.1
cond. whole, sweet. (30g)	5	.3
dried, skimmed (12g)	.8	.04
dried, whole (10g)	16	.7
evap. whole, unsweet. (30g)	5	.3
flavoured (230g)	–	–
fresh, skimmed (230g)	.04	.04
fresh, whole (230g)	2	.1
longlife, UHT (230g)	2	.1
goat's (230g)	3	.1
human (100g)	2	.3
Milkshake, flavoured (340g)	–	–
Yoghurt, flavoured (200g)	–	–
fruit, low-fat (200g)	.6	.02
natural, low-fat (200g)	.6	.02
plain (200g)	–	–
NUTS		
Almonds (10=15g)	4	10
Brazil nuts (5=20g)	16	23
Cashews, roast (10=20g)	–	–
Chestnuts (4=20g)	.5	1
Coconut, desiccated (15g)	53	1
Hazel nuts (10=15g)	3	4
Macadamia nuts (8=20g)	–	–
Peanuts, raw, in shells (5=25g)	6	10
roasted, salted (30=25g)	9	14
Pistachio nuts, shelled (25=15g)	–	–

35	Walnuts (5=20g)

SAUCES & CONDIMENTS

–	Barbecue sauce (10g)
–	Chilli sauce (–)
–	Chutney, tomato (20g)
–	Curry powder (–)
8	French dressing (15g)
–	Ginger (ground) (–)
–	Mayonnaise (20g)
–	Mustard powder (–)
–	Oxo cubes (–)
–	Pepper (–)
–	Pickles, mustard (20g)
–	sweet (20g)
–	Salad cream (25g)
–	Salt, table (–)
–	Sesame seeds (–)
–	Soy sauce (–)
–	Tartare sauce (20g)
.3	Tomato sauce (25g)
–	Vinegar (–)
–	Worcestershire sauce (–)

SOUPS (as served)

–	Chicken, condensed (230g)
–	Chicken noodle, dried (230g)
–	Minestrone, dried (230g)
–	Mushroom, canned (230g)
–	Tomato, condensed (230g)
–	Tomato, dried (230g)
–	Vegetable, canned (230g)

SUGARS, JAMS AND SPREADS

–	Fish paste (5g)
–	Honey (30g)
–	Jam, fruit, edible seeds (30g)
–	Jam, stone fruit (30g)
–	Marmalade (30g)
.9	Meat paste (5g)
14	Peanut butter (20g)
–	Sugar, white (–)
–	Syrup, golden (30g)
–	Topping, flavoured (40g)
–	Treacle, black (30g)
–	Vegemite (3g)

6	Walnuts (5=20g)

SAUCES & CONDIMENTS

–	Barbecue sauce (10g)
–	Chilli sauce (–)
–	Chutney, tomato (20g)
–	Curry powder (–)
10	French dressing (15g)
–	Ginger (ground) (–)
–	Mayonnaise (20g)
–	Mustard powder (–)
–	Oxo cubes (–)
–	Pepper (–)
–	Pickles, mustard (20g)
–	sweet (20g)
–	Salad cream (25g)
–	Salt, table (–)
–	Sesame seeds (–)
–	Soy sauce (–)
–	Tartare sauce (20g)
.9	Tomato sauce (25g)
–	Vinegar (–)
–	Worcestershire sauce (–)

SOUPS (as served)

–	Chicken, condensed (230g)
–	Chicken noodle, dried (230g)
–	Minestrone, dried (230g)
–	Mushroom, canned (230g)
–	Tomato, condensed (230g)
–	Tomato, dried (230g)
–	Vegetable, canned (230g)

SUGARS, JAMS AND SPREADS

–	Fish paste (5g)
–	Honey (30g)
–	Jam, fruit, edible seeds (30g)
–	Jam, stone fruit (30g)
–	Marmalade (30g)
4	Meat paste (5g)
11	Peanut butter (20g)
–	Sugar, white (–)
–	Syrup, golden (30g)
–	Topping, flavoured (40g)
–	Treacle, black (30g)
–	Vegemite (3g)

	Polyunsaturated Fats	Saturated Fats
SWEETS		
Boiled sweet (5g)	–	–
Butterscotch (5g)	–	–
Caramel (5g)	–	–
Carob bar (75g)	–	–
Chocolate square, milk (5g)	1	18
Fruit and honey bar (50g)	–	–
Jelly bean (5g)	–	–
Liquorice allsort (7g)	–	–
Pastille (5g)	–	–
Peppermint (4g)	–	–
Popcorn, plain unsalted (15g)	–	–
Sesame bar (50g)	–	–
Toffee, mixed (5g)	–	–
VEGETABLES		
Artichoke, globe, boiled (100g)	–	–
Asparagus, boiled (5=100g)	–	–
Bamboo shoots (50g)	–	–
Beans, French, boiled (100g)	–	–
baked, in tomato sauce (125g)	.3	.1
broad, boiled (100g)	–	–
kidney (and haricot), boiled (100g)	–	–
mung, cooked dahl (100g)	–	–
soya-, boiled (100g)	–	–
Beetroot, slices, boiled (2=30g)	–	–
canned (2=30g)	–	–
Broccoli, boiled (100g)	–	–
Brussels sprouts, boiled (7=70g)	–	–
Cabbage, raw (50g)	–	–
boiled (100g)	–	–
Carrots, raw (50g)	–	–
boiled (50g)	–	–
young, canned (50g)	–	–
Cauliflower, raw (50g)	–	–
boiled (100g)	–	–
Celeriac, boiled (3=60g)	–	–
Celery, raw (50g)	–	–
boiled (50g)	–	–
Chickpeas, cooked dahl (60g)	.04	.03
Cucumber, slices (5=30g)	–	–
Egg plant, baked (½=100g)	–	–
Endive, raw leaves (3=15g)	–	–
Leeks, boiled (4=100g)	–	–

Lentils, split, boiled (100g)	–	–
Lettuce, raw leaves (2=20g)	–	–
Marrow, boiled (100g)	–	–
Mushrooms, raw (3=30g)	.1	.3
fried (6=60g)	–	–
Onions, raw (¼=20g)	–	–
boiled (100g)	–	–
fried (70g)	–	–
spring (4=20g)	–	–
Parsley, sprigs (2=5g)	–	–
Parsnip, boiled (½=60g)	–	–
Peas, canned (60g)	.2	.03
canned, processed (60g)	.2	.03
fresh, boiled (60g)	.2	.03
frozen, boiled (60g)	.2	.03
split, boiled (60g)	.1	.03
Peppers, green, raw (¼=15g)	.1	2
boiled (50g)	.1	.2
Potato, baked (inc. skin 120g)	.01	.1
boiled (120g)	.01	.1
chips, fresh, fried (12=120g)	–	–
chips, frozen, fried (8-14=120g)	–	–
crisps (10=25g)	–	–
mashed (100g)	–	–
instant, cooked (100g)	.03	.1
new, boiled (2=100g)	.01	.1
new, canned (2=100g)	.01	.1
roast (120g)	–	–
Pumpkin (100g)	–	–
Radishes (2=20g)	–	–
Spinach, leaves, boiled (3=60g)	.1	.3
Swede, boiled (80g)	–	–
Sweetcorn, on cob, boiled (150g)	.4	.1
canned kernels (80g)	.1	.2
Sweet potato, boiled (100g)	.2	.2
Tomato, raw (120g)	–	–
canned (120g)	–	–
fried (120g)	–	–
juice, canned (120g)	–	–
Turnip, boiled (80g)	.03	.2
Yam, boiled (100g)	–	–

The alcohol content of beverages (standard glasses)

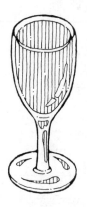

FORTIFIED WINE

GLASS: 60ml

ALCOHOL CONTENT 10·5ml – 17·5%

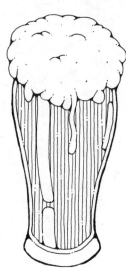

BEER

GLASS: 285ml

ALCOHOL CONTENT 11·4ml – 4%

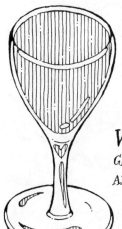

WINE

GLASS: 100ml

ALCOHOL CONTENT 11·5ml – 11·5%

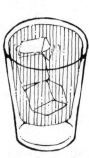

SPIRIT

GLASS: 200ml

ALCOHOL CONTENT 11·4ml

CONTAINS ONE

30ml NIP OF

SPIRITS (38%)

A L C O H O L

The usual alcohol present in food and beverages is called ethanol. It is made by fermentation of carbohydrate. It is virtually never found in freshly collected food. It has an energy value of 7 kilocalories or 29 kilojoules per gram. But, with high alcohol intakes, proportionately less of the alcohol is used to produce useful energy.

There is some evidence that a small amount of ethanol may actually protect against coronary heart disease. However, depending on other lifestyle factors, there may be a 'trade-off' in that any quantity of ethanol increases blood pressure to some extent, which increases the risk of strokes.

ALCOHOL INTAKE

When the average intake of ethanol exceeds 80 grams per day, disease of one sort or another is in due course inevitable. This situation is one of alcohol abuse. The adverse effects are seen on brain, liver, heart, muscles, blood, gut, nerves, pancreas (leading to diabetes or pancreatitis) and nutritional status. Alcohol abuse can lead to deficiencies of vitamins, including vitamin B-1, vitamin B-2, niacin, vitamin B-6, folacin and vitamin C, and to element (mineral) deficiencies, which include zinc and magnesium. These deficiencies will arise for various reasons such as failure to eat food containing these nutrients, decreased absorption or interference with nutrient usage. For some individuals, an average daily alcohol intake of 40 grams per day will adversely affect health. Probably the safest level of alcohol intake is one to two drinks a day, equivalent to 8 to 20 grams of ethanol.

The safe range of alcohol intake is 8-20 grams of ethanol per day.

FIGURE 49: THE ALCOHOL CONTENT OF BEVERAGES

BEVERAGE	(grams per 100 grams)	AVERAGE ALCOHOL CONTENT (millilitres per 100 millilitres)	(grams per 100 millilitres)
Beer, bitter	3.9	4.9	3.9
Beer, low alcohol	2.6	3.3	2.6
Cider, dry	3.8	4.8	3.7
Cider, sweet	3.7	4.6	3.7
Port	15.9	19.6	15.6
Sherry:			
Dry	15.7	19.3	15.3
Medium	14.8	18.2	14.4
Sweet	15.6	19.2	15.2
Spirits 70° proof (brandy, gin, whisky, vodka, rum)	31.7	38.1	30.2
Vermouth:			
Dry	13.9	17.2	13.7
Sweet	13.0	16.1	12.8
Wine:			
White, dry	9.1	11.3	9.0
White, medium	8.8	10.9	8.7
White, sparkling	9.9	12.3	9.8
White, sweet	10.2	12.7	10.1
Red	9.5	11.8	9.4
Rosé	8.7	10.8	8.6

Notes: 1 ml of beverage weighs approximately 1 gram. Proof spirit is used to describe the alcohol content of spirits. In Australia and the U.K., 100° proof spirit contains 57 per cent alcohol by volume, and in the U.S.A. 50 per cent alcohol.

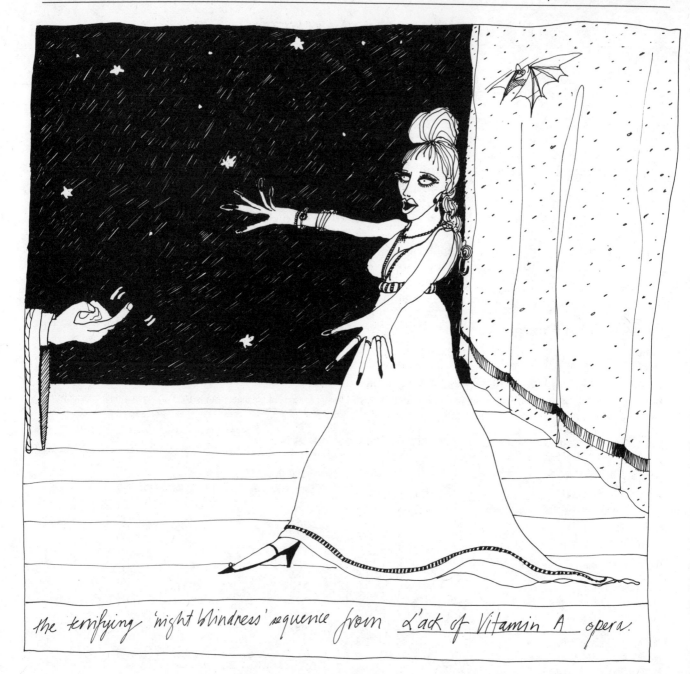

the terrifying 'night blindness' sequence from L'ack of Vitamin A opera.

FAT-SOLUBLE VITAMINS

1 1

V I T A M I N   A

Some foods contain both vitamin A itself, and other substances that can be converted to vitamin A, known as provitamin A, vitamin A precursors or carotenoids. Although it is possible to have a toxic amount of preformed vitamin A, this appears not to be the case with provitamin A, so that it is clearly safer to have more of the latter.

Vitamin A is a fat-soluble vitamin, as also are vitamins D, E and K. It is therefore necessary to have some fat in the diet for these vitamins to be adequately absorbed.

One of the most important consequences of vitamin A deficiency is dryness of the eyes eventually leading to blindness. It remains one of the main causes of blindness in the world. Night blindness is also an eye complication of early vitamin A deficiency.

The units for expressing the amount of vitamin A have changed from time to time because of the need to consider both preformed vitamin A (called retinol) and provitamin A (a group of components called carotenoids, of which beta-carotene is the most active and the most important). The present custom is to express the total amount of vitamin A activity as equivalent to so many micrograms of retinol. But some vitamin preparations may express the amount of vitamin A in different ways, so to help you compare these a list of conversion factors are given below:

1 retinol equivalent =   1 microgram retinol
                       =   6 micrograms beta-carotene
                       = 12 micrograms of other
                            provitamin A carotenoids.

The original system using international units (IU) was different, so:

1 retinol equivalent =   3.33 IU vitamin A activity
                            from retinol
                         = 10 IU vitamin A activity from
                            beta-carotene.

VITAMIN A INTAKE

Recommended dietary intake of vitamin A for adults (Australia): 750 micrograms of retinol equivalents per day.
For children and lactating women, see the table of recommended intakes shown in Figure 7.

Toxic levels of intake:
Children – greater than 3000 micrograms retinol equivalents per day
Adults – greater than 15 000 micrograms retinol equivalents per day

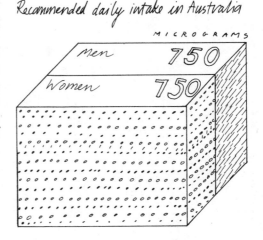

Recommended daily intake in Australia

MICROGRAMS

Men 750
Women 750

micrograms per 100 grams

BEVERAGES

Beer (240g)	0
Cider, dry, alcoholic (180g)	0
sweet, alcoholic (180g)	0
sweet, non-alcoholic (220g)	–
Cocoa powder (5g)	0
Coffee, percolated (230g)	0
Cola-type drinks (240g)	0
Cordial, diluted 1:4 (240g)	0
Drinking chocolate (10g)	0
Lemonade, carbonated drinks (240g)	0
Milo (10g)	1250
Ovaltine (10g)	1250
Port (60g)	0
Sherry, dry (60g)	0
medium (60g)	0
sweet (60g)	0
Spirits, e.g. whisky (30g)	0
Tea, infusion (230g)	0
Wine, red (100g)	0
white, dry (100g)	0
medium (100g)	0
sparkling (100g)	0
sweet (100g)	0

CEREALS, BISCUITS, CAKES, DESSERTS

Barley, pearl, boiled (–)	0
Biscuit, chocolate (20g)	0
cream-filled (20g)	–
crispbread, rye (20g)	0
wheat, starch-red. (11g)	0
gingernut (15g)	0
semi-sweet (15g)	0
short-sweet (15g)	0
Bran, wheat (8g)	0
Bread, brown, slice (25g)	0
Lebanese (pita) (¼=25g)	–
white, slice (25g)	0
wholemeal, slice (25g)	0
roll, brown (35g)	0
starch-reduced (35g)	0
white (35g)	0
Cake, fruit (60g)	120
plain (60g)	–

Egg, fried (60g)	140
omelette (100g)	190
poached (55g)	140
raw (55g)	140
scrambled (70g)	130
Macaroni cheese (180g)	90
Quiche Lorraine (150g)	160

FATS AND OILS

Butter, salted (10g)	895
Dripping, beef (–)	–
Lard (–)	Tr
Margarine (10g)	580
Vegetable oils (–)	0

FISH AND OTHER SEAFOODS

Bream, steamed (100g)	Tr
Cod, baked (100g)	Tr
fried in batter (100g)	Tr
poached (100g)	Tr
steamed (100g)	Tr
Crab, boiled (150g)	Tr
canned (90g)	Tr
Fish cakes, fried (4=100g)	Tr
fingers, fried (5=100g)	Tr
in batter, fried (120g)	20
Flounder, baked (100g)	–
Haddock, fried (100g)	Tr
steamed (100g)	Tr
Lobster, boiled (120g)	Tr
Mussels, boiled (12=120g)	–
Oysters, raw (12=120g)	75
Prawns, boiled (6=120g)	Tr
Roe, cod, fried (100g)	150
Salmon, canned (100g)	90
Sardines, canned (60g)	Tr
Scallops, steamed (10=100g)	–
Tuna, canned in oil (120g)	–
Whiting, crumbed, fried (100g)	Tr
steamed (100g)	Tr

FRUIT

Apple (inc. skin, core 100g)	0
baked, no sugar (inc. skin 110g)	0
stewed, no sugar (110g)	0
Apricots (inc. stones 3 =100g)	0

Food	Vitamin A
Cake, sponge (60g)	300
Chapati (60g)	–
Cheesecake (120g)	280
Cornflakes (30g)	0
Crumpet (50g)	–
Custard (70g)	40
Custard tart (120g)	100
Doughnut (40g)	0
Eclair (50g)	200
Flour, corn- (–)	0
plain (–)	0
self-raising (–)	0
soya, full-fat (–)	0
low-fat (–)	0
wholemeal (–)	0
Fruit pie (150g)	0
Jam tart (35g)	70
Jelly, made with water (100g)	0
Lamington (60g)	55
Lemon meringue pie (120g)	100
Meringue (15g)	0
Milk pudding (e.g. sago) (160g)	30
Muesli (30g)	0
Noodles (chow mein) (250g)	–
Pancake (75g)	40
Pasta, macaroni, boiled (150g)	0
spaghetti, boiled (120g)	0
canned in tomato sauce (120g)	0
Pastry, flaky (–)	200
short crust (–)	160
Pizza, cheese and tomato (150g)	70
Porridge (30g)	0
Rice, boiled (160g)	0
fried (120g)	–
puffed (25g)	0
Scone (30g)	150
Sponge pudding, steamed (100g)	180
Trifle (100g)	50
Wheat, breakfast biscuit (35g)	0
Yeast, dried, baker's (–)	0

EGG AND CHEESE DISHES

Food	Vitamin A
Cauliflower cheese (100g)	80
Cheese soufflé (100g)	200
Egg, boiled (55g)	140

Food	Vitamin A
Apricots, canned (100g)	0
dried (25g)	0
stewed, no sugar (inc. stones 110g)	0
Avocado pear (½ = 150g)	0
Banana (100g)	0
Blackberries (100g)	0
stewed, no sugar (100g)	0
Cantaloup (inc. skin 120g)	0
Cherries (inc. stones 20 = 100g)	0
stewed, no sugar (inc. stones 100g)	0
Currants, black (90g)	0
dried (15g)	0
red (90g)	0
Dates, dried (6 = 35g)	0
Figs (2 = 75g)	0
dried (2 = 40g)	0
Fruit salad, canned (120g)	0
Grapes, black (20 = 100g)	0
white (20 = 100g)	0
Grapefruit, whole (200g)	0
canned (100g)	0
juice, canned (120g)	0
Guavas, canned (100g)	0
Lemon, slices (2 = 15g)	0
juice (15g)	0
Loganberries (100g)	0
canned (100g)	0
stewed, no sugar (100g)	0
Lychees, canned (100g)	0
Mandarins (2 = 100g)	0
canned (50g)	0
Mango (100g)	0
canned (100g)	0
Nectarines (inc. stones 3 = 100g)	0
Olives, in brine (5 = 20g)	0
Orange, whole (130g)	0
juice, fresh (120g)	0
canned (120g)	0
Passionfruit, whole (30g)	0
Papaw (100g)	0
canned (100g)	0
Peach (inc. stones 120g)	0
canned (120g)	0
dried (25g)	0

0	Peach, stewed, no sugar (120g)
0	Pear (inc. skin, core 120g)
0	canned (120g)
0	stewed, no sugar (120g)
0	Pineapple (80g)
0	canned (80g)
0	juice, canned (120g)
0	Plums (inc. stones 3 = 100g)
0	stewed, no sugar (inc. stones 100g)
0	Prunes (inc. stones 8=80g)
0	stewed, no sugar (inc. stones 120g)
0	Quince, raw (100g)
0	Raisins, dried (20g)
0	Raspberries (100g)
0	canned (100g)
0	stewed, no sugar (100g)
0	Rhubarb, stewed, no sugar (120g)
0	Strawberries (10=100g)
0	canned (100g)
0	Sultanas, dried (15g)
0	Watermelon (260g)

MEAT AND MEAT PRODUCTS

Tr	Bacon rashers, middle, fried (2=40g)
Tr	grilled (40g)
Tr	Beef, corned, canned (90g)
6	fillet steak, grilled (130g)
Tr	mince, stewed (120g)
Tr	rump steak, fried (150g)
Tr	grilled (150g)
Tr	silverside, salted, boiled (120g)
Tr	sirloin, roast (120g)
Tr	stewing steak, stewed (120g)
Tr	topside, roast (120g)
Tr	Beefburger, frozen, fried (60g)
Tr	Beef stew (250g)
Tr	Bolognese sauce (100g)
Tr	Chicken, boiled (100g)
–	crumbed, no bone (140g)
Tr	roast (130g)
Tr	leg quarter (inc. bone 130g)
Tr	wing quarter (inc. bone 130g)
11,100	Chicken livers, fried (130g)
–	Duck, roast (100g)

180	cheese spread (10g)
30	cottage (25g)
385	cream cheese (15g)
270	Danish blue (25g)
215	edam (25g)
325	parmesan (10g)
240	processed (25g)
370	stilton (25g)
305	Swiss (25g)
460	Cream, 35% fat (30g)
190	sterilized, canned (15g)
15	Ice-cream (60g)
–	non-dairy (60g)
Tr	Milk, cow's, cond. skim, sweet. (30g)
100	cond. whole, sweet. (30g)
Tr	dried, skimmed (12g)
290	dried, whole (10g)
85	evap. whole, unsweet. (30g)
30	flavoured (230g)
Tr	fresh, skimmed (230g)
35	fresh, whole (230g)
30	longlife, UHT (230g)
40	goat's (230g)
60	human (100g)
40	Milkshake, flavoured (340g)
30	Yoghurt, flavoured (200g)
8	fruit, low-fat (200g)
8	natural, low-fat (200g)
35	plain (200g)

NUTS

0	Almonds (10=15g)
0	Brazil nuts (5=20g)
0	Cashews, roast (10=20g)
0	Chestnuts (4=20g)
0	Coconut, desiccated (15g)
0	Hazel nuts (10=15g)
0	Macadamia nuts (8=20g)
0	Peanuts, raw, in shells (5=25g)
0	roasted, salted (30=25g)
–	Pistachio nuts, shelled (25=15g)
0	Walnuts (5=20g)

SAUCES & CONDIMENTS

0	Barbecue sauce (10g)
0	Chilli sauce (–)

Vitamin A	Food
0	Gelatin (–)
Tr	Ham, canned (90g)
–	Hamburger (170g)
–	with cheese (190g)
Tr	Irish stew (250g)
Tr	Lamb, brain, boiled (150g)
Tr	chops, loin, grilled (inc. bone 120g)
Tr	cutlets, grilled (inc. bone 100g)
Tr	heart, roast (140g)
160	kidney, fried (100g)
Tr	leg, roast (120g)
26,780	liver, fried (130g)
Tr	shoulder, roast (120g)
Tr	tongue, stewed (100g)
Tr	Luncheon meat, canned (90g)
–	Meat pie (180g)
30	Moussaka (200g)
Tr	Pastie (160g)
Tr	Pork, chop, loin, grilled (100g)
Tr	leg, roast (120g)
–	sweet and sour (250g)
Tr	Pork pie (180g)
–	Rabbit, stewed (inc. bone 170g)
Tr	Salami, slices (3 = 90g)
8300	Sausage, liver (60g)
100	Sausage roll (100g)
Tr	Sausages, beef, fried (2 = 120g)
Tr	grilled (2 = 120g)
Tr	frankfurter (2 = 100g)
Tr	pork, fried (2 = 120g)
Tr	grilled (2 = 120g)
Tr	saveloy, large (2 = 150g)
0	Spring roll, fried (200g)
–	Steak and kidney pie (180g)
Tr	Stewed steak in gravy, canned (100g)
Tr	Tongue, canned (100g)
Tr	Tripe, stewed (100g)
–	Turkey, roast (120g)
Tr	Veal, cutlet, fried (110g)
Tr	fillet, roast (100g)
–	schnitzel (140g)

MILK & MILK PRODUCTS

Vitamin A	Food
215	Cheese, camembert (25g)
310	cheddar (25g)

Vitamin A	Food
0	Chutney, tomato (20g)
–	Curry powder (–)
0	French dressing (15g)
–	Ginger (ground) (–)
80	Mayonnaise (20g)
–	Mustard powder (–)
0	Oxo cubes (–)
0	Pepper (–)
0	Pickles, mustard (20g)
0	sweet (20g)
–	Salad cream (25g)
0	Salt, table (–)
0	Sesame seeds (–)
0	Soy sauce (–)
Tr	Tartare sauce (20g)
30	Tomato sauce (25g)
0	Vinegar (–)
–	Worcestershire sauce (–)

SOUPS (as served)

Vitamin A	Food
0	Chicken, condensed (230g)
0	Chicken noodle, dried (230g)
0	Minestrone, dried (230g)
0	Mushroom, canned (230g)
0	Tomato, condensed (230g)
0	Tomato, dried (230g)
0	Vegetable, canned (230g)

SUGARS, JAMS AND SPREADS

Vitamin A	Food
–	Fish paste (5g)
0	Honey (30g)
0	Jam, fruit, edible seeds (30g)
0	Jam, stone fruit (30g)
0	Marmalade (30g)
Tr	Meat paste (5g)
0	Peanut butter (20g)
0	Sugar, white (–)
0	Syrup, golden (30g)
–	Topping, flavoured (40g)
0	Treacle, black (30g)
–	Vegemite (3g)

SWEETS

Vitamin A	Food
0	Boiled sweet (5g)
0	Butterscotch (5g)
–	Caramel (5g)

Carob bar (75g)	-
Chocolate square, milk (5g)	Tr
Fruit and honey bar (50g)	-
Jelly bean (5g)	-
Liquorice allsort (7g)	0
Pastille (5g)	0
Peppermint (4g)	0
Popcorn, plain unsalted (15g)	-
Sesame bar (50g)	-
Toffee, mixed (5g)	0

VEGETABLES

Artichoke, globe, boiled (100g)	0
Asparagus, boiled (5=100g)	0
Bamboo shoots (50g)	0
Beans, French, boiled (100g)	0
baked, in tomato sauce (125g)	0
broad, boiled (100g)	0
kidney (and haricot), boiled (100g)	0
mung, cooked dahl (100g)	60
soya-, boiled (100g)	0
Beetroot, slices, boiled (2=30g)	0
canned (2=30g)	0
Broccoli, boiled (100g)	0
Brussels sprouts, boiled (7=70g)	0
Cabbage, raw (50g)	0
boiled (100g)	0
Carrots, raw (50g)	0
boiled (50g)	0
young, canned (50g)	0
Cauliflower, raw (50g)	0
boiled (100g)	0
Celeriac, boiled (3=60g)	0
Celery, raw (50g)	0
boiled (50g)	0
Chickpeas, cooked dahl (60g)	50
Cucumber, slices (5=30g)	0
Egg plant, baked (½=100g)	-
Endive, raw leaves (3=15g)	0
Leeks, boiled (4=100g)	0
Lentils, split, boiled (100g)	0
Lettuce, raw leaves (2=20g)	0
Marrow, boiled (100g)	0
Mushrooms, raw (3=30g)	0
fried (6=60g)	0

Onions, raw (¼=20g)	0
boiled (100g)	0
fried (70g)	0
spring (4=20g)	0
Parsley, sprigs (2=5g)	0
Parsnip, boiled (½=60g)	0
Peas, canned (60g)	0
canned, processed (60g)	0
fresh, boiled (60g)	0
frozen, boiled (60g)	0
split, boiled (60g)	0
Peppers, green, raw (¼=15g)	0
boiled (50g)	0
Potato, baked (inc. skin 120g)	0
boiled (120g)	0
chips, fresh, fried (12=120g)	0
chips, frozen, fried (8-14=120g)	0
crisps (10=25g)	0
mashed (100g)	Tr
instant, cooked (100g)	0
new, boiled (2=100g)	0
new, canned (2=100g)	0
roast (120g)	0
Pumpkin (100g)	0
Radishes (2=20g)	0
Spinach, leaves, boiled (3=60g)	0
Swede, boiled (80g)	0
Sweetcorn, on cob, boiled (150g)	0
canned kernels (80g)	0
Sweet potato, boiled (100g)	0
Tomato, raw (120g)	0
canned (120g)	0
fried (120g)	0
juice, canned (120g)	0
Turnip, boiled (80g)	0
Yam, boiled (100g)	0

12
PROVITAMIN A
(BETA-
CAROTENE)

There are two kinds of vitamin A. Vitamin A activity in food can come from retinol, which is preformed, or from a group of components called carotenoids, of which beta-carotene is the most active and the most important. Other components do not have as much vitamin A activity. For the majority of people, most vitamin A activity is derived from carotenoids and this is the safest way to have it to avoid vitamin A toxicity. Vitamin A supplements are more likely to contain preformed vitamin A, which in large amounts is toxic. The only adverse effect of excessive intake of carotenoids appears to be a possible yellow-orange appearance of the skin.

Of great interest is the growing evidence that a high intake of carotenoid-containing foods may be protective against certain cancers such as lung and prostate cancer. In general, green leafy vegetables are good sources of provitamin A.

PROVITAMIN A INTAKE

There is no recommended intake specifically for provitamin A. Provitamin A has about one-sixth of the biological activity of retinol, the most active form of vitamin A, so we would need six times more of provitamin A than of retinol if the provitamin were our only source of vitamin A supply. Usually a mixed diet has both forms of vitamin A, so our daily requirement of 750 micrograms of retinol equivalents is made up of some vitamin A and some provitamin A.

micrograms per 100 grams

BEVERAGES

Beer (240g)	Tr-
Cider, dry, alcoholic (180g)	Tr
sweet, alcoholic (180g)	Tr
sweet, non-alcoholic (220g)	-
Cocoa powder (5g)	40
Coffee, percolated (230g)	-
Cola-type drinks (240g)	0
Cordial, diluted 1:4 (240g)	-
Drinking chocolate (10g)	-
Lemonade, carbonated drinks (240g)	Tr
Milo (10g)	-
Ovaltine (10g)	-
Port (60g)	Tr
Sherry, dry (60g)	Tr
medium (60g)	Tr
sweet (60g)	Tr
Spirits, e.g. whisky (30g)	0
Tea, infusion (230g)	0
Wine, red (100g)	Tr
white, dry (100g)	Tr
medium (100g)	Tr
sparkling (100g)	Tr
sweet (100g)	Tr

CEREALS, BISCUITS, CAKES, DESSERTS

Barley, pearl, boiled (-)	0
Biscuit, chocolate (20g)	Tr
cream-filled (20g)	-
crispbread, rye (20g)	0
wheat, starch-red. (11g)	0
gingernut (15g)	0
semi-sweet (15g)	0
short-sweet (15g)	0
Bran, wheat (8g)	0
Bread, brown, slice (25g)	0
Lebanese (pita) (¼=25g)	-
white, slice (25g)	0
wholemeal, slice (25g)	0
roll, brown (35g)	0
starch-reduced (35g)	0
white (35g)	0
Cake, fruit (60g)	10
plain (60g)	-

Egg, fried (60g)	Tr
omelette (100g)	40
poached (55g)	Tr
raw (55g)	Tr
scrambled (70g)	80
Macaroni cheese (180g)	40
Quiche Lorraine (150g)	50

FATS AND OILS

Butter, salted (10g)	660
Dripping, beef (-)	-
Lard (-)	0
Margarine (10g)	400
Vegetable oils (-)	Tr

FISH AND OTHER SEAFOODS

Bream, steamed (100g)	0
Cod, baked (100g)	Tr
fried in batter (100g)	Tr
poached (100g)	Tr
steamed (100g)	Tr
Crab, boiled (150g)	Tr
canned (90g)	Tr
Fish cakes, fried (4=100g)	Tr
fingers, fried (5=100g)	Tr
in batter, fried (120g)	25
Flounder, baked (100g)	-
Haddock, fried (100g)	Tr
steamed (100g)	Tr
Lobster, boiled (120g)	Tr
Mussels, boiled (12=120g)	Tr
Oysters, raw (12=120g)	Tr
Prawns, boiled (6=120g)	Tr
Roe, cod, fried (100g)	Tr
Salmon, canned (100g)	Tr
Sardines, canned (60g)	Tr
Scallops, steamed (10=100g)	Tr
Tuna, canned in oil (120g)	Tr
Whiting, crumbed, fried (100g)	Tr
steamed (100g)	Tr

FRUIT

Apple (inc. skin, core 100g)	25
baked, no sugar (inc. skin 110g)	20
stewed, no sugar (110g)	20
Apricots (inc. stones 3=100g)	1380

µg	Food
1000	Apricots, canned (100g)
3600	dried (25g)
1180	stewed, no sugar (inc. stones 110g)
100	Avocado pear (½=150g)
200	Banana (100g)
100	Blackberries (100g)
85	stewed, no sugar (100g)
1180	Cantaloup (inc. skin 120g)
100	Cherries (inc. stones 20=100g)
85	stewed, no sugar (inc. stones 100g)
200	Currants, black (90g)
30	dried (15g)
70	red (90g)
50	Dates, dried (6=35g)
500	Figs (2=75g)
50	dried (2=40g)
300	Fruit salad, canned (120g)
Tr	Grapes, black (20=100g)
Tr	white (20=100g)
Tr	Grapefruit, whole (200g)
Tr	canned (100g)
Tr	juice, canned (120g)
100	Guavas, canned (100g)
Tr	Lemon, slices (2=15g)
Tr	juice (15g)
80	Loganberries (100g)
70	canned (100g)
75	stewed, no sugar (100g)
Tr	Lychees, canned (100g)
280	Mandarins (2=100g)
50	canned (50g)
1200	Mango (100g)
1200	canned (100g)
460	Nectarines (inc. stones 3=100g)
140	Olives, in brine (5=20g)
40	Orange, whole (130g)
50	juice, fresh (120g)
50	canned (120g)
4	Passionfruit, whole (30g)
790	Papaw (100g)
500	canned (100g)
440	Peach (inc. stones 120g)
250	canned (120g)
2000	dried (25g)

µg	Food
0	Cake, sponge (60g)
–	Chapati (60g)
110	Cheesecake (120g)
0	Cornflakes (30g)
–	Crumpet (50g)
20	Custard (70g)
10	Custard tart (120g)
–	Doughnut (40g)
70	Eclair (50g)
0	Flour, corn- (–)
0	plain (–)
0	self-raising (–)
0	soya, full-fat (–)
0	low-fat (–)
0	wholemeal (–)
Tr	Fruit pie (150g)
Tr	Jam tart (35g)
0	Jelly, made with water (100g)
55	Lamington (60g)
0	Lemon meringue pie (120g)
0	Meringue (15g)
20	Milk pudding (e.g. sago) (160g)
0	Muesli (30g)
–	Noodles (chow mein) (250g)
10	Pancake (75g)
0	Pasta, macaroni, boiled (150g)
0	spaghetti, boiled (120g)
0	canned in tomato sauce (120g)
0	Pastry, flaky (–)
0	short crust (–)
230	Pizza, cheese and tomato (150g)
0	Porridge (30g)
0	Rice, boiled (160g)
–	fried (120g)
0	puffed (25g)
5	Scone (30g)
Tr	Sponge pudding, steamed (100g)
60	Trifle (100g)
0	Wheat, breakfast biscuit (35g)
Tr	Yeast, dried, baker's (–)

EGG AND CHEESE DISHES

µg	Food
50	Cauliflower cheese (100g)
40	Cheese soufflé (100g)
Tr	Egg, boiled (55g)

Value	Food
740	Peach, stewed, no sugar (120g)
7	Pear (inc. skin, core 120g)
10	canned (120g)
9	stewed, no sugar (120g)
60	Pineapple (80g)
40	canned (80g)
40	juice, canned (120g)
200	Plums (inc. stones 3=100g)
170	stewed, no sugar (inc. stones 100g)
830	Prunes (inc. stones 8=80g)
460	stewed, no sugar (inc. stones 120g)
Tr	Quince, raw (100g)
30	Raisins, dried (20g)
80	Raspberries (100g)
75	canned (100g)
85	stewed, no sugar (100g)
55	Rhubarb, stewed, no sugar (120g)
30	Strawberries (10=100g)
Tr	canned (100g)
30	Sultanas, dried (15g)
10	Watermelon (260g)

MEAT AND MEAT PRODUCTS

Value	Food
Tr	Bacon rashers, middle, fried (2=40g)
Tr	grilled (40g)
Tr	Beef, corned, canned (90g)
Tr	fillet steak, grilled (130g)
Tr	mince, stewed (120g)
Tr	rump steak, fried (150g)
Tr	grilled (150g)
Tr	silverside, salted, boiled (120g)
Tr	sirloin, roast (120g)
Tr	stewing steak, stewed (120g)
Tr	topside, roast (120g)
Tr	Beefburger, frozen, fried (60g)
1600	Beef stew (250g)
1940	Bolognese sauce (100g)
Tr	Chicken, boiled (100g)
-	crumbed, no bone (140g)
Tr	roast (130g)
Tr	leg quarter (inc. bone 130g)
Tr	wing quarter (inc. bone 130g)
0	Chicken livers, fried (130g)
-	Duck, roast (100g)

Value	Food
105	cheese spread (10g)
20	cottage (25g)
220	cream cheese (15g)
170	Danish blue (25g)
130	edam (25g)
195	parmesan (10g)
120	processed (25g)
230	stilton (25g)
390	Swiss (25g)
240	Cream, 35% fat (30g)
110	sterilized, canned (15g)
0	Ice-cream (60g)
0	non-dairy (60g)
Tr	Milk, cow's, cond. skim, sweet. (30g)
50	cond. whole, sweet. (30g)
Tr	dried, skimmed (12g)
170	dried, whole (10g)
50	evap. whole, unsweet. (30g)
25	flavoured (230g)
Tr	fresh, skimmed (230g)
20	fresh, whole (230g)
20	longlife, UHT (230g)
0	goat's (230g)
0	human (100g)
35	Milkshake, flavoured (340g)
40	Yoghurt, flavoured (200g)
30	fruit, low-fat (200g)
5	natural, low-fat (200g)
45	plain (200g)

NUTS

Value	Food
0	Almonds (10=15g)
0	Brazil nuts (5=20g)
0	Cashews, roast (10=20g)
0	Chestnuts (4=20g)
0	Coconut, desiccated (15g)
0	Hazel nuts (10=15g)
0	Macadamia nuts (8=20g)
0	Peanuts, raw, in shells (5=25g)
0	roasted, salted (30=25g)
200	Pistachio nuts, shelled (25=15g)
0	Walnuts (5=20g)

SAUCES & CONDIMENTS

Value	Food
215	Barbecue sauce (10g)
5735	Chilli sauce (-)

0	Gelatin (–)
Tr	Ham, canned (90g)
–	Hamburger (170g)
–	with cheese (190g)
Tr	Irish stew (250g)
Tr	Lamb, brain, boiled (150g)
Tr	chops, loin, grilled (inc. bone 120g)
Tr	cutlets, grilled (inc. bone 100g)
Tr	heart, roast (140g)
–	kidney, fried (100g)
Tr	leg, roast (120g)
60	liver, fried (130g)
Tr	shoulder, roast (120g)
Tr	tongue, stewed (100g)
Tr	Luncheon meat, canned (90g)
–	Meat pie (180g)
65	Moussaka (200g)
Tr	Pastie (160g)
Tr	Pork, chop, loin, grilled (100g)
Tr	leg, roast (120g)
–	sweet and sour (250g)
Tr	Pork pie (180g)
–	Rabbit, stewed (inc. bone 170g)
Tr	Salami, slices (3=90g)
Tr	Sausage, liver (60g)
Tr	Sausage roll (100g)
Tr	Sausages, beef, fried (2=120g)
Tr	grilled (2=120g)
Tr	frankfurter (2=100g)
Tr	pork, fried (2=120g)
Tr	grilled (2=120g)
Tr	saveloy, large (2=150g)
1200	Spring roll, fried (200g)
Tr	Steak and kidney pie (180g)
Tr	Stewed steak in gravy, canned (100g)
Tr	Tongue, canned (100g)
Tr	Tripe, stewed (100g)
–	Turkey, roast (120g)
Tr	Veal, cutlet, fried (110g)
Tr	fillet, roast (100g)
–	schnitzel (140g)

MILK & MILK PRODUCTS

135	Cheese, camembert (25g)
205	cheddar (25g)

360	Chutney, tomato (20g)
–	Curry powder (–)
0	French dressing (15g)
–	Ginger (ground) (–)
Tr	Mayonnaise (20g)
–	Mustard powder (–)
0	Oxo cubes (–)
–	Pepper (–)
–	Pickles, mustard (20g)
–	sweet (20g)
–	Salad cream (25g)
0	Salt, table (–)
20	Sesame seeds (–)
0	Soy sauce (–)
200	Tartare sauce (20g)
1230	Tomato sauce (25g)
0	Vinegar (–)
–	Worcestershire sauce (–)

SOUPS (as served)

0	Chicken, condensed (230g)
0	Chicken noodle, dried (230g)
–	Minestrone, dried (230g)
0	Mushroom, canned (230g)
200	Tomato, condensed (230g)
–	Tomato, dried (230g)
Tr	Vegetable, canned (230g)

SUGARS, JAMS AND SPREADS

Tr	Fish paste (5g)
0	Honey (30g)
Tr	Jam, fruit, edible seeds (30g)
Tr	Jam, stone fruit (30g)
50	Marmalade (30g)
Tr	Meat paste (5g)
0	Peanut butter (20g)
0	Sugar, white (–)
0	Syrup, golden (30g)
–	Topping, flavoured (40g)
0	Treacle, black (30g)
–	Vegemite (3g)

SWEETS

0	Boiled sweet (5g)
90	Butterscotch (5g)
3	Caramel (5g)

Food	β-carotene (µg)
Carob bar (75g)	–
Chocolate square, milk (5g)	0
Fruit and honey bar (50g)	–
Jelly bean (5g)	–
Liquorice allsort (7g)	0
Pastille (5g)	0
Peppermint (4g)	0
Popcorn, plain unsalted (15g)	–
Sesame bar (50g)	–
Toffee, mixed (5g)	0

VEGETABLES

Food	β-carotene (µg)
Artichoke, globe, boiled (100g)	40
Asparagus, boiled (5=100g)	250
Bamboo shoots (50g)	10
Beans, French, boiled (100g)	400
baked, in tomato sauce (125g)	–
broad, boiled (100g)	250
kidney (and haricot), boiled (100g)	Tr
mung, cooked dahl (100g)	45
soya-, boiled (100g)	18
Beetroot, slices, boiled (2=30g)	Tr
canned (2=30g)	5
Broccoli, boiled (100g)	2500
Brussels sprouts, boiled (7=70g)	400
Cabbage, raw (50g)	300
boiled (100g)	300
Carrots, raw (50g)	12000
boiled (50g)	12000
young, canned (50g)	7000
Cauliflower, raw (50g)	30
boiled (100g)	30
Celeriac, boiled (3=60g)	0
Celery, raw (50g)	Tr
boiled (50g)	Tr
Chickpeas, cooked dahl (60g)	210
Cucumber, slices (5=30g)	Tr
Egg plant, baked (½=100g)	20
Endive, raw leaves (3=15g)	2000
Leeks, boiled (4=100g)	40
Lentils, split, boiled (100g)	20
Lettuce, raw leaves (2=20g)	1000
Marrow, boiled (100g)	30
Mushrooms, raw (3=30g)	0
fried (6=60g)	0
Onions, raw (¼=20g)	0
boiled (100g)	0
fried (70g)	0
spring (4=20g)	Tr
Parsley, sprigs (2=5g)	7000
Parsnip, boiled (½=60g)	Tr
Peas, canned (60g)	300
canned, processed (60g)	300
fresh, boiled (60g)	300
frozen, boiled (60g)	300
split, boiled (60g)	50
Peppers, green, raw (¼=15g)	200
boiled (50g)	200
Potato, baked (inc. skin 120g)	Tr
boiled (120g)	Tr
chips, fresh, fried (12=120g)	Tr
chips, frozen, fried (8-14=120g)	Tr
crisps (10=25g)	Tr
mashed (100g)	Tr
instant, cooked (100g)	Tr
new, boiled (2=100g)	Tr
new, canned (2=100g)	Tr
roast (120g)	Tr
Pumpkin (100g)	1500
Radishes (2=20g)	Tr
Spinach, leaves, boiled (3=60g)	6000
Swede, boiled (80g)	Tr
Sweetcorn, on cob, boiled (150g)	240
canned kernels (80g)	210
Sweet potato, boiled (100g)	4000
Tomato, raw (120g)	600
canned (120g)	500
fried (120g)	–
juice, canned (120g)	500
Turnip, boiled (80g)	0
Yam, boiled (100g)	10

1 3
VITAMIN D

Vitamin D (cholecalciferol) is essential for humans, but can be made in our skin under the influence of ultraviolet light from the sun. Thus we need not always obtain vitamin D from the diet.

People who are mainly dependent on dietary vitamin D, which is fat-soluble, may be deficient in the vitamin, since poor absorption of vitamin D can occur because of poor fat absorption. Also, for the full action of vitamin D it must be further metabolized in liver and kidney, which means that disorders of these organs can lead to vitamin D deficiency.

The main function of vitamin D in humans is to regulate calcium and phosphorus metabolism. Its deficiency in children leads to rickets and in adults to osteomalacia, both of which are disorders of bone. As little as 2.5 micrograms (100 international units) of vitamin D per day will prevent rickets, but 10 micrograms (400 international units) per day is usually recommended for children, in case there is inadequate sunlight, or they have dark skin (which hinders absorption of ultraviolet light through their skin), or both.

VITAMIN D INTAKE

Recommended dietary intake of vitamin D:

Children – 10 micrograms (400 international units) per day (Australia and U.S.A.)

Adults — 5 micrograms (200 international units) per day (U.S.A.). An additional 5 micrograms (200 international units) per day may be required during pregnancy and lactation.

Vitamin D toxicity can occur if several times the recommended intake is ingested. The toxicity is associated with high blood calcium levels, which adversely affect the function of many tissues.

FIGURE 50: THE VITAMIN D CONTENT OF SOME FOODS

FOOD	VITAMIN D (micrograms per 100 grams of food)
Cod liver oil	200-700
Fish (salmon, sardines, tuna)	5-12
Margarine	5-6
Eggs	1-2
Butter	.4-1.2
Cheese	.1-.3

Milk, meat, fruit and vegetables are not significant sources of this vitamin.

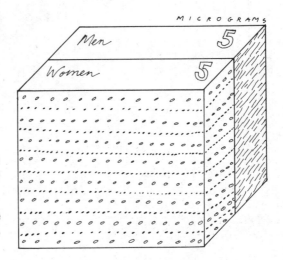

Recommended daily allowance in USA

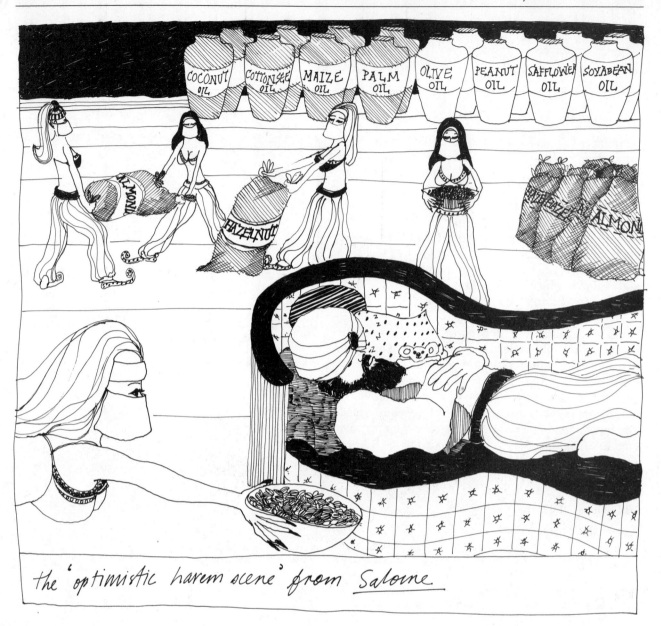

the 'optimistic harem scene' from *Salome*

V I T A M I N   E

Vitamin E originates from plants. It is found in vegetable oils such as corn, olive, palm, peanut and cotton-seed oils. Animals acquire their vitamin E from plants directly, or by eating other animals that have derived their vitamin E from plants and stored it in their liver, muscles and fat. Vitamin E is a fat-soluble vitamin like A, D and K.

Vitamin E has an important function as an 'antioxidant'. As such, it prevents the degradation of polyunsaturated fat and other compounds by oxygen. It may have some additional functions in the membranes of body cells. Although an attractive idea, there is really no good evidence that vitamin E retards the ageing process or reduces coronary heart disease. The erroneous view that it might improve libido arose because vitamin-E-deficient animals can be infertile.

It has been recommended that enough vitamin E should be present in food containing polyunsaturated fat in order to prevent oxidation (degradation) of the fat. Where up to 10 per cent of dietary energy comes from polyunsaturated fat, 10 to 20 milligrams of vitamin E per day adequately protects the fat and provides enough of the vitamin for an adult. An alternative recommendation is that the diet should contain 0.4 milligram vitamin E for each 1 gram of polyunsaturated fatty acid consumed.

Vitamin E can be found in different forms known as tocopherols or tocotrienols. Although there is some variation in their biological activity, about 1 milligram vitamin E is equivalent to 1 international unit (IU).

VITAMIN E INTAKE

Recommended daily dietary intake of vitamin E (U.S.A.):

Infants:	3-4 milligrams
Children:	5-8 milligrams
Adult men:	10 milligrams
Adult women:	8 milligrams
Pregnancy:	10 milligrams
Lactation:	11 milligrams

Toxic level of intake:

More than 1000 milligrams vitamin E per day, but, possibly, more than 400 milligrams per day.

Recommended daily intake in USA

milligrams per 100 grams

BEVERAGES
–	Beer (240g)
–	Cider, dry, alcoholic (180g)
–	sweet, alcoholic (180g)
–	sweet, non-alcoholic (220g)
.4	Cocoa powder (5g)
–	Coffee, percolated (230g)
0	Cola-type drinks (240g)
–	Cordial, diluted 1:4 (240g)
.1	Drinking chocolate (10g)
Tr	Lemonade, carbonated drinks (240g)
–	Milo (10g)
–	Ovaltine (10g)
0	Port (60g)
0	Sherry, dry (60g)
0	medium (60g)
0	sweet (60g)
0	Spirits, e.g. whisky (30g)
–	Tea, infusion (230g)
–	Wine, red (100g)
–	white, dry (100g)
–	medium (100g)
–	sparkling (100g)
–	sweet (100g)

CEREALS, BISCUITS, CAKES, DESSERTS
Tr	Barley, pearl, boiled (–)
1	Biscuit, chocolate (20g)
–	cream-filled (20g)
.5	crispbread, rye (20g)
.5	wheat, starch-red. (11g)
2	gingernut (15g)
1	semi-sweet (15g)
1	short-sweet (15g)
1.6	Bran, wheat (8g)
Tr	Bread, brown, slice (25g)
–	Lebanese (pita) (¼=25g)
Tr	white, slice (25g)
.2	wholemeal, slice (25g)
Tr	roll, brown (35g)
–	starch-reduced (35g)
Tr	white (35g)
1.4	Cake, fruit (60g)
–	plain (60g)

1.6	Egg, fried (60g)
1.5	omelette (100g)
1.6	poached (55g)
1.6	raw (55g)
1.6	scrambled (70g)
.3	Macaroni cheese (180g)
.9	Quiche Lorraine (150g)

FATS AND OILS
–	Butter, salted (10g)
.3	Dripping, beef (–)
Tr	Lard (–)
–	Margarine (10g)
※	Vegetable oils (–)

see footnote at end of chart

FISH AND OTHER SEAFOODS
–	Bream, steamed (100g)
.6	Cod, baked (100g)
–	fried in batter (100g)
.6	poached (100g)
.5	steamed (100g)
–	Crab, boiled (150g)
–	canned (90g)
–	Fish cakes, fried (4=100g)
–	fingers, fried (5=100g)
–	in batter, fried (120g)
–	Flounder, baked (100g)
–	Haddock, fried (100g)
–	steamed (100g)
1.5	Lobster, boiled (120g)
1.2	Mussels, boiled (12=120g)
.9	Oysters, raw (12=120g)
–	Prawns, boiled (6=120g)
6.9	Roe, cod, fried (100g)
1.5	Salmon, canned (100g)
1.1	Sardines, canned (60g)
–	Scallops, steamed (10=100g)
6.3	Tuna, canned in oil (120g)
–	Whiting, crumbed, fried (100g)
–	steamed (100g)

FRUIT
.2	Apple (inc. skin, core 100g)
.1	baked, no sugar (inc. skin 110g)
–	stewed, no sugar (110g)
.2	Apricots (inc. stones 3=100g)

Vitamin E	Food
–	Apricots, canned (100g)
–	dried (25g)
–	stewed, no sugar (inc. stones 110g)
3.2	Avocado pear (½=150g)
.2	Banana (100g)
3.5	Blackberries (100g)
3	stewed, no sugar (100g)
.1	Cantaloup (inc. skin 120g)
.1	Cherries (inc. stones 20=100g)
.1	stewed, no sugar (inc. stones 100g)
1	Currants, black (90g)
–	dried (15g)
.1	red (90g)
–	Dates, dried (6=35g)
–	Figs (2=75g)
–	dried (2=40g)
–	Fruit salad, canned (120g)
–	Grapes, black (20=100g)
–	white (20=100g)
.1	Grapefruit, whole (200g)
Tr	canned (100g)
Tr	juice, canned (120g)
–	Guavas, canned (100g)
–	Lemon, slices (2=15g)
–	juice (15g)
.3	Loganberries (100g)
–	canned (100g)
.3	stewed, no sugar (100g)
–	Lychees, canned (100g)
–	Mandarins (2=100g)
Tr	canned (50g)
–	Mango (100g)
–	canned (100g)
–	Nectarines (inc. stones 3=100g)
–	Olives, in brine (5=20g)
.2	Orange, whole (130g)
Tr	juice, fresh (120g)
–	canned (120g)
–	Passionfruit, whole (30g)
–	Papaw (100g)
–	canned (100g)
–	Peach (inc. stones 120g)
–	canned (120g)
–	dried (25g)

Vitamin E	Food
2.7	Cake, sponge (60g)
–	Chapati (60g)
–	Cheesecake (120g)
–	Cornflakes (30g)
–	Crumpet (50g)
.1	Custard (70g)
.8	Custard tart (120g)
–	Doughnut (40g)
1.2	Eclair (50g)
–	Flour, corn– (–)
–	plain (–)
–	self-raising (–)
–	soya, full-fat (–)
–	low-fat (–)
–	wholemeal (–)
–	Fruit pie (150g)
.6	Jam tart (35g)
0	Jelly, made with water (100g)
–	Lamington (60g)
1	Lemon meringue pie (120g)
0	Meringue (15g)
.1	Milk pudding (e.g. sago) (160g)
–	Muesli (30g)
–	Noodles (chow mein) (250g)
.3	Pancake (75g)
Tr	Pasta, macaroni, boiled (150g)
–	spaghetti, boiled (120g)
–	canned in tomato sauce (120g)
1.8	Pastry, flaky (–)
1.4	short crust (–)
.7	Pizza, cheese and tomato (150g)
.1	Porridge (30g)
.1	Rice, boiled (160g)
–	fried (120g)
–	puffed (25g)
1.3	Scone (30g)
1.6	Sponge pudding, steamed (100g)
.3	Trifle (100g)
–	Wheat, breakfast biscuit (35g)
Tr	Yeast, dried, baker's (–)

EGG AND CHEESE DISHES

Vitamin E	Food
.4	Cauliflower cheese (100g)
1.3	Cheese soufflé (100g)
1.6	Egg, boiled (55g)

Food	Vitamin E
cheese spread (10g)	–
cottage (25g)	–
cream cheese (15g)	1
Danish blue (25g)	.7
edam (25g)	.8
parmesan (10g)	.9
processed (25g)	–
stilton (25g)	1
Swiss (25g)	–
Cream, 35% fat (30g)	–
sterilized, canned (15g)	.5
Ice-cream (60g)	.4
non-dairy (60g)	1.2
Milk, cow's, cond. skim, sweet. (30g)	Tr
cond. whole, sweet. (30g)	.4
dried, skimmed (12g)	Tr
dried, whole (10g)	.6
evap. whole, unsweet. (30g)	.6
flavoured (230g)	–
fresh, skimmed (230g)	Tr
fresh, whole (230g)	.1
longlife, UHT (230g)	.09
goat's (230g)	–
human (100g)	.3
Milkshake, flavoured (340g)	–
Yoghurt, flavoured (200g)	–
fruit, low-fat (200g)	.07
natural, low-fat (200g)	.03
plain (200g)	–
NUTS	
Almonds (10=15g)	20
Brazil nuts (5=20g)	6.5
Cashews, roast (10=20g)	–
Chestnuts (4=20g)	.5
Coconut, desiccated (15g)	–
Hazel nuts (10=15g)	21
Macadamia nuts (8=20g)	–
Peanuts, raw, in shells (5=25g)	5.6
roasted, salted (30=25g)	8.1
Pistachio nuts, shelled (25=15g)	–
Walnuts (5=20g)	.8
SAUCES & CONDIMENTS	
Barbecue sauce (10g)	–
Chilli sauce (–)	–

Food	Vitamin E
Peach, stewed, no sugar (120g)	–
Pear (inc. skin, core 120g)	Tr
canned (120g)	Tr
stewed, no sugar (120g)	Tr
Pineapple (80g)	–
canned (80g)	–
juice, canned (120g)	–
Plums (inc. stones 3=100g)	.6
stewed, no sugar (inc. stones 100g)	.5
Prunes (inc. stones 8=80g)	–
stewed, no sugar (inc. stones 120g)	–
Quince, raw (100g)	–
Raisins, dried (20g)	1.2
Raspberries (100g)	.3
canned (100g)	–
stewed, no sugar (100g)	.3
Rhubarb, stewed, no sugar (120g)	.2
Strawberries (10=100g)	.2
canned (100g)	–
Sultanas, dried (15g)	.7
Watermelon (260g)	Tr
MEAT AND MEAT PRODUCTS	
Bacon rashers, middle, fried (2=40g)	.2
grilled (40g)	.1
Beef, corned, canned (90g)	.8
fillet steak, grilled (130g)	–
mince, stewed (120g)	.3
rump steak, fried (150g)	.3
grilled (150g)	.3
silverside, salted, boiled (120g)	.3
sirloin, roast (120g)	.3
stewing steak, stewed (120g)	.3
topside, roast (120g)	.3
Beefburger, frozen, fried (60g)	.6
Beef stew (250g)	.2
Bolognese sauce (100g)	1.3
Chicken, boiled (100g)	.07
crumbed, no bone (140g)	–
roast (130g)	–
leg quarter (inc. bone 130g)	.07
wing quarter (inc. bone 130g)	.06
Chicken livers, fried (130g)	.3
Duck, roast (100g)	–

–	Gelatin (–)
.08	Ham, canned (90g)
–	Hamburger (170g)
–	with cheese (190g)
.1	Irish stew (250g)
1.1	Lamb, brain, boiled (150g)
.09	chops, loin, grilled (inc. bone 120g)
.09	cutlets, grilled (inc. bone 100g)
.7	heart, roast (140g)
.4	kidney, fried (100g)
.1	leg, roast (120g)
.3	liver, fried (130g)
.1	shoulder, roast (120g)
.3	tongue, stewed (100g)
.1	Luncheon meat, canned (90g)
–	Meat pie (180g)
.3	Moussaka (200g)
1.3	Pastie (160g)
.02	Pork, chop, loin, grilled (100g)
.03	leg, roast (120g)
–	sweet and sour (250g)
.4	Pork pie (180g)
–	Rabbit, stewed (inc. bone 170g)
.3	Salami, slices (3=90g)
.1	Sausage, liver (60g)
1	Sausage roll (100g)
.3	Sausages, beef, fried (2=120g)
.2	grilled (2=120g)
.3	frankfurter (2=100g)
.3	pork, fried (2=120g)
.2	grilled (2=120g)
.08	saveloy, large (2=150g)
–	Spring roll, fried (200g)
–	Steak and kidney pie (180g)
.6	Stewed steak in gravy, canned (100g)
.3	Tongue, canned (100g)
.1	Tripe, stewed (100g)
Tr	Turkey, roast (120g)
–	Veal, cutlet, fried (110g)
–	fillet, roast (100g)
–	schnitzel (140g)

MILK & MILK PRODUCTS

.6	Cheese, camembert (25g)
.8	cheddar (25g)

.8	Chutney, tomato (20g)
–	Curry powder (–)
3.9	French dressing (15g)
–	Ginger (ground) (–)
4.9	Mayonnaise (20g)
–	Mustard powder (–)
–	Oxo cubes (–)
–	Pepper (–)
–	Pickles, mustard (20g)
–	sweet (20g)
–	Salad cream (25g)
0	Salt, table (–)
–	Sesame seeds (–)
–	Soy sauce (–)
–	Tartare sauce (20g)
1.4	Tomato sauce (25g)
0	Vinegar (–)
–	Worcestershire sauce (–)

SOUPS (as served)

–	Chicken, condensed (230g)
–	Chicken noodle, dried (230g)
–	Minestrone, dried (230g)
–	Mushroom, canned (230g)
–	Tomato, condensed (230g)
–	Tomato, dried (230g)
–	Vegetable, canned (230g)

SUGARS, JAMS AND SPREADS

.9	Fish paste (5g)
–	Honey (30g)
Tr	Jam, fruit, edible seeds (30g)
Tr	Jam, stone fruit (30g)
Tr	Marmalade (30g)
.2	Meat paste (5g)
4.7	Peanut butter (20g)
0	Sugar, white (–)
0	Syrup, golden (30g)
–	Topping, flavoured (40g)
0	Treacle, black (30g)
–	Vegemite (3g)

SWEETS

0	Boiled sweet (5g)
–	Butterscotch (5g)
–	Caramel (5g)

Food	Vitamin E
Carob bar (75g)	—
Chocolate square, milk (5g)	.5
Fruit and honey bar (50g)	—
Jelly bean (5g)	—
Liquorice allsort (7g)	0
Pastille (5g)	0
Peppermint (4g)	0
Popcorn, plain unsalted (15g)	—
Sesame bar (50g)	—
Toffee, mixed (5g)	—

VEGETABLES

Food	Vitamin E
Artichoke, globe, boiled (100g)	—
Asparagus, boiled (5 = 100g)	1.3
Bamboo shoots (50g)	—
Beans, French, boiled (100g)	.2
baked, in tomato sauce (125g)	.6
broad, boiled (100g)	Tr
kidney (and haricot), boiled (100g)	—
mung, cooked dahl (100g)	—
soya-, boiled (100g)	—
Beetroot, slices, boiled (2 = 30g)	0
canned (2 = 30g)	—
Broccoli, boiled (100g)	1.1
Brussels sprouts, boiled (7 = 70g)	.9
Cabbage, raw (50g)	.2
boiled (100g)	.2
Carrots, raw (50g)	.5
boiled (50g)	.5
young, canned (50g)	.5
Cauliflower, raw (50g)	.2
boiled (100g)	.1
Celeriac, boiled (3 = 60g)	—
Celery, raw (50g)	.2
boiled (50g)	.2
Chickpeas, cooked dahl (60g)	—
Cucumber, slices (5 = 30g)	Tr
Egg plant, baked (½ = 100g)	—
Endive, raw leaves (3 = 15g)	—
Leeks, boiled (4 = 100g)	.8
Lentils, split, boiled (100g)	—
Lettuce, raw leaves (2 = 20g)	.5
Marrow, boiled (100g)	Tr
Mushrooms, raw (3 = 30g)	Tr
fried (6 = 60g)	Tr

Food	Vitamin E
Onions, raw (¼ = 20g)	Tr
boiled (100g)	Tr
fried (70g)	—
spring (4 = 20g)	Tr
Parsley, sprigs (2 = 5g)	1.8
Parsnip, boiled (½ = 60g)	1
Peas, canned (60g)	Tr
canned, processed (60g)	Tr
fresh, boiled (60g)	Tr
frozen, boiled (60g)	Tr
split, boiled (60g)	Tr
Peppers, green, raw (¼ = 15g)	.8
boiled (50g)	.8
Potato, baked (inc. skin 120g)	.1
boiled (120g)	.1
chips, fresh, fried (12 = 120g)	.1
chips, frozen, fried (8-14 = 120g)	—
crisps (10 = 25g)	6.1
mashed (100g)	.1
instant, cooked (100g)	—
new, boiled (2 = 100g)	.1
new, canned (2 = 100g)	.1
roast (120g)	.1
Pumpkin (100g)	Tr
Radishes (2 = 20g)	0
Spinach, leaves, boiled (3 = 60g)	2
Swede, boiled (80g)	0
Sweetcorn, on cob, boiled (150g)	.5
canned kernels (80g)	.5
Sweet potato, boiled (100g)	4
Tomato, raw (120g)	1.2
canned (120g)	1.2
fried (120g)	—
juice, canned (120g)	.2
Turnip, boiled (80g)	0
Yam, boiled (100g)	—

The amount of Vitamin E in vegetable oil depends on the source of the oil:

VEGETABLE OIL	VITAMIN E	VEGETABLE OIL	VITAMIN E
Coconut	0.5	Palm	26
Cottonseed	39	Peanut	13
Maize	11	Safflower	39
Olive	5	Soyabean	10

15

V I T A M I N K

Vitamin K cannot be made by our bodies, but not all vitamin K needs to be obtained from food, because bacteria in our gut can make it (as also is the case with biotin). Probably, about half our vitamin K needs can be made by gut bacteria.

Vitamin K is involved in the formation of special liver proteins, known as coagulation factors, which, when circulating in our blood, reduce the risk of haemorrhage or bleeding. Conversely, if you are susceptible to blood clotting, medication (usually warfarin) that interferes with the formation of these vitamin-K-dependent factors may be prescribed for you. If you are taking warfarin, you need to be particularly careful not to alter your intake of vitamin-K-containing foods without close medical supervision.

Newborn babies can sometimes suffer vitamin K deficiency, as can people who do not absorb fat, since vitamin K is fat soluble. Those with liver disease may require more vitamin K.

Some proteins in bone and kidney are vitamin K dependent, so that vitamin K may have functions in these tissues as well.

VITAMIN K INTAKE

Safe and adequate daily intake of vitamin K (U.S.A.):

Infants:	10-20 micrograms
Children and adolescents:	15-100 micrograms
Adults:	70-140 micrograms

Another way of expressing vitamin K requirement is to say that about 2 micrograms per kilogram of body weight per day are needed, but half of this could come from gut bacteria.

Toxic level of intake:

Many milligrams of natural vitamin K can be ingested by healthy adults without adverse effects. Synthetic forms of vitamin K can be more of a problem in high dosages.

FIGURE 51: THE VITAMIN K CONTENT OF SOME FOODS

FOOD	VITAMIN K (micrograms per 100 grams of food)
Apples	less than 5
Asparagus	21
Beans, green	22
Beef, mince	7
Beef, liver	100
Broccoli	100
Cabbage	100
Carrots	15
Cauliflower	150
Lettuce	200
Milk, cow's	5
Milk, cow's, skim	4
Oranges	less than 5
Peas	19
Potatoes	20
Soya beans	190
Spinach	240
Strawberries	13
Wheat bran	80
Wheat germ	37

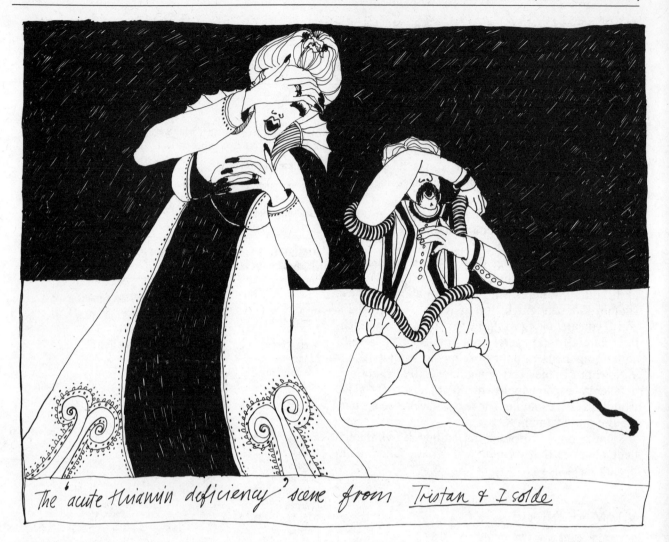

The 'acute thiamin deficiency' scene from Tristan & Isolde

1 6

V I T A M I N   B - 1   (T H I A M I N)

Whether there is a thiamin deficiency or not can depend not only on the amount of thiamin ingested, but on the presence of thiamin antagonists in food. For example, an enzyme (a natural substance that speeds up a chemical reaction), called thiaminase, occurring in raw fish can break down thiamin, and cause beri-beri in some people. One of the most significant losses of thiamin from food occurs in the milling of cereals. But thiamin is also water soluble and can be lost in cooking water. It can also be destroyed on heating and is sensitive to air or oxygen and also to alkaline conditions. In addition, alcohol can reduce the availability of thiamin to the body. For these various reasons, in both developing and developed countries, thiamin deficiency can be a problem.

Thiamin is involved in the action of certain enzymes in the body, especially one that enables carbohydrate to be used as energy. Thus, with thiamin deficiency, a number of important body functions can be disturbed. They include brain function, nerve function (especially of the legs), and heart function; these three impairments are called 'Wernicke-Korsakoff's psychosis', dry beri-beri and wet beri-beri, respectively.

VITAMIN B1 INTAKE

The requirement for thiamin relates to the amount of energy, especially carbohydrate, consumed.

Recommended daily dietary intake of thiamin (Australia):

Infants:	0.4 milligram
Children:	0.5-1.2 milligrams
Adult men:	0.8-1.1 milligrams (dependent on energy intake, the requirements for which decline with advancing years)
Adult women:	0.6-0.8 milligram (dependent on energy intake, as above)
Pregnancy:	0.8-0.9 milligram
Lactation:	1.0 milligram.

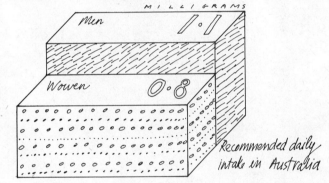

milligrams per 100 grams

BEVERAGES

Tr	Beer (240g)
Tr	Cider, dry, alcoholic (180g)
Tr	sweet, alcoholic (180g)
.02	sweet, non-alcoholic (220g)
.2	Cocoa powder (5g)
–	Coffee, percolated (230g)
0	Cola-type drinks (240g)
Tr	Cordial, diluted 1:4 (240g)
.06	Drinking chocolate (10g)
Tr	Lemonade, carbonated drinks (240g)
2	Milo (10g)
1.8	Ovaltine (10g)
Tr	Port (60g)
Tr	Sherry, dry (60g)
Tr	medium (60g)
Tr	sweet (60g)
0	Spirits, e.g. whisky (30g)
Tr	Tea, infusion (230g)
Tr	Wine, red (100g)
Tr	white, dry (100g)
Tr	medium (100g)
Tr	sparkling (100g)
Tr	sweet (100g)

CEREALS, BISCUITS, CAKES, DESSERTS

Tr	Barley, pearl, boiled (–)
.03	Biscuit, chocolate (20g)
–	cream-filled (20g)
.3	crispbread, rye (20g)
.2	wheat, starch-red. (11g)
.1	gingernut (15g)
.1	semi-sweet (15g)
.2	short-sweet (15g)
.9	Bran, wheat (8g)
.2	Bread, brown, slice (25g)
–	Lebanese (pita) (¼=25g)
.2	white, slice (25g)
.3	wholemeal, slice (25g)
.2	roll, brown (35g)
–	starch-reduced (35g)
.2	white (35g)
.08	Cake, fruit (60g)
.08	plain (60g)

.07	Egg, fried (60g)
.07	omelette (100g)
.07	poached (55g)
.09	raw (55g)
.07	scrambled (70g)
.03	Macaroni cheese (180g)
.1	Quiche Lorraine (150g)

FATS AND OILS

Tr	Butter, salted (10g)
Tr	Dripping, beef (–)
Tr	Lard (–)
–	Margarine (10g)
Tr	Vegetable oils (–)

FISH AND OTHER SEAFOODS

.06	Bream, steamed (100g)
.07	Cod, baked (100g)
–	fried in batter (100g)
.08	poached (100g)
.09	steamed (100g)
.1	Crab, boiled (150g)
Tr	canned (90g)
.06	Fish cakes, fried (4=100g)
.08	fingers, fried (5=100g)
.06	in batter, fried (120g)
.06	Flounder, baked (100g)
–	Haddock, fried (100g)
.08	steamed (100g)
.08	Lobster, boiled (120g)
–	Mussels, boiled (12=120g)
.1	Oysters, raw (12=120g)
–	Prawns, boiled (6=120g)
1.3	Roe, cod, fried (100g)
.04	Salmon, canned (100g)
.03	Sardines, canned (60g)
–	Scallops, steamed (10=100g)
.04	Tuna, canned in oil (120g)
–	Whiting, crumbed, fried (100g)
–	steamed (100g)

FRUIT

.03	Apple (inc. skin, core 100g)
.03	baked, no sugar (inc. skin 110g)
.03	stewed, no sugar (110g)
.04	Apricots (inc. stones 3=100g)

.02	Apricots, canned (100g)
Tr	dried (25g)
.03	stewed, no sugar (inc. stones 110g)
.1	Avocado pear (½=150g)
.04	Banana (100g)
.03	Blackberries (100g)
.03	stewed, no sugar (100g)
.03	Cantaloup (inc. skin 120g)
.04	Cherries (inc. stones 20=100g)
.03	stewed, no sugar (inc. stones 100g)
.03	Currants, black (90g)
.03	dried (15g)
.04	red (90g)
.07	Dates, dried (6=35g)
.06	Figs (2=75g)
.1	dried (2=40g)
.02	Fruit salad, canned (120g)
.03	Grapes, black (20=100g)
.04	white (20=100g)
.02	Grapefruit, whole (200g)
.04	canned (100g)
.04	juice, canned (120g)
.04	Guavas, canned (100g)
.05	Lemon, slices (2=15g)
.02	juice (15g)
.02	Loganberries (100g)
.01	canned (100g)
.02	stewed, no sugar (100g)
.03	Lychees, canned (100g)
.07	Mandarins (2=100g)
.07	canned (50g)
.03	Mango (100g)
.02	canned (100g)
.02	Nectarines (inc. stones 3=100g)
Tr	Olives, in brine (5=20g)
.08	Orange, whole (130g)
.08	juice, fresh (120g)
.07	canned (120g)
Tr	Passionfruit, whole (30g)
.04	Papaw (100g)
.02	canned (100g)
.02	Peach (inc. stones 120g)
.01	canned (120g)
Tr	dried (25g)

Tr	Cake, sponge (60g)
.3	Chapati (60g)
.05	Cheesecake (120g)
.9	Cornflakes (30g)
.05	Crumpet (50g)
.05	Custard (70g)
.1	Custard tart (120g)
–	Doughnut (40g)
.05	Eclair (50g)
–	Flour, corn- (–)
.2	plain (–)
.2	self-raising (–)
.8	soya, full-fat (–)
.9	low-fat (–)
.5	wholemeal (–)
.05	Fruit pie (150g)
.08	Jam tart (35g)
0	Jelly, made with water (100g)
.07	Lamington (60g)
.07	Lemon meringue pie (120g)
0	Meringue (15g)
.04	Milk pudding (e.g. sago) (160g)
–	Muesli (30g)
–	Noodles (chow mein) (250g)
.1	Pancake (75g)
.01	Pasta, macaroni, boiled (150g)
.01	spaghetti, boiled (120g)
.01	canned in tomato sauce (120g)
.1	Pastry, flaky (–)
.2	short crust (–)
.1	Pizza, cheese and tomato (150g)
.05	Porridge (30g)
.01	Rice, boiled (160g)
–	fried (120g)
.9	puffed (25g)
Tr	Scone (30g)
Tr	Sponge pudding, steamed (100g)
.05	Trifle (100g)
.9	Wheat, breakfast biscuit (35g)
2.3	Yeast, dried, baker's (–)

EGG AND CHEESE DISHES

.06	Cauliflower cheese (100g)
.07	Cheese soufflé (100g)
.08	Egg, boiled (55g)

Value	Food
.02	cheese spread (10g)
.02	cottage (25g)
.02	cream cheese (15g)
.03	Danish blue (25g)
.04	edam (25g)
.02	parmesan (10g)
.02	processed (25g)
.07	stilton (25g)
.01	Swiss (25g)
.03	Cream, 35% fat (30g)
.01	sterilized, canned (15g)
.04	Ice-cream (60g)
.04	non-dairy (60g)
.1	Milk, cow's, cond. skim, sweet. (30g)
.08	cond. whole, sweet. (30g)
.4	dried, skimmed (12g)
.3	dried, whole (10g)
.06	evap. whole, unsweet. (30g)
.04	flavoured (230g)
.04	fresh, skimmed (230g)
.04	fresh, whole (230g)
.04	longlife, UHT (230g)
.04	goat's (230g)
.02	human (100g)
.04	Milkshake, flavoured (340g)
.05	Yoghurt, flavoured (200g)
.05	fruit, low-fat (200g)
.05	natural, low-fat (200g)
.05	plain (200g)

NUTS

Value	Food
.2	Almonds (10 = 15g)
1.0	Brazil nuts (5 = 20g)
.6	Cashews, roast (10 = 20g)
.2	Chestnuts (4 = 20g)
.06	Coconut, desiccated (15g)
.4	Hazel nuts (10 = 15g)
.3	Macadamia nuts (8 = 20g)
.6	Peanuts, raw, in shells (5 = 25g)
.2	roasted, salted (30 = 25g)
.7	Pistachio nuts, shelled (25 = 15g)
.3	Walnuts (5 = 20g)

SAUCES & CONDIMENTS

Value	Food
.01	Barbecue sauce (10g)
.01	Chilli sauce (–)

Value	Food
Tr	Peach, stewed, no sugar (120g)
.02	Pear (inc. skin, core 120g)
.01	canned (120g)
.03	stewed, no sugar (120g)
.08	Pineapple (80g)
.05	canned (80g)
.06	juice, canned (120g)
.09	Plums (inc. stones 3 = 100g)
.07	stewed, no sugar (inc. stones 100g)
.08	Prunes (inc. stones 8 = 80g)
.04	stewed, no sugar (inc. stones 120g)
.02	Quince, raw (100g)
.1	Raisins, dried (20g)
.02	Raspberries (100g)
.01	canned (100g)
.02	stewed, no sugar (100g)
Tr	Rhubarb, stewed, no sugar (120g)
.02	Strawberries (10 = 100g)
.01	canned (100g)
.1	Sultanas, dried (15g)
.01	Watermelon (260g)

MEAT AND MEAT PRODUCTS

Value	Food
.4	Bacon rashers, middle, fried (2 = 40g)
.4	grilled (40g)
Tr	Beef, corned, canned (90g)
.08	fillet steak, grilled (130g)
.05	mince, stewed (120g)
.08	rump steak, fried (150g)
.08	grilled (150g)
.03	silverside, salted, boiled (120g)
.06	sirloin, roast (120g)
.03	stewing steak, stewed (120g)
.07	topside, roast (120g)
.02	Beefburger, frozen, fried (60g)
.04	Beef stew (250g)
.06	Bolognese sauce (100g)
.06	Chicken, boiled (100g)
–	crumbed, no bone (140g)
–	roast (130g)
.05	leg quarter (inc. bone 130g)
.04	wing quarter (inc. bone 130g)
.4	Chicken livers, fried (130g)
–	Duck, roast (100g)

Gelatin (–)	Tr
Ham, canned (90g)	.5
Hamburger (170g)	–
with cheese (190g)	–
Irish stew (250g)	.05
Lamb, brain, boiled (150g)	.1
chops, loin, grilled (inc. bone 120g)	.09
cutlets, grilled (inc. bone 100g)	.07
heart, roast (140g)	.5
kidney, fried (100g)	.6
leg, roast (120g)	.1
liver, fried (130g)	.3
shoulder, roast (120g)	.07
tongue, stewed (100g)	.1
Luncheon meat, canned (90g)	.07
Meat pie (180g)	–
Moussaka (200g)	.06
Pastie (160g)	.1
Pork, chop, loin, grilled (100g)	.5
leg, roast (120g)	.7
sweet and sour (250g)	–
Pork pie (180g)	.2
Rabbit, stewed (inc. bone 170g)	.04
Salami, slices (3=90g)	.2
Sausage, liver (60g)	.2
Sausage roll (100g)	.1
Sausages, beef, fried (2=120g)	Tr
grilled (2=120g)	Tr
frankfurter (2=100g)	.08
pork, fried (2=120g)	.01
grilled (2=120g)	.02
saveloy, large (2=150g)	.1
Spring roll, fried (200g)	.07
Steak and kidney pie (180g)	.1
Stewed steak in gravy, canned (100g)	Tr
Tongue, canned (100g)	.04
Tripe, stewed (100g)	Tr
Turkey, roast (120g)	–
Veal, cutlet, fried (110g)	–
fillet, roast (100g)	.06
schnitzel (140g)	.1

MILK & MILK PRODUCTS

Cheese, camembert (25g)	.05
cheddar (25g)	.04

Chutney, tomato (20g)	.04
Curry powder (–)	–
French dressing (15g)	0
Ginger (ground) (–)	–
Mayonnaise (20g)	.06
Mustard powder (–)	–
Oxo cubes (–)	–
Pepper (–)	–
Pickles, mustard (20g)	.2
sweet (20g)	.03
Salad cream (25g)	–
Salt, table (–)	0
Sesame seeds (–)	1
Soy sauce (–)	.02
Tartare sauce (20g)	.02
Tomato sauce (25g)	.08
Vinegar (–)	0
Worcestershire sauce (–)	–

SOUPS (as served)

Chicken, condensed (230g)	.01
Chicken noodle, dried (230g)	.01
Minestrone, dried (230g)	.02
Mushroom, canned (230g)	Tr
Tomato, condensed (230g)	.03
Tomato, dried (230g)	.02
Vegetable, canned (230g)	.03

SUGARS, JAMS AND SPREADS

Fish paste (5g)	.02
Honey (30g)	Tr
Jam, fruit, edible seeds (30g)	Tr
Jam, stone fruit (30g)	Tr
Marmalade (30g)	Tr
Meat paste (5g)	.03
Peanut butter (20g)	.2
Sugar, white (–)	0
Syrup, golden (30g)	Tr
Topping, flavoured (40g)	–
Treacle, black (30g)	Tr
Vegemite (3g)	11

SWEETS

Boiled sweet (5g)	0
Butterscotch (5g)	0
Caramel (5g)	.02

Value	Food
–	Carob bar (75g)
.1	Chocolate square, milk (5g)
–	Fruit and honey bar (50g)
.04	Jelly bean (5g)
0	Liquorice allsort (7g)
0	Pastille (5g)
0	Peppermint (4g)
–	Popcorn, plain unsalted (15g)
–	Sesame bar (50g)
0	Toffee, mixed (5g)

VEGETABLES

Value	Food
.03	Artichoke, globe, boiled (100g)
.05	Asparagus, boiled (5=100g)
.2	Bamboo shoots (50g)
.04	Beans, French, boiled (100g)
.07	baked, in tomato sauce (125g)
.1	broad, boiled (100g)
–	kidney (and haricot), boiled (100g)
.09	mung, cooked dahl (100g)
.2	soya-, boiled (100g)
.02	Beetroot, slices, boiled (2=30g)
.01	canned (2=30g)
.06	Broccoli, boiled (100g)
.06	Brussels sprouts, boiled (7=70g)
.06	Cabbage, raw (50g)
.03	boiled (100g)
.06	Carrots, raw (50g)
.05	boiled (50g)
.04	young, canned (50g)
.1	Cauliflower, raw (50g)
.06	boiled (100g)
.04	Celeriac, boiled (3=60g)
.03	Celery, raw (50g)
.02	boiled (50g)
.1	Chickpeas, cooked dahl (60g)
.04	Cucumber, slices (5=30g)
.04	Egg plant, baked (½=100g)
.06	Endive, raw leaves (3=15g)
.07	Leeks, boiled (4=100g)
.1	Lentils, split, boiled (100g)
.07	Lettuce, raw leaves (2=20g)
Tr	Marrow, boiled (100g)
.1	Mushrooms, raw (3=30g)
.07	fried (6=60g)
.03	Onions, raw (¼=20g)
.02	boiled (100g)
–	fried (70g)
.03	spring (4=20g)
.2	Parsley, sprigs (2=5g)
.07	Parsnip, boiled (½=60g)
.1	Peas, canned (60g)
.1	canned, processed (60g)
.3	fresh, boiled (60g)
.2	frozen, boiled (60g)
.1	split, boiled (60g)
Tr	Peppers, green, raw (¼=15g)
.01	boiled (50g)
.08	Potato, baked (inc. skin 120g)
.08	boiled (120g)
.1	chips, fresh, fried (12=120g)
.09	chips, frozen, fried (8-14=120g)
.2	crisps (10=25g)
.08	mashed (100g)
.01	instant, cooked (100g)
.1	new, boiled (2=100g)
.02	new, canned (2=100g)
.1	roast (120g)
.04	Pumpkin (100g)
.04	Radishes (2=20g)
.07	Spinach, leaves, boiled (3=60g)
.04	Swede, boiled (80g)
.2	Sweetcorn, on cob, boiled (150g)
.05	canned kernels (80g)
.08	Sweet potato, boiled (100g)
.06	Tomato, raw (120g)
.06	canned (120g)
–	fried (120g)
.06	juice, canned (120g)
.03	Turnip, boiled (80g)
.05	Yam, boiled (100g)

†Yeast, dried, brewers (–) contains 13 milligram

VITAMIN B-2 (RIBOFLAVIN)

Riboflavin, like other water-soluble vitamins, can be lost when cooking water containing the dissolved vitamin is discarded. Riboflavin can be destroyed by the action of ultraviolet radiation in sunlight. A particularly important loss of this vitamin can occur in milk packed in clear containers when they are exposed to sunlight during or after delivery. The products of this destruction can also cause a loss of vitamin C.

Riboflavin deficiency results in inflammation of the tongue and lips and also cracking and dryness of the lips and corner of the mouth (cheilosis) and other symptoms. Riboflavin deficiency in children causes growth retardation. Inadequate intakes of riboflavin would normally be associated with a deficiency of other B-group vitamins, which would result in multiple problems.

VITAMIN B-2 INTAKE

Since riboflavin forms part of enzymes (natural substances that speed chemical reactions) involved in energy metabolism, more may be needed when energy intakes are high.

Recommended daily dietary intake of riboflavin (Australia):

Infants:	0.5 milligram
Children:	0.7-1.5 milligrams
Adult men:	1.0-1.4 milligrams (dependent on energy intake, the requirement for which declines with advancing years)
Adult women:	0.8-1.0 milligram (dependent on energy intake, as above)
Pregnancy:	1.0-1.1 milligrams
Lactation:	1.2-1.3 milligrams

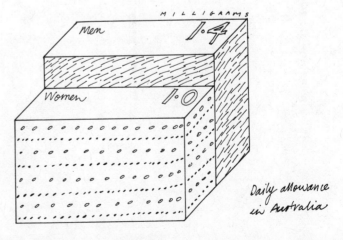

Daily allowance in Australia

milligrams per 100 grams

BEVERAGES

.03	Beer (240g)
Tr	Cider, dry, alcoholic (180g)
Tr	sweet, alcoholic (180g)
.02	sweet, non-alcoholic (220g)
.06	Cocoa powder (5g)
.01	Coffee, percolated (230g)
0	Cola-type drinks (240g)
Tr	Cordial, diluted 1:4 (240g)
.04	Drinking chocolate (10g)
Tr	Lemonade, carbonated drinks (240g)
–	Milo (10g)
2.7	Ovaltine (10g)
.01	Port (60g)
.01	Sherry, dry (60g)
.01	medium (60g)
.01	sweet (60g)
0	Spirits, e.g. whisky (30g)
.01	Tea, infusion (230g)
.02	Wine, red (100g)
.01	white, dry (100g)
.01	medium (100g)
.01	sparkling (100g)
.01	sweet (100g)

CEREALS, BISCUITS, CAKES, DESSERTS

Tr	Barley, pearl, boiled (–)
.1	Biscuit, chocolate (20g)
–	cream-filled (20g)
.1	crispbread, rye (20g)
.1	wheat, starch-red. (11g)
.03	gingernut (15g)
.08	semi-sweet (15g)
.04	short-sweet (15g)
.4	Bran, wheat (8g)
.1	Bread, brown, slice (25g)
–	Lebanese (pita) (¼=25g)
.1	white, slice (25g)
.1	wholemeal, slice (25g)
.1	roll, brown (35g)
–	starch-reduced (35g)
.1	white (35g)
.08	Cake, fruit (60g)
.1	plain (60g)

.4	Egg, fried (60g)
.3	omelette (100g)
.4	poached (55g)
.5	raw (55g)
.3	scrambled (70g)
.1	Macaroni cheese (180g)
.2	Quiche Lorraine (150g)

FATS AND OILS

Tr	Butter, salted (10g)
Tr	Dripping, beef (–)
Tr	Lard (–)
–	Margarine (10g)
Tr	Vegetable oils (–)

FISH AND OTHER SEAFOODS

.1	Bream, steamed (100g)
.07	Cod, baked (100g)
–	fried in batter (100g)
.08	poached (100g)
.09	steamed (100g)
.2	Crab, boiled (150g)
.05	canned (90g)
.06	Fish cakes, fried (4=100g)
.07	fingers, fried (5=100g)
.1	in batter, fried (120g)
.08	Flounder, baked (100g)
–	Haddock, fried (100g)
.1	steamed (100g)
.05	Lobster, boiled (120g)
–	Mussels, boiled (12=120g)
.2	Oysters, raw (12=120g)
–	Prawns, boiled (6=120g)
.9	Roe, cod, fried (100g)
.2	Salmon, canned (100g)
.3	Sardines, canned (60g)
–	Scallops, steamed (10=100g)
.1	Tuna, canned in oil (120g)
–	Whiting, crumbed, fried (100g)
–	steamed (100g)

FRUIT

.02	Apple (inc. skin, core 100g)
.01	baked, no sugar (inc. skin 110g)
.02	stewed, no sugar (110g)
.05	Apricots (inc. stones 3 = 100g)

.01 Apricots, canned (100g)
.2 dried (25g)
.04 stewed, no sugar (inc. stones 110g)
.1 Avocado pear (½=150g)
.07 Banana (100g)
.04 Blackberries (100g)
.03 stewed, no sugar (100g)
.02 Cantaloup (inc. skin 120g)
.06 Cherries (inc. stones 20=100g)
.05 stewed, no sugar (inc. stones 100g)
.06 Currants, black (90g)
.08 dried (15g)
.06 red (90g)
.04 Dates, dried (6=35g)
.05 Figs (2=75g)
.08 dried (2=40g)
.01 Fruit salad, canned (120g)
.02 Grapes, black (20=100g)
.02 white (20=100g)
.01 Grapefruit, whole (200g)
.01 canned (100g)
.01 juice, canned (120g)
.03 Guavas, canned (100g)
.04 Lemon, slices (2=15g)
.01 juice (15g)
.03 Loganberries (100g)
.02 canned (100g)
.03 stewed, no sugar (100g)
.03 Lychees, canned (100g)
.03 Mandarins (2=100g)
.02 canned (50g)
.04 Mango (100g)
.03 canned (100g)
.05 Nectarines (inc. stones 3=100g)
Tr Olives, in brine (5=20g)
.02 Orange, whole (130g)
.02 juice, fresh (120g)
.02 canned (120g)
.04 Passionfruit, whole (30g)
.04 Papaw (100g)
.02 canned (100g)
.04 Peach (inc. stones 120g)
.02 canned (120g)
.2 dried (25g)

.1 Cake, sponge (60g)
.04 Chapati (60g)
.1 Cheesecake (120g)
1.3 Cornflakes (30g)
.03 Crumpet (50g)
.2 Custard (70g)
.1 Custard tart (120g)
- Doughnut (40g)
.09 Eclair (50g)
.01 Flour, corn- (-)
.05 plain (-)
.05 self-raising (-)
.3 soya, full-fat (-)
.4 low-fat (-)
.09 wholemeal (-)
.02 Fruit pie (150g)
.01 Jam tart (35g)
0 Jelly, made with water (100g)
.09 Lamington (60g)
.08 Lemon meringue pie (120g)
.3 Meringue (15g)
.1 Milk pudding (e.g. sago) (160g)
- Muesli (30g)
- Noodles (chow mein) (250g)
.2 Pancake (75g)
.01 Pasta, macaroni, boiled (150g)
.01 spaghetti, boiled (120g)
.01 canned in tomato sauce (120g)
.01 Pastry, flaky (-)
.01 short crust (-)
.1 Pizza, cheese and tomato (150g)
.01 Porridge (30g)
.01 Rice, boiled (160g)
- fried (120g)
1.3 puffed (25g)
.08 Scone (30g)
.09 Sponge pudding, steamed (100g)
.1 Trifle (100g)
1.3 Wheat, breakfast biscuit (35g)
4 Yeast, dried, baker's (-)

EGG AND CHEESE DISHES
.1 Cauliflower cheese (100g)
.3 Cheese soufflé (100g)
.5 Egg, boiled (55g)

cheese spread (10g)	.2
cottage (25g)	.2
cream cheese (15g)	.1
Danish blue (25g)	.6
edam (25g)	.4
parmesan (10g)	.5
processed (25g)	.3
stilton (25g)	.3
Swiss (25g)	.4
Cream, 35% fat (30g)	.1
sterilized, canned (15g)	.1
Ice-cream (60g)	.2
non-dairy (60g)	.2
Milk, cow's, cond. skim, sweet. (30g)	.6
cond. whole, sweet. (30g)	.5
dried, skimmed (12g)	1.6
dried, whole (10g)	1.1
evap. whole, unsweet. (30g)	.5
flavoured (230g)	.2
fresh, skimmed (230g)	.2
fresh, whole (230g)	.2
longlife, UHT (230g)	.2
goat's (230g)	.2
human (100g)	.03
Milkshake, flavoured (340g)	.2
Yoghurt, flavoured (200g)	.2
fruit, low-fat (200g)	.2
natural, low-fat (200g)	.3
plain (200g)	.2

NUTS

Almonds (10=15g)	.9
Brazil nuts (5=20g)	.1
Cashews, roast (10=20g)	.2
Chestnuts (4=20g)	.2
Coconut, desiccated (15g)	.04
Hazel nuts (10=15g)	-
Macadamia nuts (8=20g)	.1
Peanuts, raw, in shells (5=25g)	.07
roasted, salted (30=25g)	.1
Pistachio nuts, shelled (25=15g)	-
Walnuts (5=20g)	.1

SAUCES & CONDIMENTS

Barbecue sauce (10g)	.01
Chilli sauce (–)	.09

Peach, stewed, no sugar (120g)	.06
Pear (inc. skin, core 120g)	.02
canned (120g)	.01
stewed, no sugar (120g)	.03
Pineapple (80g)	.02
canned (80g)	.02
juice, canned (120g)	.03
Plums (inc. stones 3 = 100g)	.03
stewed, no sugar (inc. stones 100g)	.03
Prunes (inc. stones 8=80g)	.2
stewed, no sugar (inc. stones 120g)	.08
Quince, raw (100g)	.02
Raisins, dried (20g)	.08
Raspberries (100g)	.03
canned (100g)	.03
stewed, no sugar (100g)	.03
Rhubarb, stewed, no sugar (120g)	.03
Strawberries (10=100g)	.03
canned (100g)	.02
Sultanas, dried (15g)	.08
Watermelon (260g)	.01

MEAT AND MEAT PRODUCTS

Bacon rashers, middle, fried (2=40g)	.2
grilled (40g)	.2
Beef, corned, canned (90g)	.2
fillet steak, grilled (130g)	.2
mince, stewed (120g)	.3
rump steak, fried (150g)	.4
grilled (150g)	.3
silverside, salted, boiled (120g)	.3
sirloin, roast (120g)	.3
stewing steak, stewed (120g)	.3
topside, roast (120g)	.3
Beefburger, frozen, fried (60g)	.2
Beef stew (250g)	.1
Bolognese sauce (100g)	.1
Chicken, boiled (100g)	.2
crumbed, no bone (140g)	-
roast (130g)	-
leg quarter (inc. bone 130g)	.1
wing quarter (inc. bone 130g)	.1
Chicken livers, fried (130g)	1.7
Duck, roast (100g)	-

Tr	Gelatin (–)
.3	Ham, canned (90g)
–	Hamburger (170g)
–	with cheese (190g)
.06	Irish stew (250g)
.2	Lamb, brain, boiled (150g)
.2	chops, loin, grilled (inc. bone 120g)
.1	cutlets, grilled (inc. bone 100g)
1.5	heart, roast (140g)
2.3	kidney, fried (100g)
.3	leg, roast (120g)
4.4	liver, fried (130g)
.2	shoulder, roast (120g)
.5	tongue, stewed (100g)
.1	Luncheon meat, canned (90g)
–	Meat pie (180g)
.2	Moussaka (200g)
.06	Pastie (160g)
.2	Pork, chop, loin, grilled (100g)
.3	leg, roast (120g)
–	sweet and sour (250g)
.09	Pork pie (180g)
.1	Rabbit, stewed (inc. bone 170g)
.2	Salami, slices (3=90g)
1.6	Sausage, liver (60g)
.04	Sausage roll (100g)
.1	Sausages, beef, fried (2=120g)
.1	grilled (2=120g)
.1	frankfurter (2=100g)
.2	pork, fried (2=120g)
.2	grilled (2=120g)
.1	saveloy, large (2=150g)
.04	Spring roll, fried (200g)
.2	Steak and kidney pie (180g)
.1	Stewed steak in gravy, canned (100g)
.4	Tongue, canned (100g)
.08	Tripe, stewed (100g)
–	Turkey, roast (120g)
–	Veal, cutlet, fried (110g)
.3	fillet, roast (100g)
.2	schnitzel (140g)

MILK & MILK PRODUCTS

.6	Cheese, camembert (25g)
.5	cheddar (25g)

.05	Chutney, tomato (20g)
–	Curry powder (–)
0	French dressing (15g)
–	Ginger (ground) (–)
.1	Mayonnaise (20g)
–	Mustard powder (–)
–	Oxo cubes (–)
–	Pepper (–)
.01	Pickles, mustard (20g)
.01	sweet (20g)
–	Salad cream (25g)
0	Salt, table (–)
.2	Sesame seeds (–)
.3	Soy sauce (–)
.03	Tartare sauce (20g)
.05	Tomato sauce (25g)
0	Vinegar (–)
–	Worcestershire sauce (–)

SOUPS (as served)

.02	Chicken, condensed (230g)
Tr	Chicken noodle, dried (230g)
.01	Minestrone, dried (230g)
.05	Mushroom, canned (230g)
.03	Tomato, condensed (230g)
.02	Tomato, dried (230g)
.02	Vegetable, canned (230g)

SUGARS, JAMS AND SPREADS

.2	Fish paste (5g)
.05	Honey (30g)
Tr	Jam, fruit, edible seeds (30g)
Tr	Jam, stone fruit (30g)
Tr	Marmalade (30g)
.3	Meat paste (5g)
.1	Peanut butter (20g)
0	Sugar, white (–)
Tr	Syrup, golden (30g)
–	Topping, flavoured (40g)
Tr	Treacle, black (30g)
16	Vegemite (3g)

SWEETS

0	Boiled sweet (5g)
Tr	Butterscotch (5g)
.2	Caramel (5g)

-	Carob bar (75g)
.2	Chocolate square, milk (5g)
-	Fruit and honey bar (50g)
.1	Jelly bean (5g)
0	Liquorice allsort (7g)
0	Pastille (5g)
0	Peppermint (4g)
.06	Popcorn, plain unsalted (15g)
-	Sesame bar (50g)
0	Toffee, mixed (5g)

VEGETABLES

.01	Artichoke, globe, boiled (100g)
.04	Asparagus, boiled (5 = 100g)
.07	Bamboo shoots (50g)
.07	Beans, French, boiled (100g)
.05	baked, in tomato sauce (125g)
.04	broad, boiled (100g)
-	kidney (and haricot), boiled (100g)
.04	mung, cooked dahl (100g)
.1	soya-, boiled (100g)
.04	Beetroot, slices, boiled (2 = 30g)
.02	canned (2 = 30g)
.2	Broccoli, boiled (100g)
.1	Brussels sprouts, boiled (7 = 70g)
.05	Cabbage, raw (50g)
.03	boiled (100g)
.05	Carrots, raw (50g)
.04	boiled (50g)
.02	young, canned (50g)
.1	Cauliflower, raw (50g)
.06	boiled (100g)
.04	Celeriac, boiled (3 = 60g)
.03	Celery, raw (50g)
.02	boiled (50g)
.05	Chickpeas, cooked dahl (60g)
.04	Cucumber, slices (5 = 30g)
.04	Egg plant, baked (½ = 100g)
.1	Endive, raw leaves (3 = 15g)
.03	Leeks, boiled (4 = 100g)
.04	Lentils, split, boiled (100g)
.08	Lettuce, raw leaves (2 = 20g)
Tr	Marrow, boiled (100g)
.4	Mushrooms, raw (3 = 30g)
.4	fried (6 = 60g)

.05	Onions, raw (¼ = 20g)
.04	boiled (100g)
-	fried (70g)
.05	spring (4 = 20g)
.3	Parsley, sprigs (2 = 5g)
.06	Parsnip, boiled (½ = 60g)
.1	Peas, canned (60g)
.04	canned, processed (60g)
.1	fresh, boiled (60g)
.07	frozen, boiled (60g)
.06	split, boiled (60g)
.03	Peppers, green, raw (¼ = 15g)
.02	boiled (50g)
.03	Potato, baked (inc. skin 120g)
.03	boiled (120g)
.04	chips, fresh, fried (12 = 120g)
.02	chips, frozen, fried (8-14 = 120g)
.07	crisps (10 = 25g)
.04	mashed (100g)
.03	instant, cooked (100g)
.03	new, boiled (2 = 100g)
.03	new, canned (2 = 100g)
.04	roast (120g)
.04	Pumpkin (100g)
.02	Radishes (2 = 20g)
.2	Spinach, leaves, boiled (3 = 60g)
.03	Swede, boiled (80g)
.08	Sweetcorn, on cob, boiled (150g)
.08	canned kernels (80g)
.04	Sweet potato, boiled (100g)
.04	Tomato, raw (120g)
.03	canned (120g)
-	fried (120g)
.03	juice, canned (120g)
.04	Turnip, boiled (80g)
.01	Yam, boiled (100g)

NIACIN

Niacin can be obtained from food or made in our bodies from the amino acid, tryptophan. Tryptophan is a constituent of protein, although not all proteins are good sources of tryptophan. To obtain 1 milligram of niacin, we need 60 milligrams of tryptophan. Thus, if both niacin and tryptophan in food are taken into account, the niacin equivalent (in milligrams) in a food can be worked out. However, not all niacin in food may be equally available to the body, because some is rather tightly bound to other food constituents and not easily released.

Since niacin is water soluble, losses can occur by discarding water containing the dissolved vitamin.

Those at particular risk of niacin deficiency are the socio-economically deprived, those with a high consumption of corn, which is low in both tryptophan and niacin, and alcohol abusers (see 'Alcohol' on page 105). Pellagra is a condition resulting from niacin deficiency, in which there are symptoms of dermatitis in skin exposed to the sun, diarrhoea and dementia. With lesser degrees of deficiency, general weakness, loss of appetite and indigestion can occur, but these symptoms can also occur in many other circumstances.

NIACIN INTAKE

Recommended daily dietary intake of niacin (Australia):

Infants:	7 milligrams niacin equivalents
Children:	9-20 milligrams niacin equivalents
Adult men:	14-18 milligrams niacin equivalents (related to energy intake, which declines with advancing years)
Adult women:	10-13 milligrams niacin equivalents (related to energy intake, as above)
Pregnancy:	13-14 milligrams niacin equivalents
Lactation:	16-17 milligrams niacin equivalents

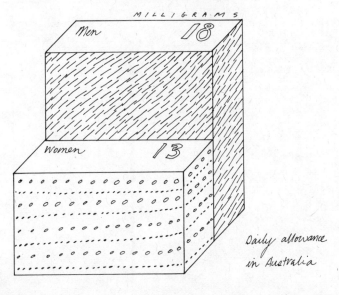

Daily allowance in Australia

milligrams per 100 grams

BEVERAGES

	mg/100g
Beer (240g)	.3
Cider, dry, alcoholic (180g)	0
sweet, alcoholic (180g)	0
sweet, non-alcoholic (220g)	.2
Cocoa powder (5g)	1.5
Coffee, percolated (230g)	.7
Cola-type drinks (240g)	0
Cordial, diluted 1:4 (240g)	Tr
Drinking chocolate (10g)	.5
Lemonade, carbonated drinks (240g)	Tr
Milo (10g)	–
Ovaltine (10g)	18
Port (60g)	.1
Sherry, dry (60g)	.1
medium (60g)	.1
sweet (60g)	.1
Spirits, e.g. whisky (30g)	0
Tea, infusion (230g)	.1
Wine, red (100g)	.1
white, dry (100g)	.1
medium (100g)	.1
sparkling (100g)	.1
sweet (100g)	.1

CEREALS, BISCUITS, CAKES, DESSERTS

	mg/100g
Barley, pearl, boiled (–)	0
Biscuit, chocolate (20g)	.5
cream-filled (20g)	–
crispbread, rye (20g)	1
wheat, starch-red. (11g)	4
gingernut (15g)	1
semi-sweet (15g)	2
short-sweet (15g)	1
Bran, wheat (8g)	29.5
Bread, brown, slice (25g)	2.5
Lebanese (pita) (¼=25g)	–
white, slice (25g)	1
wholemeal, slice (25g)	2.5
roll, brown (35g)	2.5
starch-reduced (35g)	–
white (35g)	1.5
Cake, fruit (60g)	.5
plain (60g)	.5

	mg/100g
Egg, fried (60g)	.1
omelette (100g)	.1
poached (55g)	.1
raw (55g)	.1
scrambled (70g)	.1
Macaroni cheese (180g)	.2
Quiche Lorraine (150g)	1

FATS AND OILS

	mg/100g
Butter, salted (10g)	Tr
Dripping, beef (–)	Tr
Lard (–)	Tr
Margarine (10g)	–
Vegetable oils (–)	Tr

FISH AND OTHER SEAFOODS

	mg/100g
Bream, steamed (100g)	3
Cod, baked (100g)	1.5
fried in batter (100g)	–
poached (100g)	1.5
steamed (100g)	2
Crab, boiled (150g)	2.5
canned (90g)	1
Fish cakes, fried (4=100g)	1
fingers, fried (5=100g)	1.5
in batter, fried (120g)	2
Flounder, baked (100g)	2.5
Haddock, fried (100g)	–
steamed (100g)	5
Lobster, boiled (120g)	1.5
Mussels, boiled (12=120g)	1
Oysters, raw (12=120g)	1.5
Prawns, boiled (6=120g)	–
Roe, cod, fried (100g)	1.5
Salmon, canned (100g)	7
Sardines, canned (60g)	7
Scallops, steamed (10=100g)	–
Tuna, canned in oil (120g)	13
Whiting, crumbed, fried (100g)	–
steamed (100g)	–

FRUIT

	mg/100g
Apple (inc. skin, core 100g)	.1
baked, no sugar (inc. skin 110g)	.1
stewed, no sugar (110g)	.1
Apricots (inc. stones 3=100g)	.5

Food	Niacin
Apricots, canned (100g)	.3
dried (25g)	3
stewed, no sugar (inc. stones 110g)	.4
Avocado pear (½=150g)	1
Banana (100g)	.6
Blackberries (100g)	.4
stewed, no sugar (100g)	.3
Cantaloup (inc. skin 120g)	.3
Cherries (inc. stones 20=100g)	.3
stewed, no sugar (inc. stones 100g)	.3
Currants, black (90g)	.3
dried (15g)	.5
red (90g)	.1
Dates, dried (6=35g)	2
Figs (2=75g)	.4
dried (2=40g)	1.5
Fruit salad, canned (120g)	.3
Grapes, black (20=100g)	.2
white (20=100g)	.3
Grapefruit, whole (200g)	.1
canned (100g)	.2
juice, canned (120g)	.2
Guavas, canned (100g)	.9
Lemon, slices (2=15g)	.2
juice (15g)	.1
Loganberries (100g)	.4
canned (100g)	.3
stewed, no sugar (100g)	.4
Lychees, canned (100g)	.2
Mandarins (2=100g)	.2
canned (50g)	.2
Mango (100g)	.3
canned (100g)	.2
Nectarines (inc. stones 3=100g)	.9
Olives, in brine (5=20g)	Tr
Orange, whole (130g)	.2
juice, fresh (120g)	.2
canned (120g)	.2
Passionfruit, whole (30g)	.6
Papaw (100g)	.3
canned (100g)	.2
Peach (inc. stones 120g)	.9
canned (120g)	.6
dried (25g)	5.5

Food	Niacin
Cake, sponge (60g)	.5
Chapati (60g)	1.5
Cheesecake (120g)	.5
Cornflakes (30g)	9
Crumpet (50g)	.4
Custard (70g)	.1
Custard tart (120g)	.6
Doughnut (40g)	–
Eclair (50g)	.5
Flour, corn– (–)	Tr
plain (–)	1.5
self-raising (–)	1.5
soya, full-fat (–)	2
low-fat (–)	2.5
wholemeal (–)	5.6
Fruit pie (150g)	.5
Jam tart (35g)	.5
Jelly, made with water (100g)	0
Lamington (60g)	.2
Lemon meringue pie (120g)	.5
Meringue (15g)	.1
Milk pudding (e.g. sago) (160g)	.1
Muesli (30g)	–
Noodles (chow mein) (250g)	–
Pancake (75g)	.5
Pasta, macaroni, boiled (150g)	.3
spaghetti, boiled (120g)	.3
canned in tomato sauce (120g)	.3
Pastry, flaky (–)	1
short crust (–)	1.5
Pizza, cheese and tomato (150g)	1
Porridge (30g)	0
Rice, boiled (160g)	.3
fried (120g)	–
puffed (25g)	9
Scone (30g)	1
Sponge pudding, steamed (100g)	.5
Trifle (100g)	.2
Wheat, breakfast biscuit (35g)	9
Yeast, dried, baker's (–)	36

EGG AND CHEESE DISHES

Food	Niacin
Cauliflower cheese (100g)	.4
Cheese soufflé (100g)	.2
Egg, boiled (55g)	.1

cheese spread (10g)	.1
cottage (25g)	.1
cream cheese (15g)	.1
Danish blue (25g)	.9
edam (25g)	.1
parmesan (10g)	.3
processed (25g)	.1
stilton (25g)	–
Swiss (25g)	.1
Cream, 35% fat (30g)	.1
sterilized, canned (15g)	.1
Ice-cream (60g)	.1
non-dairy (60g)	.1
Milk, cow's, cond. skim, sweet. (30g)	.3
cond. whole, sweet. (30g)	.2
dried, skimmed (12g)	1.2
dried, whole (10g)	.6
evap. whole, unsweet. (30g)	.3
flavoured (230g)	.1
fresh, skimmed (230g)	.1
fresh, whole (230g)	.1
longlife, UHT (230g)	.1
goat's (230g)	.2
human (100g)	.2
Milkshake, flavoured (340g)	.2
Yoghurt, flavoured (200g)	.1
fruit, low-fat (200g)	.1
natural, low-fat (200g)	.1
plain (200g)	.1

NUTS

Almonds (10=15g)	2
Brazil nuts (5=20g)	1.5
Cashews, roast (10=20g)	2
Chestnuts (4=20g)	.2
Coconut, desiccated (15g)	.6
Hazel nuts (10=15g)	.9
Macadamia nuts (8=20g)	1
Peanuts, raw, in shells (5=25g)	11
roasted, salted (30=25g)	16
Pistachio nuts, shelled (25=15g)	1
Walnuts (5=20g)	1

SAUCES & CONDIMENTS

Barbecue sauce (10g)	.3
Chilli sauce (–)	.6

Peach, stewed, no sugar (120g)	2
Pear (inc. skin, core 120g)	.1
canned (120g)	.2
stewed, no sugar (120g)	.2
Pineapple (80g)	.2
canned (80g)	.2
juice, canned (120g)	.7
Plums (inc. stones 3=100g)	.3
stewed, no sugar (inc. stones 100g)	.3
Prunes (inc. stones 8=80g)	1
stewed, no sugar (inc. stones 120g)	.7
Quince, raw (100g)	.2
Raisins, dried (20g)	.5
Raspberries (100g)	.4
canned (100g)	.3
stewed, no sugar (100g)	.4
Rhubarb, stewed, no sugar (120g)	.3
Strawberries (10=100g)	.4
canned (100g)	.3
Sultanas, dried (15g)	.5
Watermelon (260g)	.1

MEAT AND MEAT PRODUCTS

Bacon rashers, middle, fried (2=40g)	5
grilled (40g)	4.5
Beef, corned, canned (90g)	2.5
fillet steak, grilled (130g)	6
mince, stewed (120g)	4.5
rump steak, fried (150g)	5.5
grilled (150g)	5.5
silverside, salted, boiled (120g)	3.5
sirloin, roast (120g)	5
stewing steak, stewed (120g)	3.5
topside, roast (120g)	5.5
Beefburger, frozen, fried (60g)	4
Beef stew (250g)	1.5
Bolognese sauce (100g)	1.5
Chicken, boiled (100g)	6.5
crumbed, no bone (140g)	–
roast (130g)	–
leg quarter (inc. bone 130g)	5
wing quarter (inc. bone 130g)	4
Chicken livers, fried (130g)	10.5
Duck, roast (100g)	–

Value	Food
Tr	Gelatin (–)
4	Ham, canned (90g)
–	Hamburger (170g)
–	with cheese (190g)
1.5	Irish stew (250g)
2	Lamb, brain, boiled (150g)
4	chops, loin, grilled (inc. bone 120g)
3	cutlets, grilled (inc. bone 100g)
9	heart, roast (140g)
9.5	kidney, fried (100g)
5.5	leg, roast (120g)
15	liver, fried (130g)
3	shoulder, roast (120g)
3.5	tongue, stewed (100g)
2	Luncheon meat, canned (90g)
–	Meat pie (180g)
1.5	Moussaka (200g)
2	Pastie (160g)
4.5	Pork, chop, loin, grilled (100g)
5	leg, roast (120g)
–	sweet and sour (250g)
2	Pork pie (180g)
4.3	Rabbit, stewed (inc. bone 170g)
4.5	Salami, slices (3=90g)
4.5	Sausage, liver (60g)
–	Sausage roll (100g)
7	Sausages, beef, fried (2=120g)
5.5	grilled (2=120g)
1.5	frankfurter (2=100g)
4.5	pork, fried (2=120g)
4	grilled (2=120g)
2	saveloy, large (2=150g)
1	Spring roll, fried (200g)
2	Steak and kidney pie (180g)
2.5	Stewed steak in gravy, canned (100g)
2.5	Tongue, canned (100g)
0	Tripe, stewed (100g)
–	Turkey, roast (120g)
–	Veal, cutlet, fried (110g)
7	fillet, roast (100g)
6	schnitzel (140g)

MILK & MILK PRODUCTS

Value	Food
.8	Cheese, camembert (25g)
.1	cheddar (25g)

Value	Food
.5	Chutney, tomato (20g)
–	Curry powder (–)
0	French dressing (15g)
–	Ginger (ground) (–)
Tr	Mayonnaise (20g)
–	Mustard powder (–)
–	Oxo cubes (–)
–	Pepper (–)
.2	Pickles, mustard (20g)
.2	sweet (20g)
–	Salad cream (25g)
0	Salt, table (–)
5	Sesame seeds (–)
.4	Soy sauce (–)
Tr	Tartare sauce (20g)
1	Tomato sauce (25g)
0	Vinegar (–)
–	Worcestershire sauce (–)

SOUPS (as served)

Value	Food
.3	Chicken, condensed (230g)
.1	Chicken noodle, dried (230g)
.2	Minestrone, dried (230g)
.3	Mushroom, canned (230g)
.5	Tomato, condensed (230g)
.2	Tomato, dried (230g)
.4	Vegetable, canned (230g)

SUGARS, JAMS AND SPREADS

Value	Food
4	Fish paste (5g)
.2	Honey (30g)
Tr	Jam, fruit, edible seeds (30g)
Tr	Jam, stone fruit (30g)
Tr	Marmalade (30g)
4	Meat paste (5g)
15	Peanut butter (20g)
0	Sugar, white (30g)
Tr	Syrup, golden (30g)
–	Topping, flavoured (40g)
Tr	Treacle, black (30g)
110	Vegemite (3g)

SWEETS

Value	Food
0	Boiled sweet (5g)
Tr	Butterscotch (5g)
.2	Caramel (5g)

–	Carob bar (75g)
.2	Chocolate square, milk (5g)
–	Fruit and honey bar (50g)
.1	Jelly bean (5g)
0	Liquorice allsort (7g)
0	Pastille (5g)
0	Peppermint (4g)
1	Popcorn, plain unsalted (15g)
–	Sesame bar (50g)
0	Toffee, mixed (5g)

VEGETABLES

.4	Artichoke, globe, boiled (100g)
.4	Asparagus, boiled (5=100g)
.6	Bamboo shoots (50g)
.3	Beans, French, boiled (100g)
.5	baked, in tomato sauce (125g)
3	broad, boiled (100g)
–	kidney (and haricot), boiled (100g)
.4	mung, cooked dahl (100g)
.6	soya-, boiled (100g)
.1	Beetroot, slices, boiled (2=30g)
.1	canned (2=30g)
.6	Broccoli, boiled (100g)
.4	Brussels sprouts, boiled (7=70g)
.3	Cabbage, raw (50g)
.2	boiled (100g)
.6	Carrots, raw (50g)
.4	boiled (50g)
.3	young, canned (50g)
.6	Cauliflower, raw (50g)
.4	boiled (100g)
.5	Celeriac, boiled (3=60g)
.3	Celery, raw (50g)
.2	boiled (50g)
.5	Chickpeas, cooked dahl (60g)
.2	Cucumber, slices (5=30g)
.5	Egg plant, baked (½=100g)
.4	Endive, raw leaves (3=15g)
.4	Leeks, boiled (4=100g)
.4	Lentils, split, boiled (100g)
.3	Lettuce, raw leaves (2=20g)
.2	Marrow, boiled (100g)
4	Mushrooms, raw (3=30g)
3.5	fried (6=60g)

.2	Onions, raw (¼=20g)
.1	boiled (100g)
–	fried (70g)
.2	spring (4=20g)
1	Parsley, sprigs (2=5g)
.7	Parsnip, boiled (½=60g)
–	Peas, canned (60g)
.5	canned, processed (60g)
1.5	fresh, boiled (60g)
1.5	frozen, boiled (60g)
1	split, boiled (60g)
.7	Peppers, green, raw (¼=15g)
.6	boiled (50g)
1	Potato, baked (inc. skin 120g)
.8	boiled (120g)
1	chips, fresh, fried (12=120g)
2	chips, frozen, fried (8-14=120g)
4.5	crisps (10=25g)
.8	mashed (100g)
1	instant, cooked (100g)
1	new, boiled (2=100g)
.7	new, canned (2=100g)
1	roast (120g)
.4	Pumpkin (100g)
.2	Radishes (2=20g)
.4	Spinach, leaves, boiled (3=60g)
.8	Swede, boiled (80g)
1.5	Sweetcorn, on cob, boiled (150g)
1	canned kernels (80g)
.6	Sweet potato, boiled (100g)
.7	Tomato, raw (120g)
.7	canned (120g)
–	fried (120g)
.7	juice, canned (120g)
.4	Turnip, boiled (80g)
.5	Yam, boiled (100g)

VITAMIN B - 6

You may see vitamin B-6 called by different names. They are different forms of the vitamin, but they have the same function in our bodies. The forms of vitamin B-6 found in food are pyridoxine, mainly in vegetables, and pyridoxal and pyridoxamine, mainly in foods from animal sources. Vitamin B-6 is water soluble and can be lost by discarding water in which it is dissolved. It is also sensitive to light, air or oxygen and to alkaline conditions.

Vitamin B-6 is involved in the functioning of some enzymes (natural substances that speed up chemical reactions), especially those involved in protein metabolism, the formation of chemicals for transmission of impulses in brain and nerves, and in red blood cell formation.

With early deficiency of vitamin B-6, ill-defined symptoms such as sleeplessness, irritability and weakness may occur, but, of course, their presence may be for other reasons. If you have been on high-dosage vitamin B-6, you may develop these symptoms during its withdrawal as your body readjusts to more normal intakes. A bigger vitamin B-6 deficiency may lead to depression, convulsions, abnormal nerve functions (especially in the limbs), dermatitis, cracking of skin at the corner of the mouth and the lips, a smooth tongue, and anaemia.

Those at risk from vitamin B-6 deficiency include alcohol abusers. Certain medication, such as the oral contraceptive pill and isoniazid, which is used to treat tuberculosis, may increase vitamin B-6 requirement. In some metabolic diseases the requirement of vitamin B-6 is increased.

VITAMIN B-6 INTAKE

Recommended daily dietary intake of vitamin B-6 (Australia):

Infants:	0.3-0.5 milligrams
Children:	0.6-2.2 milligrams
Adult men:	1.0-1.9 milligrams
Adult women:	0.8-1.4 milligrams
Pregnancy:	1.0-1.5 milligrams
Lactation:	1.6-2.2 milligrams

milligrams per 100 grams

BEVERAGES
- .02 Beer (240g)
- .01 Cider, dry, alcoholic (180g)
- .01 sweet, alcoholic (180g)
- − sweet, non-alcoholic (220g)
- .05 Cocoa powder (5g)
- − Coffee, percolated (230g)
- − Cola-type drinks (240g)
- − Cordial, diluted 1:4 (240g)
- .02 Drinking chocolate (10g)
- Tr Lemonade, carbonated drinks (240g)
- − Milo (10g)
- − Ovaltine (10g)
- .01 Port (60g)
- .01 Sherry, dry (60g)
- .01 medium (60g)
- .01 sweet (60g)
- 0 Spirits, e.g. whisky (30g)
- − Tea, infusion (230g)
- .02 Wine, red (100g)
- .02 white, dry (100g)
- .01 medium (100g)
- .02 sparkling (100g)
- .01 sweet (100g)

CEREALS, BISCUITS, CAKES, DESSERTS
- Tr Barley, pearl, boiled (−)
- .04 Biscuit, chocolate (20g)
- − cream-filled (20g)
- .3 crispbread, rye (20g)
- .2 wheat, starch-red. (11g)
- .05 gingernut (15g)
- .05 semi-sweet (15g)
- .05 short-sweet (15g)
- 1.4 Bran, wheat (8g)
- .1 Bread, brown, slice (25g)
- − Lebanese (pita) (¼=25g)
- .04 white, slice (25g)
- .1 wholemeal, slice (25g)
- .2 roll, brown (35g)
- − starch-reduced (35g)
- .1 white (35g)
- .1 Cake, fruit (60g)
- − plain (60g)

- .1 Egg, fried (60g)
- .1 omelette (100g)
- .1 poached (55g)
- .1 raw (55g)
- .1 scrambled (70g)
- .03 Macaroni cheese (180g)
- .1 Quiche Lorraine (150g)

FATS AND OILS
- Tr Butter, salted (10g)
- Tr Dripping, beef (−)
- Tr Lard (−)
- Tr Margarine (10g)
- Tr Vegetable oils (−)

FISH AND OTHER SEAFOODS
- − Bream, steamed (100g)
- .4 Cod, baked (100g)
- − fried in batter (100g)
- .4 poached (100g)
- .4 steamed (100g)
- .4 Crab, boiled (150g)
- − canned (90g)
- − Fish cakes, fried (4=100g)
- .2 fingers, fried (5=100g)
- − in batter, fried (120g)
- − Flounder, baked (100g)
- − Haddock, fried (100g)
- .3 steamed (100g)
- − Lobster, boiled (120g)
- − Mussels, boiled (12=120g)
- .03 Oysters, raw (12=120g)
- − Prawns, boiled (6=120g)
- .3 Roe, cod, fried (100g)
- .5 Salmon, canned (100g)
- .4 Sardines, canned (60g)
- − Scallops, steamed (10=100g)
- .4 Tuna, canned in oil (120g)
- − Whiting, crumbed, fried (100g)
- − steamed (100g)

FRUIT
- .02 Apple (inc. skin, core 100g)
- .01 baked, no sugar (inc. skin 110g)
- .02 stewed, no sugar (110g)
- .05 Apricots (inc. stones 3=100g)

Food	Vitamin B-6
Apricots, canned (100g)	.05
dried (25g)	.2
stewed, no sugar (inc. stones 110g)	.04
Avocado pear (½=150g)	.4
Banana (100g)	.5
Blackberries (100g)	.05
stewed, no sugar (100g)	.03
Cantaloup (inc. skin 120g)	.04
Cherries (inc. stones 20=100g)	.04
stewed, no sugar (inc. stones 100g)	.02
Currants, black (90g)	.1
dried (15g)	.3
red (90g)	.05
Dates, dried (6=35g)	.2
Figs (2=75g)	.1
dried (2=40g)	.2
Fruit salad, canned (120g)	.01
Grapes, black (20=100g)	.1
white (20=100g)	.1
Grapefruit, whole (200g)	.01
canned (100g)	.02
juice, canned (120g)	.01
Guavas, canned (100g)	–
Lemon, slices (2=15g)	.1
juice (15g)	.05
Loganberries (100g)	.06
canned (100g)	.04
stewed, no sugar (100g)	.05
Lychees, canned (100g)	–
Mandarins (2=100g)	–
canned (50g)	.03
Mango (100g)	–
canned (100g)	–
Nectarines (inc. stones 3=100g)	.02
Olives, in brine (5=20g)	.02
Orange, whole (130g)	.05
juice, fresh (120g)	.04
canned (120g)	.04
Passionfruit, whole (30g)	–
Papaw (100g)	–
canned (100g)	–
Peach (inc. stones 120g)	.02
canned (120g)	.02
dried (25g)	.1

Food	Vitamin B-6
Cake, sponge (60g)	.05
Chapati (60g)	.2
Cheesecake (120g)	.02
Cornflakes (30g)	–
Crumpet (50g)	–
Custard (70g)	.05
Custard tart (120g)	.05
Doughnut (40g)	–
Eclair (50g)	.04
Flour, corn- (-)	–
plain (-)	.2
self-raising (-)	.2
soya, full-fat (-)	.6
low-fat (-)	.7
wholemeal (-)	.5
Fruit pie (150g)	–
Jam tart (35g)	.04
Jelly, made with water (100g)	0
Lamington (60g)	–
Lemon meringue pie (120g)	.05
Meringue (15g)	Tr
Milk pudding (e.g. sago) (160g)	.05
Muesli (30g)	–
Noodles (chow mein) (250g)	–
Pancake (75g)	.1
Pasta, macaroni, boiled (150g)	–
spaghetti, boiled (120g)	.01
canned in tomato sauce (120g)	.01
Pastry, flaky (-)	.05
short crust (-)	.1
Pizza, cheese and tomato (150g)	.1
Porridge (30g)	.01
Rice, boiled (160g)	.05
fried (120g)	–
puffed (25g)	–
Scone (30g)	.1
Sponge pudding, steamed (100g)	.05
Trifle (100g)	.05
Wheat, breakfast biscuit (35g)	–
Yeast, dried, baker's (-)	2

EGG AND CHEESE DISHES

Food	Vitamin B-6
Cauliflower cheese (100g)	.1
Cheese soufflé (100g)	.05
Egg, boiled (55g)	.1

Food	Vitamin B-6
cheese spread (10g)	–
cottage (25g)	.01
cream cheese (15g)	.01
Danish blue (25g)	.2
edam (25g)	.1
parmesan (10g)	.1
processed (25g)	–
stilton (25g)	–
Swiss (25g)	–
Cream, 35% fat (30g)	–
sterilized, canned (15g)	.01
Ice-cream (60g)	.02
non-dairy (60g)	.02
Milk, cow's, cond. skim, sweet. (30g)	.02
cond. whole, sweet. (30g)	.02
dried, skimmed (12g)	.3
dried, whole (10g)	.2
evap. whole, unsweet. (30g)	.04
flavoured (230g)	–
fresh, skimmed (230g)	.04
fresh, whole (230g)	.04
longlife, UHT (230g)	.04
goat's (230g)	.04
human (100g)	.01
Milkshake, flavoured (340g)	–
Yoghurt, flavoured (200g)	–
fruit, low-fat (200g)	.04
natural, low-fat (200g)	.04
plain (200g)	–

NUTS

Food	Vitamin B-6
Almonds (10=15g)	.1
Brazil nuts (5=20g)	.2
Cashews, roast (10=20g)	–
Chestnuts (4=20g)	.3
Coconut, desiccated (15g)	–
Hazel nuts (10=15g)	.6
Macadamia nuts (8=20g)	–
Peanuts, raw, in shells (5=25g)	.4
roasted, salted (30=25g)	.4
Pistachio nuts, shelled (25=15g)	–
Walnuts (5=20g)	.7

SAUCES & CONDIMENTS

Food	Vitamin B-6
Barbecue sauce (10g)	–
Chilli sauce (–)	–

Food	Vitamin B-6
Peach, stewed, no sugar (120g)	.03
Pear (inc. skin, core 120g)	.01
canned (120g)	.01
stewed, no sugar (120g)	.02
Pineapple (80g)	.1
canned (80g)	.05
juice, canned (120g)	.1
Plums (inc. stones 3=100g)	.05
stewed, no sugar (inc. stones 100g)	.03
Prunes (inc. stones 8=80g)	.2
stewed, no sugar (inc. stones 120g)	.1
Quince, raw (100g)	–
Raisins, dried (20g)	.3
Raspberries (100g)	.05
canned (100g)	.04
stewed, no sugar (100g)	.05
Rhubarb, stewed, no sugar (120g)	.02
Strawberries (10=100g)	.05
canned (100g)	.03
Sultanas, dried (15g)	.3
Watermelon (260g)	.04

MEAT AND MEAT PRODUCTS

Food	Vitamin B-6
Bacon rashers, middle, fried (2=40g)	.3
grilled (40g)	.3
Beef, corned, canned (90g)	.05
fillet steak, grilled (130g)	–
mince, stewed (120g)	.3
rump steak, fried (150g)	.3
grilled (150g)	.3
silverside, salted, boiled (120g)	.3
sirloin, roast (120g)	.3
stewing steak, stewed (120g)	.3
topside, roast (120g)	.3
Beefburger, frozen, fried (60g)	.2
Beef stew (250g)	.1
Bolognese sauce (100g)	.2
Chicken, boiled (100g)	.4
crumbed, no bone (140g)	–
roast (130g)	–
leg quarter (inc. bone 130g)	.2
wing quarter (inc. bone 130g)	.1
Chicken livers, fried (130g)	.5
Duck, roast (100g)	–

Food	B-6
Gelatin (–)	Tr
Ham, canned (90g)	.2
Hamburger (170g)	–
with cheese (190g)	–
Irish stew (250g)	.1
Lamb, brain, boiled (150g)	.1
chops, loin, grilled (inc. bone 120g)	.1
cutlets, grilled (inc. bone 100g)	.1
heart, roast (140g)	.4
kidney, fried (100g)	.3
leg, roast (120g)	.2
liver, fried (130g)	.5
shoulder, roast (120g)	.2
tongue, stewed (100g)	.1
Luncheon meat, canned (90g)	.02
Meat pie (180g)	–
Moussaka (200g)	.2
Pastie (160g)	.1
Pork, chop, loin, grilled (100g)	.2
leg, roast (120g)	.3
sweet and sour (250g)	–
Pork pie (180g)	.05
Rabbit, stewed (inc. bone 170g)	.3
Salami, slices (3=90g)	.2
Sausage, liver (60g)	.1
Sausage roll (100g)	–
Sausages, beef, fried (2=120g)	.05
grilled (2=120g)	.05
frankfurter (2=100g)	.03
pork, fried (2=120g)	.05
grilled (2=120g)	.05
saveloy, large (2=150g)	.05
Spring roll, fried (200g)	–
Steak and kidney pie (180g)	.05
Stewed steak in gravy, canned (100g)	.05
Tongue, canned (100g)	.04
Tripe, stewed (100g)	.02
Turkey, roast (120g)	–
Veal, cutlet, fried (110g)	–
fillet, roast (100g)	.3
schnitzel (140g)	–

MILK & MILK PRODUCTS

Food	B-6
Cheese, camembert (25g)	.2
cheddar (25g)	.1

Food	B-6
Chutney, tomato (20g)	.1
Curry powder (–)	–
French dressing (15g)	0
Ginger (ground) (–)	–
Mayonnaise (20g)	.1
Mustard powder (–)	–
Oxo cubes (–)	–
Pepper (–)	–
Pickles, mustard (20g)	–
sweet (20g)	–
Salad cream (25g)	–
Salt, table (–)	0
Sesame seeds (–)	–
Soy sauce (–)	–
Tartare sauce (20g)	–
Tomato sauce (25g)	.1
Vinegar (–)	0
Worcestershire sauce (–)	–

SOUPS (as served)

Food	B-6
Chicken, condensed (230g)	–
Chicken noodle, dried (230g)	–
Minestrone, dried (230g)	–
Mushroom, canned (230g)	.01
Tomato, condensed (230g)	–
Tomato, dried (230g)	–
Vegetable, canned (230g)	.05

SUGARS, JAMS AND SPREADS

Food	B-6
Fish paste (5g)	–
Honey (30g)	–
Jam, fruit, edible seeds (30g)	Tr
Jam, stone fruit (30g)	Tr
Marmalade (30g)	Tr
Meat paste (5g)	.1
Peanut butter (20g)	.5
Sugar, white (–)	0
Syrup, golden (30g)	Tr
Topping, flavoured (40g)	–
Treacle, black (30g)	Tr
Vegemite (3g)	3

SWEETS

Food	B-6
Boiled sweet (5g)	0
Butterscotch (5g)	–
Caramel (5g)	–

.1	Onions, raw (¼=20g)
.05	boiled (100g)
–	fried (70g)
.1	spring (4=20g)
.2	Parsley, sprigs (2=5g)
.05	Parsnip, boiled (½=60g)
.05	Peas, canned (60g)
.03	canned, processed (60g)
.1	fresh, boiled (60g)
.05	frozen, boiled (60g)
–	split, boiled (60g)
.2	Peppers, green, raw (¼=15g)
.1	boiled (50g)
.1	Potato, baked (inc. skin 120g)
.2	boiled (120g)
.2	chips, fresh, fried (12=120g)
.4	chips, frozen, fried (8-14=120g)
.9	crisps (10=25g)
.2	mashed (100g)
.2	instant, cooked (100g)
.2	new, boiled (2=100g)
.2	new, canned (2=100g)
.2	roast (120g)
.05	Pumpkin (100g)
.1	Radishes (2=20g)
.2	Spinach, leaves, boiled (3=60g)
.1	Swede, boiled (80g)
.2	Sweetcorn, on cob, boiled (150g)
.2	canned kernels (80g)
.1	Sweet potato, boiled (100g)
.1	Tomato, raw (120g)
.1	canned (120g)
–	fried (120g)
.1	juice, canned (120g)
.05	Turnip, boiled (80g)
–	Yam, boiled (100g)

–	Carob bar (75g)
.02	Chocolate square, milk (5g)
–	Fruit and honey bar (50g)
–	Jelly bean (5g)
0	Liquorice allsort (7g)
0	Pastille (5g)
0	Peppermint (4g)
–	Popcorn, plain unsalted (15g)
–	Sesame bar (50g)
0	Toffee, mixed (5g)

VEGETABLES

.03	Artichoke, globe, boiled (100g)
.02	Asparagus, boiled (5=100g)
–	Bamboo shoots (50g)
.05	Beans, French, boiled (100g)
.1	baked, in tomato sauce (125g)
–	broad, boiled (100g)
–	kidney (and haricot), boiled (100g)
.1	mung, cooked dahl (100g)
–	soya-, boiled (100g)
.03	Beetroot, slices, boiled (2=30g)
–	canned (2=30g)
.1	Broccoli, boiled (100g)
.2	Brussels sprouts, boiled (7=70g)
.2	Cabbage, raw (50g)
.1	boiled (100g)
.2	Carrots, raw (50g)
.1	boiled (50g)
.02	young, canned (50g)
.2	Cauliflower, raw (50g)
.1	boiled (100g)
.1	Celeriac, boiled (3=60g)
.1	Celery, raw (50g)
.05	boiled (50g)
–	Chickpeas, cooked dahl (60g)
.04	Cucumber, slices (5=30g)
–	Egg plant, baked (½=100g)
–	Endive, raw leaves (3=15g)
.2	Leeks, boiled (4=100g)
.1	Lentils, split, boiled (100g)
.05	Lettuce, raw leaves (2=20g)
.03	Marrow, boiled (100g)
.1	Mushrooms, raw (3=30g)
.05	fried (6=60g)

20
VITAMIN B-12
(CYANO-COBALAMIN)

Animals ultimately acquire vitamin B-12 from micro-organisms; people eating animal products are unlikely to suffer any deficiency. People in traditional vegetarian cultures probably obtained most of their vitamin B-12 through microbial contamination of food. Small amounts may also be obtained from water through its association with soil micro-organisms, and from bacteria normally living in the mouth. With newer, more hygienic practices, vitamin B-12 deficiency sometimes now occurs in people on a vegetarian diet, especially the infants of vegetarian mothers. It has been suggested that a few plants, like comfrey, might be sources of vitamin B-12. But, in the case of comfrey, to eat enough of it to obtain the recommended amount of vitamin B-12 would be to risk toxicity and liver damage.

One reason why vitamin B-12 deficiency is rare is that the liver stores in our bodies can last for as long as 5 years or more.

Vitamin B-12 is water soluble and can be lost in cooking water. It is not sensitive to heat, light, air or oxygen, but can be destroyed by alkaline conditions.

Vitamin B-12 and folacin are involved together in the formation of the genetic material in the nuclei of body cells (DNA), and in the formation of RNA, which is another important chemical involved in protein synthesis. The chief features of vitamin B-12 deficiency are anaemia and disordered function of the central nervous system. A condition called pernicious anaemia results from an inability to absorb vitamin B-12 rather than through dietary deficiency. Hence, in this condition, vitamin B-12 injections are given.

It is worth noting that vitamin B-12 contains cobalt and our bodies' need for cobalt is a need for vitamin B-12.

VITAMIN B-12 INTAKE

Recommended daily dietary intake of vitamin B-12 (Australia):

Infants:	0.3 microgram
Children:	0.9-2.0 micrograms
Adult men:	2.0 micrograms
Adult women:	2.0 micrograms
Pregnancy:	3.0 micrograms
Lactation:	2.5 micrograms

daily allowance in Australia

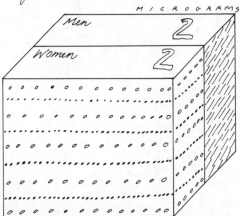

153

micrograms per 100 grams

BEVERAGES

.25	Beer (240g)
–	Cider, dry, alcoholic (180g)
–	sweet, alcoholic (180g)
–	sweet, non-alcoholic (220g)
0	Cocoa powder (5g)
0	Coffee, percolated (230g)
0	Cola-type drinks (240g)
–	Cordial, diluted 1:4 (240g)
0	Drinking chocolate (10g)
0	Lemonade, carbonated drinks (240g)
–	Milo (10g)
–	Ovaltine (10g)
Tr	Port (60g)
Tr	Sherry, dry (60g)
Tr	medium (60g)
Tr	sweet (60g)
0	Spirits, e.g. whisky (30g)
0	Tea, infusion (230g)
Tr	Wine, red (100g)
Tr	white, dry (100g)
Tr	medium (100g)
Tr	sparkling (100g)
Tr	sweet (100g)

CEREALS, BISCUITS, CAKES, DESSERTS

0	Barley, pearl, boiled (–)
0	Biscuit, chocolate (20g)
–	cream-filled (20g)
0	crispbread, rye (20g)
0	wheat, starch-red. (11g)
0	gingernut (15g)
0	semi-sweet (15g)
0	short-sweet (15g)
0	Bran, wheat (8g)
0	Bread, brown, slice (25g)
–	Lebanese (pita) (¼=25g)
0	white, slice (25g)
0	wholemeal, slice (25g)
0	roll, brown (35g)
0	starch-reduced (35g)
0	white (35g)
Tr	Cake, fruit (60g)
0	plain (60g)

1.7	Egg, fried (60g)
1.5	omelette (100g)
1.7	poached (55g)
1.7	raw (55g)
1.4	scrambled (70g)
Tr	Macaroni cheese (180g)
Tr	Quiche Lorraine (150g)

FATS AND OILS

Tr	Butter, salted (10g)
Tr	Dripping, beef (–)
Tr	Lard (–)
Tr	Margarine (10g)
0	Vegetable oils (–)

FISH AND OTHER SEAFOODS

–	Bream, steamed (100g)
2	Cod, baked (100g)
–	fried in batter (100g)
2	poached (100g)
3	steamed (100g)
Tr	Crab, boiled (150g)
Tr	canned (90g)
–	Fish cakes, fried (4=100g)
2	fingers, fried (5=100g)
–	in batter, fried (120g)
–	Flounder, baked (100g)
–	Haddock, fried (100g)
1	steamed (100g)
1	Lobster, boiled (120g)
–	Mussels, boiled (12=120g)
15	Oysters, raw (12=120g)
–	Prawns, boiled (6=120g)
11	Roe, cod, fried (100g)
4	Salmon, canned (100g)
23	Sardines, canned (60g)
–	Scallops, steamed (10=100g)
5	Tuna, canned in oil (120g)
–	Whiting, crumbed, fried (100g)
–	steamed (100g)

FRUIT

0	Apple (inc. skin, core 100g)
0	baked, no sugar (inc. skin 110g)
0	stewed, no sugar (110g)
0	Apricots (inc. stones 3=100g)

0	Apricots, canned (100g)
0	dried (25g)
0	stewed, no sugar (inc. stones 110g)
0	Avocado pear (½=150g)
0	Banana (100g)
0	Blackberries (100g)
0	stewed, no sugar (100g)
0	Cantaloup (inc. skin 120g)
0	Cherries (inc. stones 20=100g)
0	stewed, no sugar (inc. stones 100g)
0	Currants, black (90g)
0	dried (15g)
0	red (90g)
0	Dates, dried (6=35g)
0	Figs (2=75g)
0	dried (2=40g)
0	Fruit salad, canned (120g)
0	Grapes, black (20=100g)
0	white (20=100g)
0	Grapefruit, whole (200g)
0	canned (100g)
0	juice, canned (120g)
0	Guavas, canned (100g)
0	Lemon, slices (2=15g)
0	juice (15g)
0	Loganberries (100g)
0	canned (100g)
0	stewed, no sugar (100g)
0	Lychees, canned (100g)
–	Mandarins (2=100g)
0	canned (50g)
0	Mango (100g)
0	canned (100g)
0	Nectarines (inc. stones 3=100g)
0	Olives, in brine (5=20g)
0	Orange, whole (130g)
0	juice, fresh (120g)
0	canned (120g)
0	Passionfruit, whole (30g)
–	Papaw (100g)
0	Peach (inc. stones 120g)
0	canned (120g)
0	dried (25g)

Tr	Cake, sponge (60g)
0	Chapati (60g)
Tr	Cheesecake (120g)
–	Cornflakes (30g)
–	Crumpet (50g)
Tr	Custard (70g)
Tr	Custard tart (120g)
0	Doughnut (40g)
Tr	Eclair (50g)
–	Flour, corn- (–)
0	plain (–)
0	self-raising (–)
0	soya, full-fat (–)
0	low-fat (–)
0	wholemeal (–)
0	Fruit pie (150g)
0	Jam tart (35g)
0	Jelly, made with water (100g)
–	Lamington (60g)
Tr	Lemon meringue pie (120g)
Tr	Meringue (15g)
Tr	Milk pudding (e.g. sago) (160g)
–	Muesli (30g)
–	Noodles (chow mein) (250g)
Tr	Pancake (75g)
0	Pasta, macaroni, boiled (150g)
0	spaghetti, boiled (120g)
0	canned in tomato sauce (120g)
0	Pastry, flaky (–)
0	short crust (–)
Tr	Pizza, cheese and tomato (150g)
0	Porridge (30g)
0	Rice, boiled (160g)
–	fried (120g)
–	puffed (25g)
Tr	Scone (30g)
Tr	Sponge pudding, steamed (100g)
Tr	Trifle (100g)
–	Wheat, breakfast biscuit (35g)
Tr	Yeast, dried, baker's (–)

EGG AND CHEESE DISHES

Tr	Cauliflower cheese (100g)
1	Cheese soufflé (100g)
1.7	Egg, boiled (55g)

Food	µg
cheese spread (10g)	—
cottage (25g)	.5
cream cheese (15g)	Tr
Danish blue (25g)	1.2
edam (25g)	1.4
parmesan (10g)	1.5
processed (25g)	—
stilton (25g)	—
Swiss (25g)	—
Cream, 35% fat (30g)	—
sterilized, canned (15g)	Tr
Ice-cream (60g)	Tr
non-dairy (60g)	Tr
Milk, cow's, cond. skim, sweet. (30g)	.5
cond. whole, sweet. (30g)	.5
dried, skimmed (12g)	3
dried, whole (10g)	2
evap. whole, unsweet. (30g)	Tr
flavoured (230g)	—
fresh, skimmed (230g)	Tr
fresh, whole (230g)	Tr
longlife, UHT (230g)	Tr
goat's (230g)	Tr
human (100g)	Tr
Milkshake, flavoured (340g)	—
Yoghurt, flavoured (200g)	—
fruit, low-fat (200g)	Tr
natural, low-fat (200g)	Tr
plain (200g)	—

NUTS

Food	µg
Almonds (10=15g)	0
Brazil nuts (5=20g)	0
Cashews, roast (10=20g)	—
Chestnuts (4=20g)	0
Coconut, desiccated (15g)	0
Hazel nuts (10=15g)	0
Macadamia nuts (8=20g)	—
Peanuts, raw, in shells (5=25g)	0
roasted, salted (30=25g)	0
Pistachio nuts, shelled (25=15g)	—
Walnuts (5=20g)	0

SAUCES & CONDIMENTS

Food	µg
Barbecue sauce (10g)	—
Chilli sauce (–)	—

Food	µg
Peach, stewed, no sugar (120g)	0
Pear (inc. skin, core 120g)	0
canned (120g)	0
stewed, no sugar (120g)	0
Pineapple (80g)	0
canned (80g)	0
juice, canned (120g)	0
Plums (inc. stones 3 = 100g)	0
stewed, no sugar (inc. stones 100g)	0
Prunes (inc. stones 8 = 80g)	0
stewed, no sugar (inc. stones 120g)	0
Quince, raw (100g)	0
Raisins, dried (20g)	0
Raspberries (100g)	0
canned (100g)	0
stewed, no sugar (100g)	0
Rhubarb, stewed, no sugar (120g)	0
Strawberries (10=100g)	0
canned (100g)	0
Sultanas, dried (15g)	0
Watermelon (260g)	0

MEAT AND MEAT PRODUCTS

Food	µg
Bacon rashers, middle, fried (2 = 40g)	Tr
grilled (40g)	Tr
Beef, corned, canned (90g)	2
fillet steak, grilled (130g)	—
mince, stewed (120g)	2
rump steak, fried (150g)	2
grilled (150g)	2
silverside, salted, boiled (120g)	2
sirloin, roast (120g)	2
stewing steak, stewed (120g)	2
topside, roast (120g)	2
Beefburger, frozen, fried (60g)	2
Beef stew (250g)	1
Bolognese sauce (100g)	1
Chicken, boiled (100g)	Tr
crumbed, no bone (140g)	—
roast (130g)	Tr
leg quarter (inc. bone 130g)	Tr
wing quarter (inc. bone 130g)	Tr
Chicken livers, fried (130g)	49
Duck, roast (100g)	—

Gelatin (–)	0
Ham, canned (90g)	Tr
Hamburger (170g)	–
with cheese (190g)	–
Irish stew (250g)	1
Lamb, brain, boiled (150g)	8
chops, loin, grilled (inc. bone 120g)	2
cutlets, grilled (inc. bone 100g)	1
heart, roast (140g)	14
kidney, fried (100g)	79
leg, roast (120g)	2
liver, fried (130g)	81
shoulder, roast (120g)	2
tongue, stewed (100g)	7
Luncheon meat, canned (90g)	1
Meat pie (180g)	–
Moussaka (200g)	1
Pastie (160g)	1
Pork, chop, loin, grilled (100g)	1
leg, roast (120g)	1
sweet and sour (250g)	–
Pork pie (180g)	1
Rabbit, stewed (inc. bone 170g)	6
Salami, slices (3=90g)	1
Sausage, liver (60g)	8
Sausage roll (100g)	Tr
Sausages, beef, fried (2=120g)	1
grilled (2=120g)	1
frankfurter (2=100g)	1
pork, fried (2=120g)	1
grilled (2=120g)	1
saveloy, large (2=150g)	Tr
Spring roll, fried (200g)	–
Steak and kidney pie (180g)	2
Stewed steak in gravy, canned (100g)	1
Tongue, canned (100g)	5
Tripe, stewed (100g)	Tr
Turkey, roast (120g)	–
Veal, cutlet, fried (110g)	1
fillet, roast (100g)	1
schnitzel (140g)	–

MILK & MILK PRODUCTS

Cheese, camembert (25g)	1.2
cheddar (25g)	1.5

Chutney, tomato (20g)	0
Curry powder (–)	–
French dressing (15g)	0
Ginger (ground) (–)	–
Mayonnaise (20g)	1
Mustard powder (–)	–
Oxo cubes (–)	–
Pepper (–)	0
Pickles, mustard (20g)	0
sweet (20g)	0
Salad cream (25g)	–
Salt, table (–)	0
Sesame seeds (–)	–
Soy sauce (–)	–
Tartare sauce (20g)	–
Tomato sauce (25g)	0
Vinegar (–)	0
Worcestershire sauce (–)	–

SOUPS (as served)

Chicken, condensed (230g)	0
Chicken noodle, dried (230g)	0
Minestrone, dried (230g)	0
Mushroom, canned (230g)	0
Tomato, condensed (230g)	0
Tomato, dried (230g)	0
Vegetable, canned (230g)	0

SUGARS, JAMS AND SPREADS

Fish paste (5g)	–
Honey (30g)	0
Jam, fruit, edible seeds (30g)	0
Jam, stone fruit (30g)	0
Marmalade (30g)	0
Meat paste (5g)	3
Peanut butter (20g)	0
Sugar, white (–)	0
Syrup, golden (30g)	0
Topping, flavoured (40g)	–
Treacle, black (30g)	0
Vegemite (3g)	Tr

SWEETS

Boiled sweet (5g)	0
Butterscotch (5g)	–
Caramel (5g)	–

Food	B-12
Carob bar (75g)	–
Chocolate square, milk (5g)	Tr
Fruit and honey bar (50g)	–
Jelly bean (5g)	–
Liquorice allsort (7g)	0
Pastille (5g)	0
Peppermint (4g)	0
Popcorn, plain unsalted (15g)	–
Sesame bar (50g)	–
Toffee, mixed (5g)	0

VEGETABLES

Food	B-12
Artichoke, globe, boiled (100g)	0
Asparagus, boiled (5=100g)	0
Bamboo shoots (50g)	–
Beans, French, boiled (100g)	0
baked, in tomato sauce (125g)	0
broad, boiled (100g)	0
kidney (and haricot), boiled (100g)	0
mung, cooked dahl (100g)	0
soya-, boiled (100g)	–
Beetroot, slices, boiled (2=30g)	0
canned (2=30g)	–
Broccoli, boiled (100g)	0
Brussels sprouts, boiled (7=70g)	0
Cabbage, raw (50g)	0
boiled (100g)	0
Carrots, raw (50g)	0
boiled (50g)	0
young, canned (50g)	0
Cauliflower, raw (50g)	0
boiled (100g)	0
Celeriac, boiled (3=60g)	0
Celery, raw (50g)	0
boiled (50g)	0
Chickpeas, cooked dahl (60g)	0
Cucumber, slices (5=30g)	0
Egg plant, baked (½=100g)	0
Endive, raw leaves (3=15g)	–
Leeks, boiled (4=100g)	0
Lentils, split, boiled (100g)	0
Lettuce, raw leaves (2=20g)	0
Marrow, boiled (100g)	0
Mushrooms, raw (3=30g)	0
fried (6=60g)	0
Onions, raw (¼=20g)	0
boiled (100g)	0
fried (70g)	0
spring (4=20g)	0
Parsley, sprigs (2=5g)	0
Parsnip, boiled (½=60g)	0
Peas, canned (60g)	0
canned, processed (60g)	0
fresh, boiled (60g)	0
frozen, boiled (60g)	0
split, boiled (60g)	0
Peppers, green, raw (¼=15g)	0
boiled (50g)	0
Potato, baked (inc. skin 120g)	0
boiled (120g)	0
chips, fresh, fried (12=120g)	0
chips, frozen, fried (8-14=120g)	0
crisps (10=25g)	0
mashed (100g)	0
instant, cooked (100g)	0
new, boiled (2=100g)	0
new, canned (2=100g)	0
roast (120g)	0
Pumpkin (100g)	0
Radishes (2=20g)	0
Spinach, leaves, boiled (3=60g)	0
Swede, boiled (80g)	0
Sweetcorn, on cob, boiled (150g)	0
canned kernels (80g)	0
Sweet potato, boiled (100g)	0
Tomato, raw (120g)	0
canned (120g)	0
fried (120g)	0
juice, canned (120g)	0
Turnip, boiled (80g)	0
Yam, boiled (100g)	0

F O L A C I N

Folacin is present in many forms in food. It is sometimes referred to as folic acid. Food folacin values are often presented as 'free folacin' and 'total folacin'. Free folacin is the folacin without a chain of amino acids attached. This is important for you to know because the recommendations for folacin intake in some countries, for example the U.S.A. and the U.K., are based on total folacin, and, in other countries, such as Australia, on free folacin alone.

The availability to the body of folacin in food depends not only on the form, but also on other food properties, such as acidity, the amount of dietary fibre and the amount of carbohydrate.

Folacin is water soluble and easily lost in discarded cooking water. It is also sensitive to heat, to air or oxygen and to alkaline conditions.

Folacin, like vitamin B-12, is involved in the formation of the genetic material of newly forming cells and in protein formation. The consequences of deficiency include anaemia and defective lining of the gut, adversely affecting absorption of many nutrients. Since the number of blood platelets (which play a part in blood clotting) can be low with folacin deficiency, a tendency to prolonged bleeding can also occur.

Those at risk from folacin deficiency include users of certain medications (see Figure 20), pregnant women, the elderly and alcohol abusers.

FOLACIN INTAKE

Recommended daily dietary intake of folacin:

	'FREE' AUSTRALIA micrograms	'TOTAL' U.S.A. micrograms
Infants:	60	30-45
Children:	100-200	100-300
Adult men:	200	400
Adult women:	200	400
Pregnancy:	400	800
Lactation:	300	500

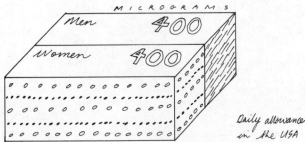

Daily allowance in the USA

micrograms per 100 grams

BEVERAGES

Food	µg
Beer (240g)	4
Cider, dry, alcoholic (180g)	–
sweet, alcoholic (180g)	–
sweet, non-alcoholic (220g)	–
Cocoa powder (5g)	38
Coffee, percolated (230g)	–
Cola-type drinks (240g)	0
Cordial, diluted 1:4 (240g)	–
Drinking chocolate (10g)	10
Lemonade, carbonated drinks (240g)	Tr
Milo (10g)	–
Ovaltine (10g)	–
Port (60g)	.1
Sherry, dry (60g)	.1
medium (60g)	.1
sweet (60g)	.1
Spirits, e.g. whisky (30g)	0
Tea, infusion (230g)	–
Wine, red (100g)	.2
white, dry (100g)	.2
medium (100g)	.2
sparkling (100g)	.1
sweet (100g)	.1

CEREALS, BISCUITS, CAKES, DESSERTS

Food	µg
Barley, pearl, boiled (–)	–
Biscuit, chocolate (20g)	–
cream-filled (20g)	–
crispbread, rye (20g)	40
wheat, starch-red. (11g)	–
gingernut (15g)	–
semi-sweet (15g)	–
short-sweet (15g)	–
Bran, wheat (8g)	260
Bread, brown, slice (25g)	36
Lebanese (pita) (¼=25g)	–
white, slice (25g)	27
wholemeal, slice (25g)	39
roll, brown (35g)	36
starch-reduced (35g)	–
white (35g)	27
Cake, fruit (60g)	4
plain (60g)	–

EGGS

Food	µg
Egg, fried (60g)	17
omelette (100g)	15
poached (55g)	16
raw (55g)	25
scrambled (70g)	15
Macaroni cheese (180g)	3
Quiche Lorraine (150g)	8

FATS AND OILS

Food	µg
Butter, salted (10g)	Tr
Dripping, beef (–)	Tr
Lard (–)	Tr
Margarine (10g)	Tr
Vegetable oils (–)	Tr

FISH AND OTHER SEAFOODS

Food	µg
Bream, steamed (100g)	–
Cod, baked (100g)	12
fried in batter (100g)	–
poached (100g)	14
steamed (100g)	12
Crab, boiled (150g)	20
canned (90g)	–
Fish cakes, fried (4=100g)	–
fingers, fried (5=100g)	16
in batter, fried (120g)	–
Flounder, baked (100g)	–
Haddock, fried (100g)	–
steamed (100g)	16
Lobster, boiled (120g)	17
Mussels, boiled (12=120g)	–
Oysters, raw (12=120g)	–
Prawns, boiled (6=120g)	–
Roe, cod, fried (100g)	–
Salmon, canned (100g)	12
Sardines, canned (60g)	7
Scallops, steamed (10=100g)	17
Tuna, canned in oil (120g)	15
Whiting, crumbed, fried (100g)	–
steamed (100g)	–

FRUIT

Food	µg
Apple (inc. skin, core 100g)	4
baked, no sugar (inc. skin 110g)	2
stewed, no sugar (110g)	2
Apricots (inc. stones 3=100g)	5

Value	Food
7	Cake, sponge (60g)
15	Chapati (60g)
3	Cheesecake (120g)
–	Cornflakes (30g)
–	Crumpet (50g)
5	Custard (70g)
6	Custard tart (120g)
–	Doughnut (40g)
5	Eclair (50g)
–	Flour, corn– (–)
22	plain (–)
19	self-raising (–)
–	soya, full-fat (–)
–	low-fat (–)
57	wholemeal (–)
–	Fruit pie (150g)
4	Jam tart (35g)
0	Jelly, made with water (100g)
–	Lamington (60g)
5	Lemon meringue pie (120g)
Tr	Meringue (15g)
4	Milk pudding (e.g. sago) (160g)
–	Muesli (30g)
–	Noodles (chow mein) (250g)
6	Pancake (75g)
–	Pasta, macaroni, boiled (150g)
2	spaghetti, boiled (120g)
2	canned in tomato sauce (120g)
7	Pastry, flaky (–)
8	short crust (–)
24	Pizza, cheese and tomato (150g)
6	Porridge (30g)
6	Rice, boiled (160g)
–	fried (120g)
–	puffed (25g)
8	Scone (30g)
7	Sponge pudding, steamed (100g)
6	Trifle (100g)
–	Wheat, breakfast biscuit (35g)
4000	Yeast, dried, baker's (–)

EGG AND CHEESE DISHES

Value	Food
13	Cauliflower cheese (100g)
12	Cheese soufflé (100g)
22	Egg, boiled (55g)

Value	Food
5	Apricots, canned (100g)
14	dried (25g)
2	stewed, no sugar (inc. stones 110g)
66	Avocado pear (½=150g)
22	Banana (100g)
–	Blackberries (100g)
–	stewed, no sugar (100g)
18	Cantaloup (inc. skin 120g)
7	Cherries (inc. stones 20=100g)
3	stewed, no sugar (inc. stones 100g)
–	Currants, black (90g)
11	dried (15g)
–	red (90g)
21	Dates, dried (6=35g)
–	Figs (2=75g)
9	dried (2=40g)
4	Fruit salad, canned (120g)
5	Grapes, black (20=100g)
6	white (20=100g)
6	Grapefruit, whole (200g)
4	canned (100g)
6	juice, canned (120g)
–	Guavas, canned (100g)
–	Lemon, slices (2=15g)
7	juice (15g)
–	Loganberries (100g)
–	canned (100g)
–	stewed, no sugar (100g)
–	Lychees, canned (100g)
–	Mandarins (2=100g)
8	canned (50g)
–	Mango (100g)
–	canned (100g)
5	Nectarines (inc. stones 3 = 100g)
–	Olives, in brine (5=20g)
28	Orange, whole (130g)
37	juice, fresh (120g)
7	canned (120g)
–	Passionfruit, whole (30g)
–	Papaw (100g)
–	canned (100g)
3	Peach (inc. stones 120g)
3	canned (120g)
14	dried (25g)

cheese spread (10g)	–
cottage (25g)	9
cream cheese (15g)	5
Danish blue (25g)	50
edam (25g)	20
parmesan (10g)	20
processed (25g)	2
stilton (25g)	–
Swiss (25g)	–
Cream, 35% fat (30g)	–
sterilized, canned (15g)	Tr
Ice-cream (60g)	Tr
non-dairy (60g)	Tr
Milk, cow's, cond. skim, sweet. (30g)	10
cond. whole, sweet. (30g)	8
dried, skimmed (12g)	21
dried, whole (10g)	40
evap. whole, unsweet. (30g)	7
flavoured (230g)	–
fresh, skimmed (230g)	5
fresh, whole (230g)	5
longlife, UHT (230g)	5
goat's (230g)	1
human (100g)	5
Milkshake, flavoured (340g)	–
Yoghurt, flavoured (200g)	–
fruit, low-fat (200g)	3
natural, low-fat (200g)	2
plain (200g)	–

NUTS

Almonds (10=15g)	96
Brazil nuts (5=20g)	–
Cashews, roast (10=20g)	–
Chestnuts (4=20g)	–
Coconut, desiccated (15g)	–
Hazel nuts (10=15g)	72
Macadamia nuts (8=20g)	–
Peanuts, raw, in shells (5=25g)	76
roasted, salted (30=25g)	–
Pistachio nuts, shelled (25=15g)	–
Walnuts (5=20g)	66

SAUCES & CONDIMENTS

Barbecue sauce (10g)	–
Chilli sauce (–)	–

Peach, stewed, no sugar (120g)	2
Pear (inc. skin, core 120g)	8
canned (120g)	5
stewed, no sugar (120g)	5
Pineapple (80g)	11
canned (80g)	–
juice, canned (120g)	–
Plums (inc. stones 3=100g)	3
stewed, no sugar (inc. stones 100g)	1
Prunes (inc. stones 8=80g)	3
stewed, no sugar (inc. stones 120g)	Tr
Quince, raw (100g)	–
Raisins, dried (20g)	4
Raspberries (100g)	–
canned (100g)	–
stewed, no sugar (100g)	–
Rhubarb, stewed, no sugar (120g)	4
Strawberries (10=100g)	20
canned (100g)	20
Sultanas, dried (15g)	4
Watermelon (260g)	2

MEAT AND MEAT PRODUCTS

Bacon rashers, middle, fried (2=40g)	1
grilled (40g)	1
Beef, corned, canned (90g)	2
fillet steak, grilled (130g)	–
mince, stewed (120g)	16
rump steak, fried (150g)	15
grilled (150g)	15
silverside, salted, boiled (120g)	15
sirloin, roast (120g)	14
stewing steak, stewed (120g)	16
topside, roast (120g)	15
Beefburger, frozen, fried (60g)	15
Beef stew (250g)	5
Bolognese sauce (100g)	10
Chicken, boiled (100g)	8
crumbed, no bone (140g)	–
roast (130g)	–
leg quarter (inc. bone 130g)	6
wing quarter (inc. bone 130g)	5
Chicken livers, fried (130g)	500
Duck, roast (100g)	–

Tr	Gelatin (–)
Tr	Ham, canned (90g)
–	Hamburger (170g)
–	with cheese (190g)
5	Irish stew (250g)
6	Lamb, brain, boiled (150g)
2	chops, loin, grilled (inc. bone 120g)
2	cutlets, grilled (inc. bone 100g)
4	heart, roast (140g)
79	kidney, fried (100g)
3	leg, roast (120g)
240	liver, fried (130g)
3	shoulder, roast (120g)
4	tongue, stewed (100g)
1	Luncheon meat, canned (90g)
–	Meat pie (180g)
8	Moussaka (200g)
3	Pastie (160g)
6	Pork, chop, loin, grilled (100g)
6	leg, roast (120g)
–	sweet and sour (250g)
3	Pork pie (180g)
2	Rabbit, stewed (inc. bone 170g)
3	Salami, slices (3=90g)
19	Sausage, liver (60g)
–	Sausage roll (100g)
2	Sausages, beef, fried (2=120g)
4	grilled (2=120g)
1	frankfurter (2=100g)
2	pork, fried (2=120g)
3	grilled (2=120g)
1	saveloy, large (2=150g)
–	Spring roll, fried (200g)
8	Steak and kidney pie (180g)
4	Stewed steak in gravy, canned (100g)
2	Tongue, canned (100g)
1	Tripe, stewed (100g)
–	Turkey, roast (120g)
–	Veal, cutlet, fried (110g)
4	fillet, roast (100g)
–	schnitzel (140g)

MILK & MILK PRODUCTS

60	Cheese, camembert (25g)
20	cheddar (25g)

11	Chutney, tomato (20g)
–	Curry powder (–)
0	French dressing (15g)
–	Ginger (ground) (–)
14	Mayonnaise (20g)
–	Mustard powder (–)
–	Oxo cubes (–)
–	Pepper (–)
–	Pickles, mustard (20g)
–	sweet (20g)
–	Salad cream (25g)
0	Salt, table (–)
–	Sesame seeds (–)
–	Soy sauce (–)
–	Tartare sauce (20g)
15	Tomato sauce (25g)
0	Vinegar (–)
–	Worcestershire sauce (–)

SOUPS (as served)

–	Chicken, condensed (230g)
–	Chicken noodle, dried (230g)
–	Minestrone, dried (230g)
–	Mushroom, canned (230g)
–	Tomato, condensed (230g)
–	Tomato, dried (230g)
10	Vegetable, canned (230g)

SUGARS, JAMS AND SPREADS

–	Fish paste (5g)
–	Honey (30g)
Tr	Jam, fruit, edible seeds (30g)
Tr	Jam, stone fruit (30g)
5	Marmalade (30g)
9	Meat paste (5g)
53	Peanut butter (20g)
0	Sugar, white (–)
Tr	Syrup, golden (30g)
–	Topping, flavoured (40g)
Tr	Treacle, black (30g)
–	Vegemite (3g)

SWEETS

0	Boiled sweet (5g)
–	Butterscotch (5g)
–	Caramel (5g)

Food	Folacin
Carob bar (75g)	–
Chocolate square, milk (5g)	10
Fruit and honey bar (50g)	–
Jelly bean (5g)	–
Liquorice allsort (7g)	0
Pastille (5g)	0
Peppermint (4g)	0
Popcorn, plain unsalted (15g)	–
Sesame bar (50g)	–
Toffee, mixed (5g)	0

VEGETABLES

Food	Folacin
Artichoke, globe, boiled (100g)	13
Asparagus, boiled (5=100g)	15
Bamboo shoots (50g)	–
Beans, French, boiled (100g)	28
baked, in tomato sauce (125g)	29
broad, boiled (100g)	–
kidney (and haricot), boiled (100g)	–
mung, cooked dahl (100g)	20
soya-, boiled (100g)	–
Beetroot, slices, boiled (2=30g)	50
canned (2=30g)	–
Broccoli, boiled (100g)	110
Brussels sprouts, boiled (7=70g)	87
Cabbage, raw (50g)	90
boiled (100g)	35
Carrots, raw (50g)	15
boiled (50g)	8
young, canned (50g)	7
Cauliflower, raw (50g)	39
boiled (100g)	49
Celeriac, boiled (3=60g)	–
Celery, raw (50g)	12
boiled (50g)	6
Chickpeas, cooked dahl (60g)	37
Cucumber, slices (5=30g)	16
Egg plant, baked (½=100g)	–
Endive, raw leaves (3=15g)	330
Leeks, boiled (4=100g)	–
Lentils, split, boiled (100g)	5
Lettuce, raw leaves (2=20g)	34
Marrow, boiled (100g)	6
Mushrooms, raw (3=30g)	23
fried (6=60g)	20
Onions, raw (¼=20g)	16
boiled (100g)	8
fried (70g)	–
spring (4=20g)	40
Parsley, sprigs (2=5g)	–
Parsnip, boiled (½=60g)	30
Peas, canned (60g)	52
canned, processed (60g)	3
fresh, boiled (60g)	–
frozen, boiled (60g)	78
split, boiled (60g)	–
Peppers, green, raw (¼=15g)	11
boiled (50g)	11
Potato, baked (inc. skin 120g)	8
boiled (120g)	10
chips, fresh, fried (12=120g)	10
chips, frozen, fried (8-14=120g)	11
crisps (10=25g)	20
mashed (100g)	10
instant, cooked (100g)	5
new, boiled (2=100g)	10
new, canned (2=100g)	11
roast (120g)	7
Pumpkin (100g)	13
Radishes (2=20g)	24
Spinach, leaves, boiled (3=60g)	140
Swede, boiled (80g)	21
Sweetcorn, on cob, boiled (150g)	33
canned kernels (80g)	32
Sweet potato, boiled (100g)	25
Tomato, raw (120g)	28
canned (120g)	25
fried (120g)	–
juice, canned (120g)	13
Turnip, boiled (80g)	10
Yam, boiled (100g)	6

2 2
PANTOTHENIC
ACID

Pantothenic acid is widely distributed in nature and is present in a wide variety of foods. Deficiency is, therefore, very rare. It is water soluble, heat sensitive and can be degraded in both acid and alkaline conditions.

The vitamin forms part of two key body chemicals and therefore has many and varied functions.

PANTOTHENIC ACID INTAKE

Safe and adequate daily intake of pantothenic acid (U.S.A.):

Infants:	2-3 milligrams
Children:	3-7 milligrams
Adults:	4-7 milligrams

milligrams per 100 grams

BEVERAGES
.1	Beer (240g)
.04	Cider, dry, alcoholic (180g)
.03	sweet, alcoholic (180g)
–	sweet, non-alcoholic (220g)
–	Cocoa powder (5g)
–	Coffee, percolated (230g)
0	Cola-type drinks (240g)
–	Cordial, diluted 1:4 (240g)
–	Drinking chocolate (10g)
Tr	Lemonade, carbonated drinks (240g)
–	Milo (10g)
–	Ovaltine (10g)
–	Port (60g)
–	Sherry, dry (60g)
–	medium (60g)
–	sweet (60g)
0	Spirits, e.g. whisky (30g)
Tr	Tea, infusion (230g)
.04	Wine, red (100g)
.03	white, dry (100g)
.03	medium (100g)
.03	sparkling (100g)
.03	sweet (100g)

CEREALS, BISCUITS, CAKES, DESSERTS
–	Barley, pearl, boiled (–)
–	Biscuit, chocolate (20g)
–	cream-filled (20g)
1.0	crispbread, rye (20g)
–	wheat, starch-red. (11g)
–	gingernut (15g)
–	semi-sweet (15g)
–	short-sweet (15g)
2.5	Bran, wheat (8g)
.3	Bread, brown, slice (25g)
–	Lebanese (pita) (¼=25g)
.3	white, slice (25g)
.6	wholemeal, slice (25g)
.6	roll, brown (35g)
–	starch-reduced (35g)
.3	white (35g)
.2	Cake, fruit (60g)
–	plain (60g)

1.5	Egg, fried (60g)
1.5	omelette (100g)
1.5	poached (55g)
2	raw (55g)
1.5	scrambled (70g)
.2	Macaroni cheese (180g)
.5	Quiche Lorraine (150g)

FATS AND OILS
Tr	Butter, salted (10g)
Tr	Dripping, beef (–)
Tr	Lard (–)
Tr	Margarine (10g)
Tr	Vegetable oils (–)

FISH AND OTHER SEAFOODS
–	Bream, steamed (100g)
.2	Cod, baked (100g)
–	fried in batter (100g)
.2	poached (100g)
.2	steamed (100g)
.5	Crab, boiled (150g)
–	canned (90g)
–	Fish cakes, fried (4=100g)
–	fingers, fried (5=100g)
–	in batter, fried (120g)
–	Flounder, baked (100g)
–	Haddock, fried (100g)
.2	steamed (100g)
1.5	Lobster, boiled (120g)
–	Mussels, boiled (12=120g)
.5	Oysters, raw (12=120g)
–	Prawns, boiled (6=120g)
2.5	Roe, cod, fried (100g)
.5	Salmon, canned (100g)
.4	Sardines, canned (60g)
.1	Scallops, steamed (10=100g)
.4	Tuna, canned in oil (120g)
–	Whiting, crumbed, fried (100g)
–	steamed (100g)

FRUIT
.08	Apple (inc. skin, core 100g)
.06	baked, no sugar (inc. skin 110g)
.08	stewed, no sugar (110g)
.3	Apricots (inc. stones 3=100g)

Food	Pantothenic acid
Apricots, canned (100g)	.1
dried (25g)	.7
stewed, no sugar (inc. stones 110g)	.2
Avocado pear (½=150g)	1
Banana (100g)	.3
Blackberries (100g)	.3
stewed, no sugar (100g)	.2
Cantaloup (inc. skin 120g)	.1
Cherries (inc. stones 20=100g)	.2
stewed, no sugar (inc. stones 100g)	.2
Currants, black (90g)	.4
dried (15g)	.1
red (90g)	.06
Dates, dried (6=35g)	.8
Figs (2=75g)	.3
dried (2=40g)	.4
Fruit salad, canned (120g)	.04
Grapes, black (20=100g)	.04
white (20=100g)	.05
Grapefruit, whole (200g)	.1
canned (100g)	.1
juice, canned (120g)	.1
Guavas, canned (100g)	-
Lemon, slices (2=15g)	.2
juice (15g)	.1
Loganberries (100g)	.2
canned (100g)	.2
stewed, no sugar (100g)	.2
Lychees, canned (100g)	-
Mandarins (2=100g)	-
canned (50g)	.2
Mango (100g)	.2
canned (100g)	-
Nectarines (inc. stones 3=100g)	.1
Olives, in brine (5=20g)	.02
Orange, whole (130g)	.2
juice, fresh (120g)	.2
canned (120g)	.1
Passionfruit, whole (30g)	-
Papaw (100g)	-
canned (100g)	.2
Peach (inc. stones 120g)	.1
canned (120g)	.05
dried (25g)	.3

Food	Pantothenic acid
Cake, sponge (60g)	.5
Chapati (60g)	.5
Cheesecake (120g)	-
Cornflakes (30g)	-
Crumpet (50g)	-
Custard (70g)	.4
Custard tart (120g)	.4
Doughnut (40g)	-
Eclair (50g)	.3
Flour, corn- (-)	-
plain (-)	.3
self-raising (-)	.3
soya, full-fat (-)	2
low-fat (-)	2
wholemeal (-)	1
Fruit pie (150g)	-
Jam tart (35g)	.1
Jelly, made with water (100g)	0
Lamington (60g)	-
Lemon meringue pie (120g)	.3
Meringue (15g)	.2
Milk pudding (e.g. sago) (160g)	.3
Muesli (30g)	-
Noodles (chow mein) (250g)	-
Pancake (75g)	.5
Pasta, macaroni, boiled (150g)	Tr
spaghetti, boiled (120g)	Tr
canned in tomato sauce (120g)	Tr
Pastry, flaky (-)	.1
short crust (-)	.2
Pizza, cheese and tomato (150g)	.3
Porridge (30g)	.1
Rice, boiled (160g)	.2
fried (120g)	-
puffed (25g)	-
Scone (30g)	.2
Sponge pudding, steamed (100g)	.3
Trifle (100g)	.4
Wheat, breakfast biscuit (35g)	-
Yeast, dried, baker's (-)	11

EGG AND CHEESE DISHES

Food	Pantothenic acid
Cauliflower cheese (100g)	.4
Cheese soufflé (100g)	.5
Egg, boiled (55g)	1.5

.1	Peach, stewed, no sugar (120g)
.05	Pear (inc. skin, core 120g)
.02	canned (120g)
.05	stewed, no sugar (120g)
.2	Pineapple (80g)
.1	canned (80g)
.1	juice, canned (120g)
.2	Plums (inc. stones 3=100g)
.2	stewed, no sugar (inc. stones 100g)
.5	Prunes (inc. stones 8=80g)
.2	stewed, no sugar (inc. stones 120g)
–	Quince, raw (100g)
.1	Raisins, dried (20g)
.2	Raspberries (100g)
.2	canned (100g)
.2	stewed, no sugar (100g)
.06	Rhubarb, stewed, no sugar (120g)
.3	Strawberries (10=100g)
.2	canned (100g)
.1	Sultanas, dried (15g)
1	Watermelon (260g)

MEAT AND MEAT PRODUCTS

.3	Bacon rashers, middle, fried (2=40g)
.5	grilled (40g)
.4	Beef, corned, canned (90g)
–	fillet steak, grilled (130g)
1	mince, stewed (120g)
1	rump steak, fried (150g)
1	grilled (150g)
1	silverside, salted, boiled (120g)
.5	sirloin, roast (120g)
1	stewing steak, stewed (120g)
1	topside, roast (120g)
.5	Beefburger, frozen, fried (60g)
.3	Beef stew (250g)
.4	Bolognese sauce (100g)
1	Chicken, boiled (100g)
–	crumbed, no bone (140g)
–	roast (130g)
.5	leg quarter (inc. bone 130g)
.5	wing quarter (inc. bone 130g)
5.5	Chicken livers, fried (130g)
–	Duck, roast (100g)

–	cheese spread (10g)
–	cottage (25g)
–	cream cheese (15g)
2	Danish blue (25g)
.3	edam (25g)
.3	parmesan (10g)
–	processed (25g)
–	stilton (25g)
–	Swiss (25g)
–	Cream, 35% fat (30g)
.3	sterilized, canned (15g)
–	Ice-cream (60g)
–	non-dairy (60g)
1	Milk, cow's, cond. skim, sweet. (30g)
1	cond. whole, sweet. (30g)
3.5	dried, skimmed (12g)
2.5	dried, whole (10g)
1	evap. whole, unsweet. (30g)
–	flavoured (230g)
.4	fresh, skimmed (230g)
.4	fresh, whole (230g)
.4	longlife, UHT (230g)
.3	goat's (230g)
.3	human (100g)
–	Milkshake, flavoured (340g)
–	Yoghurt, flavoured (200g)
–	fruit, low-fat (200g)
–	natural, low-fat (200g)
–	plain (200g)

NUTS

2.5	Almonds (10=15g)
.2	Brazil nuts (5=20g)
–	Cashews, roast (10=20g)
.5	Chestnuts (4=20g)
–	Coconut, desiccated (15g)
1	Hazel nuts (10=15g)
–	Macadamia nuts (8=20g)
2	Peanuts, raw, in shells (5=25g)
2	roasted, salted (30=25g)
–	Pistachio nuts, shelled (25=15g)
.9	Walnuts (5=20g)

SAUCES & CONDIMENTS

–	Barbecue sauce (10g)
–	Chilli sauce (–)

Value	Food
Tr	Gelatin (–)
.5	Ham, canned (90g)
–	Hamburger (170g)
–	with cheese (190g)
.3	Irish stew (250g)
1.5	Lamb, brain, boiled (150g)
.4	chops, loin, grilled (inc. bone 120g)
.3	cutlets, grilled (inc. bone 100g)
4	heart, roast (140g)
5	kidney, fried (100g)
.5	leg, roast (120g)
7.5	liver, fried (130g)
.5	shoulder, roast (120g)
1	tongue, stewed (100g)
.5	Luncheon meat, canned (90g)
–	Meat pie (180g)
.5	Moussaka (200g)
.5	Pastie (160g)
1	Pork, chop, loin, grilled (100g)
1	leg, roast (120g)
–	sweet and sour (250g)
.5	Pork pie (180g)
.4	Rabbit, stewed (inc. bone 170g)
1	Salami, slices (3=90g)
1.5	Sausage, liver (60g)
–	Sausage roll (100g)
.5	Sausages, beef, fried (2=120g)
.5	grilled (2=120g)
.4	frankfurter (2=100g)
.5	pork, fried (2=120g)
.5	grilled (2=120g)
.4	saveloy, large (2=150g)
–	Spring roll, fried (200g)
.3	Steak and kidney pie (180g)
.3	Stewed steak in gravy, canned (100g)
.4	Tongue, canned (100g)
.2	Tripe, stewed (100g)
–	Turkey, roast (120g)
–	Veal, cutlet, fried (110g)
.5	fillet, roast (100g)
–	schnitzel (140g)

MILK & MILK PRODUCTS

Value	Food
1.5	Cheese, camembert (25g)
.3	cheddar (25g)

Value	Food
.2	Chutney, tomato (20g)
–	Curry powder (15g)
0	French dressing (15g)
–	Ginger (ground) (–)
1	Mayonnaise (20g)
–	Mustard powder (–)
–	Oxo cubes (–)
–	Pepper (–)
–	Pickles, mustard (20g)
–	sweet (20g)
–	Salad cream (25g)
0	Salt, table (–)
–	Sesame seeds (–)
–	Soy sauce (–)
–	Tartare sauce (20g)
.3	Tomato sauce (25g)
0	Vinegar (–)
–	Worcestershire sauce (–)

SOUPS (as served)

Value	Food
–	Chicken, condensed (230g)
–	Chicken noodle, dried (230g)
–	Minestrone, dried (230g)
–	Mushroom, canned (230g)
–	Tomato, condensed (230g)
–	Tomato, dried (230g)
–	Vegetable, canned (230g)

SUGARS, JAMS AND SPREADS

Value	Food
–	Fish paste (5g)
–	Honey (30g)
Tr	Jam, fruit, edible seeds (30g)
Tr	Jam, stone fruit (30g)
Tr	Marmalade (30g)
.3	Meat paste (5g)
2	Peanut butter (20g)
0	Sugar, white (–)
Tr	Syrup, golden (30g)
–	Topping, flavoured (40g)
Tr	Treacle, black (30g)
8.9	Vegemite (3g)

SWEETS

Value	Food
0	Boiled sweet (5g)
–	Butterscotch (5g)
–	Caramel (5g)

	Food	mg
–	Carob bar (75g)	
.5	Chocolate square, milk (5g)	
–	Fruit and honey bar (50g)	
–	Jelly bean (5g)	
0	Liquorice allsort (7g)	
0	Pastille (5g)	
0	Peppermint (4g)	
–	Popcorn, plain unsalted (15g)	
–	Sesame bar (50g)	
0	Toffee, mixed (5g)	

VEGETABLES

	Food	mg
.09	Artichoke, globe, boiled (100g)	
.07	Asparagus, boiled (5=100g)	
–	Bamboo shoots (50g)	
.07	Beans, French, boiled (100g)	
–	baked, in tomato sauce (125g)	
4	broad, boiled (100g)	
–	kidney (and haricot), boiled (100g)	
–	mung, cooked dahl (100g)	
–	soya-, boiled (100g)	
.1	Beetroot, slices, boiled (2=30g)	
–	canned (2=30g)	
.7	Broccoli, boiled (100g)	
.3	Brussels sprouts, boiled (7=70g)	
.2	Cabbage, raw (50g)	
.2	boiled (100g)	
.3	Carrots, raw (50g)	
.2	boiled (50g)	
.1	young, canned (50g)	
.5	Cauliflower, raw (50g)	
.4	boiled (100g)	
–	Celeriac, boiled (3=60g)	
.4	Celery, raw (50g)	
.3	boiled (50g)	
–	Chickpeas, cooked dahl (60g)	
.3	Cucumber, slices (5=30g)	
–	Egg plant, baked (½=100g)	
–	Endive, raw leaves (3=15g)	
.1	Leeks, boiled (4=100g)	
.3	Lentils, split, boiled (100g)	
.2	Lettuce, raw leaves (2=20g)	
.07	Marrow, boiled (100g)	
2	Mushrooms, raw (3=30g)	
1.5	fried (6=60g)	

	Food	mg
.1	Onions, raw (¼=20g)	
.1	boiled (100g)	
–	fried (70g)	
.1	spring (4=20g)	
.3	Parsley, sprigs (2=5g)	
.4	Parsnip, boiled (½=60g)	
.2	Peas, canned (60g)	
.08	canned, processed (60g)	
.3	fresh, boiled (60g)	
.3	frozen, boiled (60g)	
–	split, boiled (60g)	
.2	Peppers, green, raw (¼=15g)	
.2	boiled (50g)	
.2	Potato, baked (inc. skin 120g)	
.2	boiled (120g)	
.2	chips, fresh, fried (12=120g)	
–	chips, frozen, fried (8-14=120g)	
–	crisps (10=25g)	
.2	mashed (100g)	
.2	instant, cooked (100g)	
.2	new, boiled (2=100g)	
–	new, canned (2=100g)	
.2	roast (120g)	
.4	Pumpkin (100g)	
.2	Radishes (2=20g)	
.2	Spinach, leaves, boiled (3=60g)	
.07	Swede, boiled (80g)	
.4	Sweetcorn, on cob, boiled (150g)	
.2	canned kernels (80g)	
.5	Sweet potato, boiled (100g)	
.3	Tomato, raw (120g)	
–	canned (120g)	
.2	fried (120g)	
.2	juice, canned (120g)	
.1	Turnip, boiled (80g)	
.4	Yam, boiled (100g)	

2 3
B I O T I N

Biotin deficiency was first recognized not because of inadequate amounts in the diet, but because of the effects of a chemical called avidin, which is found in raw eggs. Avidin binds and inactivates biotin. Biotin can be made by gut bacteria and absorbed from the large bowel, so that not all biotin needs to be obtained from food. Theoretically, antibiotics that affect gut bacteria could reduce the amount of biotin available.

Biotin is water soluble, sensitive to air and oxygen and also to alkaline conditions.

The vitamin acts as part of enzyme (natural substances that speed up chemical reactions in the body) systems involved in building up chemicals containing carbon and oxygen, such as fats and glucose.

Infants may be at risk from biotin deficiency, which shows up as a 'seborrhoeic dermatitis' that responds to biotin. Also, some infants have a metabolic disorder requiring extra biotin. There has been some suggestion that 'cot deaths' or the sudden infant death syndrome may be due, in some cases, to an inadequate intake of biotin.

The biotin in human milk averages about 10 micrograms per 1000 kilocalories (4200 kilojoules) and in infant formulae is usually at least 15 micrograms per 1000 kilocalories. However, a higher concentration of biotin may be preferable for infant formulae because nutrients can be more biologically available to the infant from human milk than from infant formulae.

BIOTIN INTAKE

Safe and adequate daily intake of biotin (U.S.A.):

Infants:	35-50 micrograms
Children:	65-120 micrograms
Adolescents:	100-200 micrograms
Adults:	100-200 micrograms

micrograms per 100 grams

BEVERAGES

Food	µg
Beer (240g)	.5
Cider, dry, alcoholic (180g)	.6
sweet, alcoholic (180g)	.6
sweet, non-alcoholic (220g)	–
Cocoa powder (5g)	–
Coffee, percolated (230g)	–
Cola-type drinks (240g)	0
Cordial, diluted 1:4 (240g)	–
Drinking chocolate (10g)	–
Lemonade, carbonated drinks (240g)	Tr
Milo (10g)	–
Ovaltine (10g)	–
Port (60g)	–
Sherry, dry (60g)	–
medium (60g)	–
sweet (60g)	–
Spirits, e.g. whisky (30g)	0
Tea, infusion (230g)	–
Wine, red (100g)	–
white, dry (100g)	–
medium (100g)	–
sparkling (100g)	–
sweet (100g)	–

CEREALS, BISCUITS, CAKES, DESSERTS

Food	µg
Barley, pearl, boiled (–)	Tr
Biscuit, chocolate (20g)	–
cream-filled (20g)	–
crispbread, rye (20g)	7
wheat, starch-red. (11g)	–
gingernut (15g)	–
semi-sweet (15g)	–
short-sweet (15g)	–
Bran, wheat (8g)	14
Bread, brown, slice (25g)	3
Lebanese (pita) (¼=25g)	–
white, slice (25g)	1
wholemeal, slice (25g)	6
roll, brown (35g)	3
starch-reduced (35g)	–
white (35g)	1
Cake, fruit (60g)	4
plain (60g)	–

FRUIT

Food	µg
Apple (inc. skin, core 100g)	.2
baked, no sugar (inc. skin 110g)	.2
stewed, no sugar (110g)	–
Apricots (inc. stones 3=100g)	.3

Food	µg
Egg, fried (60g)	25
omelette (100g)	22
poached (55g)	25
raw (55g)	25
scrambled (70g)	20
Macaroni cheese (180g)	1
Quiche Lorraine (150g)	7

FATS AND OILS

Food	µg
Butter, salted (10g)	Tr
Dripping, beef (–)	Tr
Lard (–)	Tr
Margarine (10g)	Tr
Vegetable oils (–)	Tr

FISH AND OTHER SEAFOODS

Food	µg
Bream, steamed (100g)	–
Cod, baked (100g)	3
fried in batter (100g)	–
poached (100g)	3
steamed (100g)	3
Crab, boiled (150g)	Tr
canned (90g)	Tr
Fish cakes, fried (4=100g)	–
fingers, fried (5=100g)	–
in batter, fried (120g)	–
Flounder, baked (100g)	–
Haddock, fried (100g)	–
steamed (100g)	6
Lobster, boiled (120g)	5
Mussels, boiled (12=120g)	–
Oysters, raw (12=120g)	10
Prawns, boiled (6=120g)	–
Roe, cod, fried (100g)	15
Salmon, canned (100g)	5
Sardines, canned (60g)	4
Scallops, steamed (10=100g)	Tr
Tuna, canned in oil (120g)	3
Whiting, crumbed, fried (100g)	–
steamed (100g)	–

Food	Biotin
Cake, sponge (60g)	8
Chapati (60g)	2
Cheesecake (120g)	-
Cornflakes (30g)	-
Crumpet (50g)	-
Custard (70g)	2
Custard tart (120g)	4
Doughnut (40g)	-
Eclair (50g)	4
Flour, corn- (–)	-
plain (–)	1
self-raising (–)	1
soya, full-fat (–)	-
low-fat (–)	-
wholemeal (–)	7
Fruit pie (150g)	-
Jam tart (35g)	1
Jelly, made with water (100g)	0
Lamington (60g)	-
Lemon meringue pie (120g)	5
Meringue (15g)	Tr
Milk pudding (e.g. sago) (160g)	2
Muesli (30g)	-
Noodles (chow mein) (250g)	-
Pancake (75g)	5
Pasta, macaroni, boiled (150g)	Tr
spaghetti, boiled (120g)	Tr
canned in tomato sauce (120g)	Tr
Pastry, flaky (–)	Tr
short crust (–)	1
Pizza, cheese and tomato (150g)	3
Porridge (30g)	2
Rice, boiled (160g)	1
fried (120g)	-
puffed (25g)	-
Scone (30g)	2
Sponge pudding, steamed (100g)	5
Trifle (100g)	3
Wheat, breakfast biscuit (35g)	-
Yeast, dried, baker's (–)	200

EGG AND CHEESE DISHES

Food	Biotin
Cauliflower cheese (100g)	2
Cheese soufflé (100g)	10
Egg, boiled (55g)	25

Fruit	Biotin
Apricots, canned (100g)	-
dried (25g)	-
stewed, no sugar (inc. stones 110g)	-
Avocado pear (½=150g)	3
Banana (100g)	-
Blackberries (100g)	.4
stewed, no sugar (100g)	.3
Cantaloup (inc. skin 120g)	-
Cherries (inc. stones 20=100g)	.3
stewed, no sugar (inc. stones 100g)	.3
Currants, black (90g)	2
dried (15g)	-
red (90g)	3
Dates, dried (6=35g)	-
Figs (2=75g)	-
dried (2=40g)	-
Fruit salad, canned (120g)	.1
Grapes, black (20=100g)	.2
white (20=100g)	.3
Grapefruit, whole (200g)	.5
canned (100g)	1
juice, canned (120g)	1
Guavas, canned (100g)	-
Lemon, slices (2=15g)	.5
juice (15g)	.3
Loganberries (100g)	-
canned (100g)	-
stewed, no sugar (100g)	-
Lychees, canned (100g)	-
Mandarins (2=100g)	-
canned (50g)	.8
Mango (100g)	-
canned (100g)	-
Nectarines (inc. stones 3=100g)	-
Olives, in brine (5=20g)	Tr
Orange, whole (130g)	.8
juice, fresh (120g)	.8
Passionfruit, whole (30g)	-
Papaw (100g)	-
canned (100g)	-
Peach (inc. stones 120g)	.2
canned (120g)	.2
dried (25g)	-

Food	Biotin
Peach, stewed, no sugar (120g)	–
Pear (inc. skin, core 120g)	.1
canned (120g)	Tr
stewed, no sugar (120g)	.1
Pineapple (80g)	Tr
canned (80g)	Tr
juice, canned (120g)	-
Plums (inc. stones 3=100g)	.1
stewed, no sugar (inc. stones 100g)	.1
Prunes (inc. stones 8=80g)	Tr
stewed, no sugar (inc. stones 120g)	Tr
Quince, raw (100g)	-
Raisins, dried (20g)	-
Raspberries (100g)	2
canned (100g)	-
stewed, no sugar (100g)	2
Rhubarb, stewed, no sugar (120g)	-
Strawberries (10=100g)	1
canned (100g)	1
Sultanas, dried (15g)	-
Watermelon (260g)	-

MEAT AND MEAT PRODUCTS

Food	Biotin
Bacon rashers, middle, fried (2=40g)	2
grilled (40g)	2
Beef, corned, canned (90g)	2
fillet steak, grilled (130g)	-
mince, stewed (120g)	Tr
rump steak, fried (150g)	Tr
grilled (150g)	Tr
silverside, salted, boiled (120g)	Tr
sirloin, roast (120g)	Tr
stewing steak, stewed (120g)	Tr
topside, roast (120g)	Tr
Beefburger, frozen, fried (60g)	2
Beef stew (250g)	Tr
Bolognese sauce (100g)	Tr
Chicken, boiled (100g)	4
crumbed, no bone (140g)	-
roast (130g)	-
leg quarter (inc. bone 130g)	2
wing quarter (inc. bone 130g)	2
Chicken livers, fried (130g)	170
Duck, roast (100g)	-

Food	Biotin
cheese spread (10g)	–
cottage (25g)	–
cream cheese (15g)	–
Danish blue (25g)	2
edam (25g)	2
parmesan (10g)	2
processed (25g)	–
stilton (25g)	–
Swiss (25g)	–
Cream, 35% fat (30g)	–
sterilized, canned (15g)	1
Ice-cream (60g)	–
non-dairy (60g)	–
Milk, cow's, cond. skim, sweet. (30g)	4
cond. whole, sweet. (30g)	3
dried, skimmed (12g)	16
dried, whole (10g)	10
evap. whole, unsweet. (30g)	3
flavoured (230g)	–
fresh, skimmed (230g)	2
fresh, whole (230g)	2
longlife, UHT (230g)	2
goat's (230g)	2
human (100g)	.7
Milkshake, flavoured (340g)	–
Yoghurt, flavoured (200g)	–
fruit, low-fat (200g)	–
natural, low-fat (200g)	–
plain (200g)	–

NUTS

Food	Biotin
Almonds (10=15g)	.4
Brazil nuts (5=20g)	–
Cashews, roast (10=20g)	–
Chestnuts (4=20g)	1
Coconut, desiccated (15g)	–
Hazel nuts (10=15g)	–
Macadamia nuts (8=20g)	–
Peanuts, raw, in shells (5=25g)	–
roasted, salted (30=25g)	–
Pistachio nuts, shelled (25=15g)	–
Walnuts (5=20g)	2

SAUCES & CONDIMENTS

Food	Biotin
Barbecue sauce (10g)	–
Chilli sauce (–)	–

Food	Biotin
Gelatin (–)	Tr
Ham, canned (90g)	1
Hamburger (170g)	–
with cheese (190g)	–
Irish stew (250g)	1
Lamb, brain, boiled (150g)	3
chops, loin, grilled (inc. bone 120g)	1
cutlets, grilled (inc. bone 100g)	1
heart, roast (140g)	8
kidney, fried (100g)	42
leg, roast (120g)	1
liver, fried (130g)	41
shoulder, roast (120g)	1
tongue, stewed (100g)	2
Luncheon meat, canned (90g)	Tr
Meat pie (180g)	–
Moussaka (200g)	2
Pastie (160g)	1
Pork, chop, loin, grilled (100g)	2
leg, roast (120g)	2
sweet and sour (250g)	–
Pork pie (180g)	1
Rabbit, stewed (inc. bone 170g)	Tr
Salami, slices (3=90g)	3
Sausage, liver (60g)	7
Sausage roll (100g)	1
Sausages, beef, fried (2=120g)	2
grilled (2=120g)	2
frankfurter (2=100g)	2
pork, fried (2=120g)	3
grilled (2=120g)	3
saveloy, large (2=150g)	Tr
Spring roll, fried (200g)	–
Steak and kidney pie (180g)	1
Stewed steak in gravy, canned (100g)	1
Tongue, canned (100g)	2
Tripe, stewed (100g)	2
Turkey, roast (120g)	–
Veal, cutlet, fried (110g)	Tr
fillet, roast (100g)	Tr
schnitzel (140g)	–

MILK & MILK PRODUCTS

Food	Biotin
Cheese, camembert (25g)	6
cheddar (25g)	2

Food	Biotin
Chutney, tomato (20g)	1
Curry powder (–)	–
French dressing (15g)	0
Ginger (ground) (–)	–
Mayonnaise (20g)	12
Mustard powder (–)	–
Oxo cubes (–)	–
Pepper (–)	–
Pickles, mustard (20g)	Tr
sweet (20g)	Tr
Salad cream (25g)	–
Salt, table (–)	0
Sesame seeds (–)	–
Soy sauce (–)	–
Tartare sauce (20g)	–
Tomato sauce (25g)	2
Vinegar (–)	0
Worcestershire sauce (–)	–

SOUPS (as served)

Food	Biotin
Chicken, condensed (230g)	–
Chicken noodle, dried (230g)	–
Minestrone, dried (230g)	–
Mushroom, canned (230g)	–
Tomato, canned (230g)	–
Tomato, condensed (230g)	–
Tomato, dried (230g)	–
Vegetable, canned (230g)	–

SUGARS, JAMS AND SPREADS

Food	Biotin
Fish paste (5g)	–
Honey (30g)	–
Jam, fruit, edible seeds (30g)	Tr
Jam, stone fruit (30g)	Tr
Marmalade (30g)	Tr
Meat paste (5g)	3
Peanut butter (20g)	–
Sugar, white (–)	0
Syrup, golden (30g)	Tr
Topping, flavoured (40g)	–
Treacle, black (30g)	Tr
Vegemite (3g)	Tr

SWEETS

Food	Biotin
Boiled sweet (5g)	0
Butterscotch (5g)	–
Caramel (5g)	–

Food	Biotin
Carob bar (75g)	-
Chocolate square, milk (5g)	3
Fruit and honey bar (50g)	-
Jelly bean (5g)	-
Liquorice allsort (7g)	0
Pastille (5g)	0
Peppermint (4g)	0
Popcorn, plain unsalted (15g)	-
Sesame bar (50g)	-
Toffee, mixed (5g)	0

VEGETABLES

Food	Biotin
Artichoke, globe, boiled (100g)	2
Asparagus, boiled (5=100g)	.2
Bamboo shoots (50g)	-
Beans, French, boiled (100g)	1
baked, in tomato sauce (125g)	-
broad, boiled (100g)	2
kidney (and haricot), boiled (100g)	-
mung, cooked dahl (100g)	-
soya-, boiled (100g)	Tr
Beetroot, slices, boiled (2=30g)	1
canned (2=30g)	-
Broccoli, boiled (100g)	.3
Brussels sprouts, boiled (7=70g)	.3
Cabbage, raw (50g)	.1
boiled (100g)	Tr
Carrots, raw (50g)	.6
boiled (50g)	.4
young, canned (50g)	.4
Cauliflower, raw (50g)	2
boiled (100g)	1
Celeriac, boiled (3=60g)	-
Celery, raw (50g)	.1
boiled (50g)	Tr
Chickpeas, cooked dahl (60g)	-
Cucumber, slices (5=30g)	.4
Egg plant, baked (½=100g)	-
Endive, raw leaves (3=15g)	-
Leeks, boiled (4=100g)	1
Lentils, split, boiled (100g)	-
Lettuce, raw leaves (2=20g)	.7
Marrow, boiled (100g)	-
Mushrooms, raw (3=30g)	-
fried (6=60g)	-

Food	Biotin
Onions, raw (¼=20g)	.9
boiled (100g)	.6
fried (70g)	-
spring (4=20g)	.9
Parsley, sprigs (2=5g)	.4
Parsnip, boiled (½=60g)	Tr
Peas, canned (60g)	.4
canned, processed (60g)	Tr
fresh, boiled (60g)	.4
frozen, boiled (60g)	.4
split, boiled (60g)	-
Peppers, green, raw (¼=15g)	-
boiled (50g)	-
Potato, baked (inc. skin 120g)	Tr
boiled (120g)	Tr
chips, fresh, fried (12=120g)	Tr
chips, frozen, fried (8-14=120g)	Tr
crisps (10=25g)	-
mashed (100g)	Tr
instant, cooked (100g)	.1
new, boiled (2=100g)	Tr
new, canned (2=100g)	Tr
roast (120g)	Tr
Pumpkin (100g)	4
Radishes (2=20g)	-
Spinach, leaves, boiled (3=60g)	1
Swede, boiled (80g)	Tr
Sweetcorn, on cob, boiled (150g)	-
canned kernels (80g)	-
Sweet potato, boiled (100g)	-
Tomato, raw (120g)	2
canned (120g)	2
fried (120g)	-
juice, canned (120g)	1
Turnip, boiled (80g)	Tr
Yam, boiled (100g)	-

2 4

VITAMIN C

Probably the first disease to be recognized as being caused by a nutritional deficiency was scurvy, when it was found that certain foods could prevent the disease. Scurvy was described by the Egyptians and Greeks, but it was Bachstrom in Leiden in 1734 who maintained that it was due to a lack of fresh vegetables in the diet. In 1795, the British Admiralty adopted James Lind's recommendations for citrus fruit to prevent seaboard scurvy and, thereafter, British sailors were nicknamed 'limeys'.

In scurvy, the connective tissues of the body are defective; the tissues are fragile, and bleeding occurs into the skin, from the gums and into deeper tissues. Wound healing is also poor. Changes in brain and nerve function occur, with mood and personality changes. Muscle weakness and proneness to infection may occur. Our bodies' ability to detoxify certain chemicals may also be reduced in scurvy. It seems likely that there may be lesser degrees of vitamin C deficiency than the extreme of scurvy.

Vitamin C (or ascorbic acid, as it is also called) can be lost from foods because of its water solubility, and sensitivity to heat, air or oxygen. The addition of alkalis, such as bicarbonate of soda, and the use of copper cookware can also destroy it.

People at risk from vitamin C deficiency include those who avoid fruit and vegetables, those with poor cooking practices (see page 35), the elderly, alcohol abusers and cigarette smokers.

VITAMIN C INTAKE

Recommendations about vitamin C intake were first concerned with the prevention of scurvy. Recommended intakes of about 30 milligrams per day do not usually 'saturate' the body tissues with vitamin C and, indeed, this may not be necessary. But to saturate body tissues, no more than 100 to 130 milligrams per day are required. With intakes above this, our bodies adapt by increasing breakdown of vitamin C or excreting it in the urine. From a mixed diet it would be difficult to have more than about 400 to 500 milligrams of vitamin C per day.

It has been suggested that daily intakes of vitamin C in excess of 500 milligrams may be of benefit. There is some evidence that amounts of this kind may reduce the symptoms of the common cold. This raises the question of non-nutritional or drug-like properties of the vitamin. The possible adverse effects must also be considered. These include: 'rebound scurvy', which may occur if you are coming off high-dosage vitamin C; increased excretion of oxalic acid in the urine which may lead to 'stones' in the urinary tract; an increased absorption of iron in those susceptible to iron overload; increased absorption of toxic metals, such as mercury; and interactions with certain medications, for example warfarin, aspirin, antidepressants and the contraceptive pill.

VITAMIN C INTAKE

Recommended daily dietary intake of vitamin C:

	AUSTRALIA milligrams	U.S.A. milligrams
Infants:	30	35
Children:	30-50	45
Adult men:	30	60
Adult women:	30	60
Pregnancy:	60	80
Lactation:	60	100

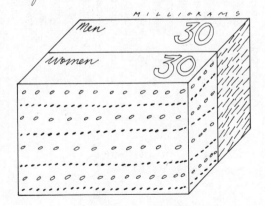

Daily allowance in Australia

milligrams per 100 grams

BEVERAGES	
Beer (240g)	0
Cider, dry, alcoholic (180g)	0
sweet, alcoholic (180g)	0
sweet, non-alcoholic (220g)	2
Cocoa powder (5g)	0
Coffee, percolated (230g)	0
Cola-type drinks (240g)	0
Cordial, diluted 1:4 (240g)	–
Drinking chocolate (10g)	0
Lemonade, carbonated drinks (240g)	Tr
Milo (10g)	–
Ovaltine (10g)	48
Port (60g)	0
Sherry, dry (60g)	0
medium (60g)	0
sweet (60g)	0
Spirits, e.g. whisky (30g)	0
Tea, infusion (230g)	0
Wine, red (100g)	0
white, dry (100g)	0
medium (100g)	0
sparkling (100g)	0
sweet (100g)	0
CEREALS, BISCUITS, CAKES, DESSERTS	
Barley, pearl, boiled (–)	0
Biscuit, chocolate (20g)	0
cream-filled (20g)	–
crispbread, rye (20g)	0
wheat, starch-red. (11g)	0
gingernut (15g)	0
semi-sweet (15g)	0
short-sweet (15g)	0
Bran, wheat (8g)	0
Bread, brown, slice (25g)	0
Lebanese (pita) (¼=25g)	–
white, slice (25g)	0
wholemeal, slice (25g)	0
roll, brown (35g)	0
starch-reduced (35g)	0
white (35g)	0
Cake, fruit (60g)	0
plain (60g)	0

Egg, fried (60g)	0
omelette (100g)	0
poached (55g)	0
raw (55g)	0
scrambled (70g)	Tr
Macaroni cheese (180g)	Tr
Quiche Lorraine (150g)	Tr
FATS AND OILS	
Butter, salted (10g)	Tr
Dripping, beef (–)	0
Lard (–)	0
Margarine (10g)	0
Vegetable oils (–)	0
FISH AND OTHER SEAFOODS	
Bream, steamed (100g)	Tr
Cod, baked (100g)	Tr
fried in batter (100g)	Tr
poached (100g)	Tr
steamed (100g)	Tr
Crab, boiled (150g)	Tr
canned (90g)	Tr
Fish cakes, fried (4=100g)	Tr
fingers, fried (5=100g)	Tr
in batter, fried (120g)	–
Flounder, baked (100g)	Tr
Haddock, fried (100g)	Tr
steamed (100g)	Tr
Lobster, boiled (120g)	Tr
Mussels, boiled (12=120g)	Tr
Oysters, raw (12=120g)	Tr
Prawns, boiled (6=120g)	Tr
Roe, cod, fried (100g)	26
Salmon, canned (100g)	Tr
Sardines, canned (60g)	Tr
Scallops, steamed (10=100g)	Tr
Tuna, canned in oil (120g)	Tr
Whiting, crumbed, fried (100g)	Tr
steamed (100g)	Tr
FRUIT	
Apple (inc. skin, core 100g)	6
baked, no sugar (inc. skin 110g)	2
stewed, no sugar (110g)	4
Apricots (inc. stones 3=100g)	6

Food	Vitamin C
Apricots, canned (100g)	2
dried (25g)	Tr
stewed, no sugar (inc. stones 110g)	5
Avocado pear (½ = 150g)	15
Banana (100g)	10
Blackberries (100g)	20
stewed, no sugar (100g)	15
Cantaloup (inc. skin 120g)	15
Cherries (inc. stones 20 = 100g)	4
stewed, no sugar (inc. stones 100g)	3
Currants, black (90g)	200
dried (15g)	0
red (90g)	40
Dates, dried (6 = 35g)	0
Figs (2 = 75g)	2
dried (2 = 40g)	0
Fruit salad, canned (120g)	3
Grapes, black (20 = 100g)	3
white (20 = 100g)	4
Grapefruit, whole (200g)	19
canned (100g)	30
juice, canned (120g)	28
Guavas, canned (100g)	180
Lemon, slices (2 = 15g)	80
juice (15g)	50
Loganberries (100g)	35
canned (100g)	25
stewed, no sugar (100g)	29
Lychees, canned (100g)	8
Mandarins (2 = 100g)	30
canned (50g)	14
Mango (100g)	30
canned (100g)	10
Nectarines (inc. stones 3 = 100g)	7
Olives, in brine (5 = 20g)	0
Orange, whole (130g)	38
juice, fresh (120g)	50
canned (120g)	35
Passionfruit, whole (30g)	8
Papaw (100g)	65
canned (100g)	15
Peach (inc. stones 120g)	7
canned (120g)	4
dried (25g)	Tr

Food	Vitamin C
Cake, sponge (60g)	0
Chapati (60g)	0
Cheesecake (120g)	2
Cornflakes (30g)	0
Crumpet (50g)	-
Custard (70g)	Tr
Custard tart (120g)	Tr
Doughnut (40g)	0
Eclair (50g)	Tr
Flour, corn- (-)	0
plain (-)	0
self-raising (-)	0
soya, full-fat (-)	0
low-fat (-)	0
wholemeal (-)	0
Fruit pie (150g)	Tr
Jam tart (35g)	4
Jelly, made with water (100g)	0
Lamington (60g)	Tr
Lemon meringue pie (120g)	5
Meringue (15g)	0
Milk pudding (e.g. sago) (160g)	Tr
Muesli (30g)	-
Noodles (chow mein) (250g)	-
Pancake (75g)	Tr
Pasta, macaroni, boiled (150g)	0
spaghetti, boiled (120g)	0
canned in tomato sauce (120g)	Tr
Pastry, flaky (-)	Tr
short crust (-)	0
Pizza, cheese and tomato (150g)	3
Porridge (30g)	0
Rice, boiled (160g)	0
fried (120g)	-
puffed (25g)	-
Scone (30g)	Tr
Sponge pudding, steamed (100g)	Tr
Trifle (100g)	1
Wheat, breakfast biscuit (35g)	-
Yeast, dried, baker's (-)	Tr

EGG AND CHEESE DISHES

Food	Vitamin C
Cauliflower cheese (100g)	8
Cheese soufflé (100g)	Tr
Egg, boiled (55g)	0

Food	Vitamin C
cheese spread (10g)	0
cottage (25g)	0
cream cheese (15g)	0
Danish blue (25g)	0
edam (25g)	0
parmesan (10g)	0
processed (25g)	0
stilton (25g)	0
Swiss (25g)	0
Cream, 35% fat (30g)	1
sterilized, canned (15g)	Tr
Ice-cream (60g)	Tr
non-dairy (60g)	0
Milk, cow's, cond. skim, sweet. (30g)	2
cond. whole, sweet. (30g)	2
dried, skimmed (12g)	6
dried, whole (10g)	6
evap. whole, unsweet. (30g)	1
flavoured (230g)	1
fresh, skimmed (230g)	2
fresh, whole (230g)	2
longlife, UHT (230g)	2
goat's (230g)	2
human (100g)	4
Milkshake, flavoured (340g)	1
Yoghurt, flavoured (200g)	1
fruit, low-fat (200g)	2
natural, low-fat (200g)	1
plain (200g)	1

NUTS

Food	Vitamin C
Almonds (10=15g)	Tr
Brazil nuts (5=20g)	Tr
Cashews, roast (10=20g)	–
Chestnuts (4=20g)	Tr
Coconut, desiccated (15g)	0
Hazel nuts (10=15g)	Tr
Macadamia nuts (8=20g)	0
Peanuts, raw, in shells (5=25g)	Tr
roasted, salted (30=25g)	Tr
Pistachio nuts, shelled (25=15g)	0
Walnuts (5=20g)	Tr

SAUCES & CONDIMENTS

Food	Vitamin C
Barbecue sauce (10g)	5
Chilli sauce (–)	30

Food	Vitamin C
Peach, stewed, no sugar (120g)	Tr
Pear (inc. skin, core 120g)	2
canned (120g)	1
stewed, no sugar (120g)	3
Pineapple (80g)	25
canned (80g)	12
juice, canned (120g)	20
Plums (inc. stones 3=100g)	3
stewed, no sugar (inc. stones 100g)	3
Prunes (inc. stones 8=80g)	Tr
stewed, no sugar (inc. stones 120g)	Tr
Quince, raw (100g)	15
Raisins, dried (20g)	0
Raspberries (100g)	25
canned (100g)	7
stewed, no sugar (100g)	23
Rhubarb, stewed, no sugar (120g)	8
Strawberries (10=100g)	60
canned (100g)	21
Sultanas, dried (15g)	0
Watermelon (260g)	3

MEAT AND MEAT PRODUCTS

Food	Vitamin C
Bacon rashers, middle, fried (2=40g)	0
grilled (40g)	0
Beef, corned, canned (90g)	0
fillet steak, grilled (130g)	0
mince, stewed (120g)	0
rump steak, fried (150g)	0
grilled (150g)	0
silverside, salted, boiled (120g)	0
sirloin, roast (120g)	0
stewing steak, stewed (120g)	0
topside, roast (120g)	0
Beefburger, frozen, fried (60g)	0
Beef stew (250g)	Tr
Bolognese sauce (100g)	5
Chicken, boiled (100g)	0
crumbed, no bone (140g)	–
roast (130g)	0
leg quarter (inc. bone 130g)	0
wing quarter (inc. bone 130g)	.0
Chicken livers, fried (130g)	13
Duck, roast (100g)	–

0	Gelatin (–)
0	Ham, canned (90g)
–	Hamburger (170g)
–	with cheese (190g)
4	Irish stew (250g)
17	Lamb, brain, boiled (150g)
0	chops, loin, grilled (inc. bone 120g)
0	cutlets, grilled (inc. bone 100g)
11	heart, roast (140g)
9	kidney, fried (100g)
0	leg, roast (120g)
12	liver, fried (130g)
0	shoulder, roast (120g)
6	tongue, stewed (100g)
0	Luncheon meat, canned (90g)
–	Meat pie (180g)
4	Moussaka (200g)
0	Pastie (160g)
0	Pork, chop, loin, grilled (100g)
0	leg, roast (120g)
–	sweet and sour (250g)
0	Pork pie (180g)
0	Rabbit, stewed (inc. bone 170g)
0	Salami, slices (3 = 90g)
Tr	Sausage, liver (60g)
–	Sausage roll (100g)
0	Sausages, beef, fried (2 = 120g)
0	grilled (2 = 120g)
0	frankfurter (2 = 100g)
0	pork, fried (2 = 120g)
0	grilled (2 = 120g)
0	saveloy, large (2 = 150g)
2	Spring roll, fried (200g)
0	Steak and kidney pie (180g)
0	Stewed steak in gravy, canned (100g)
0	Tongue, canned (100g)
3	Tripe, stewed (100g)
0	Turkey, roast (120g)
0	Veal, cutlet, fried (110g)
0	fillet, roast (100g)
0	schnitzel (140g)

MILK & MILK PRODUCTS

0	Cheese, camembert (25g)
0	cheddar (25g)

8	Chutney, tomato (20g)
–	Curry powder (–)
0	French dressing (15g)
–	Ginger (ground) (–)
0	Mayonnaise (20g)
0	Mustard powder (–)
0	Oxo cubes (–)
0	Pepper (–)
Tr	Pickles, mustard (20g)
–	sweet (20g)
0	Salad cream (25g)
0	Salt, table (–)
0	Sesame seeds (–)
0	Soy sauce (–)
3	Tartare sauce (20g)
10	Tomato sauce (25g)
0	Vinegar (–)
–	Worcestershire sauce (–)

SOUPS (as served)

0	Chicken, condensed (230g)
0	Chicken noodle, dried (230g)
0	Minestrone, dried (230g)
0	Mushroom, canned (230g)
Tr	Tomato, condensed (230g)
Tr	Tomato, dried (230g)
Tr	Vegetable, canned (230g)

SUGARS, JAMS AND SPREADS

Tr	Fish paste (5g)
Tr	Honey (30g)
10	Jam, fruit, edible seeds (30g)
Tr	Jam, stone fruit (30g)
10	Marmalade (30g)
0	Meat paste (5g)
Tr	Peanut butter (20g)
0	Sugar, white (–)
0	Syrup, golden (30g)
–	Topping, flavoured (40g)
0	Treacle, black (30g)
–	Vegemite (3g)

SWEETS

0	Boiled sweet (5g)
0	Butterscotch (5g)
Tr	Caramel (5g)

Food	Vitamin C
Carob bar (75g)	–
Chocolate square, milk (5g)	0
Fruit and honey bar (50g)	–
Jelly bean (5g)	0
Liquorice allsort (7g)	0
Pastille (5g)	0
Peppermint (4g)	0
Popcorn, plain unsalted (15g)	0
Sesame bar (50g)	–
Toffee, mixed (5g)	0

VEGETABLES

Food	Vitamin C
Artichoke, globe, boiled (100g)	3
Asparagus, boiled (5=100g)	10
Bamboo shoots (50g)	4
Beans, French, boiled (100g)	5
baked, in tomato sauce (125g)	Tr
broad, boiled (100g)	15
kidney (and haricot), boiled (100g)	0
mung, cooked dahl (100g)	Tr
soya-, boiled (100g)	–
Beetroot, slices, boiled (2=30g)	5
canned (2=30g)	3
Broccoli, boiled (100g)	34
Brussels sprouts, boiled (7=70g)	40
Cabbage, raw (50g)	60
boiled (100g)	15
Carrots, raw (50g)	6
boiled (50g)	4
young, canned (50g)	3
Cauliflower, raw (50g)	60
boiled (100g)	20
Celeriac, boiled (3=60g)	4
Celery, raw (50g)	7
boiled (50g)	5
Chickpeas, cooked dahl (60g)	3
Cucumber, slices (5=30g)	8
Egg plant, baked (½=100g)	3
Endive, raw leaves (3=15g)	12
Leeks, boiled (4=100g)	15
Lentils, split, boiled (100g)	Tr
Lettuce, raw leaves (2=20g)	15
Marrow, boiled (100g)	2
Mushrooms, raw (3=30g)	3
fried (6=60g)	1
Onions, raw (¼=20g)	10
boiled (100g)	6
fried (70g)	–
spring (4=20g)	25
Parsley, sprigs (2=5g)	150
Parsnip, boiled (½=60g)	10
Peas, canned (60g)	8
canned, processed (60g)	Tr
fresh, boiled (60g)	15
frozen, boiled (60g)	13
split, boiled (60g)	Tr
Peppers, green, raw (¼=15g)	100
boiled (50g)	60
Potato, baked (inc. skin 120g)	8
boiled (120g)	9
chips, fresh, fried (12=120g)	10
chips, frozen, fried (8-14=120g)	4
crisps (10=25g)	17
mashed (100g)	8
instant, cooked (100g)	3
new, boiled (2=100g)	18
new, canned (2=100g)	17
roast (120g)	10
Pumpkin (100g)	5
Radishes (2=20g)	25
Spinach, leaves, boiled (3=60g)	25
Swede, boiled (80g)	17
Sweetcorn, on cob, boiled (150g)	9
canned kernels (80g)	5
Sweet potato, boiled (100g)	15
Tomato, raw (120g)	20
canned (120g)	18
fried (120g)	10
juice, canned (120g)	20
Turnip, boiled (80g)	17
Yam, boiled (100g)	2

ELEMENTS
2 5
S O D I U M

Sodium occurs naturally in many foods and is also added in the form of salt or other sodium-containing substances. Common salt or table salt is a chemical compound of sodium and chlorine and is called sodium chloride. The sodium content of food has important implications for health. Salt contains about 40 per cent sodium, and a teaspoon of salt, which weighs about 5 grams, contains about 2 grams of sodium.

Rock salt and sea salt are almost entirely sodium chloride, with only traces of other elements (minerals). In contrast to pepper, which loses flavour once ground, there is no advantage in freshly grinding salt prior to its use. Iodized salt contains about 0.03 milligram of iodine per gram of salt. It is intended as a supplement for people whose diet is deficient in iodine. Recent findings in the U.S.A. indicate that the level of iodine in the diet has increased and that the widespread use of this salt is unnecessary.

Varying amounts of sodium are added to food, but not always in the form of salt. Common food additives, such as baking soda, some preservatives, and monosodium glutamate (MSG), also contribute to the total amount of sodium we consume.

SALT AND HIGH BLOOD PRESSURE

Probably one-fifth of the population, because of genetic predisposition, may be increasing their risk of high blood pressure (hypertension) by having a high intake of sodium. People who have a high intake of sodium have a high incidence of hypertension and stroke. High blood pressure is rarely seen in those who consume less than 1.2 grams (1200 milligrams) of sodium per day. In Australia, on the other hand, where the sodium intake can be in the region of 4 to 8 grams per day, about one in five adult Australians has high blood pressure. Salt is not necessarily the only important factor leading to high blood pressure, but in some cases it is. There are sound reasons why Australians should reduce their sodium intake. But sodium is an essential nutrient, and we need a certain amount for normal body function. A safe intake is considered to be between 0.9 and 2.3 grams of sodium per day, although in special circumstances, such as excessive sweating and diarrhoea, higher levels may be needed.

There is usually no need to increase salt intake in hot climates to avoid cramps, fainting and other symptoms because the body's hormones will adjust over a few days and conserve body sodium. Excessive heat presents other risks and should, in any case, be avoided.

HOW CAN WE CONTROL OUR SALT INTAKE?

Some people find it hard to reduce their intake of sodium. We all have the ability to taste salt, but the extent to which we like our food salted can be modified by experience. The amount of salt we consume cannot be wholly controlled by the moderate use of the salt shaker at the dinner table. This use only accounts for about one-third of our daily intake. Up to half of our salt intake is from processed food, with the balance occurring naturally in food and water. The amount consumed in processed food is difficult to control, although with highly salted foods, taste is a reliable guide. Some items that do not taste highly salted can contribute significant quantities of sodium to our diet because of the amounts we consume. Examples include bread, tomato sauce, and cakes and biscuits. Many 'take-away' foods, such as fish and chips, hamburgers and Chinese food, are highly salted. Bottled mineral waters can contribute a significant amount of sodium. An indication of sodium content is usually given on the label.

An increase in potassium intake seems to offset the adverse effect that sodium has on blood pressure. Foods that contain significant amounts of potassium and also low levels of sodium are fresh and frozen fruits and vegetables. But there is no justification for the unrestricted use of potassium salts as substitutes for sodium, as this would present new problems. Potassium supplements and salt substitutes can be potentially hazardous to health and should only be used under medical supervision.

SODIUM INTAKE

Recommended safe and adequate daily intake of sodium (Australia):

Adults:	0.9-2.3 grams
Infants:	0.1-0.6 grams
Children:	0.3-2.3 grams

milligrams per 100 grams

BEVERAGES

Value	Food
9	Beer (240g)
7	Cider, dry, alcoholic (180g)
7	sweet, alcoholic (180g)
4	sweet, non-alcoholic (220g)
950	Cocoa powder (5g)
Tr	Coffee, percolated (230g)
8	Cola-type drinks (240g)
–	Cordial, diluted 1:4 (240g)
250	Drinking chocolate (10g)
7	Lemonade, carbonated drinks (240g)
500	Milo (10g)
250	Ovaltine (10g)
4	Port (60g)
10	Sherry, dry (60g)
6	medium (60g)
10	sweet (60g)
Tr	Spirits, e.g. whisky (30g)
Tr	Tea, infusion (230g)
10	Wine, red (100g)
4	white, dry (100g)
20	medium (100g)
4	sparkling (100g)
10	sweet (100g)

CEREALS, BISCUITS, CAKES, DESSERTS

Value	Food
1	Barley, pearl, boiled (–)
160	Biscuit, chocolate (20g)
–	cream-filled (20g)
220	crispbread, rye (20g)
610	wheat, starch-red. (11g)
330	gingernut (15g)
410	semi-sweet (15g)
360	short-sweet (15g)
30	Bran, wheat (8g)
540	Bread, brown, slice (25g)
360	Lebanese (pita) (¼=25g)
510	white, slice (25g)
530	wholemeal, slice (25g)
640	roll, brown (35g)
650	starch-reduced (35g)
630	white (35g)
250	Cake, fruit (60g)
380	plain (60g)

Value	Food
220	Egg, fried (60g)
1030	omelette (100g)
110	poached (55g)
140	raw (55g)
1050	scrambled (70g)
280	Macaroni cheese (180g)
610	Quiche Lorraine (150g)

FATS AND OILS

Value	Food
840	Butter, salted (10g)
5	Dripping, beef (–)
2	Lard (–)
840	Margarine (10g)
Tr	Vegetable oils (–)

FISH AND OTHER SEAFOODS

Value	Food
115	Bream, steamed (100g)
340	Cod, baked (100g)
100	fried in batter (100g)
110	poached (100g)
100	steamed (100g)
370	Crab, boiled (150g)
550	canned (90g)
500	Fish cakes, fried (4=100g)
350	fingers, fried (5=100g)
470	in batter, fried (120g)
235	Flounder, baked (100g)
180	Haddock, fried (100g)
120	steamed (100g)
330	Lobster, boiled (120g)
210	Mussels, boiled (12=120g)
510	Oysters, raw (12=120g)
1590	Prawns, boiled (6=120g)
130	Roe, cod, fried (100g)
570	Salmon, canned (100g)
540	Sardines, canned (60g)
270	Scallops, steamed (10=100g)
420	Tuna, canned in oil (120g)
200	Whiting, crumbed, fried (100g)
130	steamed (100g)

FRUIT

Value	Food
2	Apple (inc. skin, core 100g)
2	baked, no sugar (inc. skin 110g)
2	stewed, no sugar (110g)
Tr	Apricots (inc. stones 3=100g)

Sodium (mg)	Food
350	Cake, sponge (60g)
130	Chapati (60g)
260	Cheesecake (120g)
1170	Cornflakes (30g)
–	Crumpet (50g)
80	Custard (70g)
250	Custard tart (120g)
60	Doughnut (40g)
160	Eclair (50g)
1	Flour, corn- (–)
2	plain (–)
730	self-raising (–)
1	soya, full-fat (–)
1	low-fat (–)
3	wholemeal (–)
210	Fruit pie (150g)
230	Jam tart (35g)
6	Jelly, made with water (100g)
140	Lamington (60g)
200	Lemon meringue pie (120g)
110	Meringue (15g)
60	Milk pudding (e.g. sago) (160g)
270	Muesli (30g)
410	Noodles (chow mein) (250g)
50	Pancake (75g)
8	Pasta, macaroni, boiled (150g)
2	spaghetti, boiled (120g)
500	canned in tomato sauce (120g)
470	Pastry, flaky (–)
480	short crust (–)
340	Pizza, cheese and tomato (150g)
220	Porridge (30g)
2	Rice, boiled (160g)
500	fried (120g)
970	puffed (25g)
800	Scone (30g)
310	Sponge pudding, steamed (100g)
50	Trifle (100g)
250	Wheat, breakfast biscuit (35g)
50	Yeast, dried, baker's (–)

EGG AND CHEESE DISHES

Sodium (mg)	Food
250	Cauliflower cheese (100g)
420	Cheese soufflé (100g)
140	Egg, boiled (55g)

Sodium (mg)	Food
1	Apricots, canned (100g)
60	dried (25g)
Tr	stewed, no sugar (inc. stones 110g)
2	Avocado pear (½ = 150g)
1	Banana (100g)
4	Blackberries (100g)
3	stewed, no sugar (100g)
9	Cantaloup (inc. skin 120g)
2	Cherries (inc. stones 20 = 100g)
3	stewed, no sugar (inc. stones 100g)
3	Currants, black (90g)
20	dried (15g)
2	red (90g)
5	Dates, dried (6 = 35g)
2	Figs (2 = 75g)
90	dried (2 = 40g)
2	Fruit salad, canned (120g)
1	Grapes, black (20 = 100g)
2	white (20 = 100g)
1	Grapefruit, whole (200g)
10	canned (100g)
3	juice, canned (120g)
7	Guavas, canned (100g)
6	Lemon, slices (2 = 15g)
2	juice (15g)
3	Loganberries (100g)
1	canned (100g)
3	stewed, no sugar (100g)
2	Lychees, canned (100g)
2	Mandarins (2 = 100g)
9	canned (50g)
7	Mango (100g)
3	canned (100g)
8	Nectarines (inc. stones 3 = 100g)
1800	Olives, in brine (5 = 20g)
2	Orange, whole (130g)
2	juice, fresh (120g)
4	canned (120g)
10	Passionfruit, whole (30g)
3	Papaw (100g)
8	canned (100g)
2	Peach (inc. stones 120g)
1	canned (120g)
6	dried (25g)

1170	cheese spread (10g)
450	cottage (25g)
300	cream cheese (15g)
1420	Danish blue (25g)
980	edam (25g)
760	parmesan (10g)
1360	processed (25g)
1150	stilton (25g)
155	Swiss (25g)
70	Cream, 35% fat (30g)
60	sterilized, canned (15g)
80	Ice-cream (60g)
70	non-dairy (60g)
180	Milk, cow's, cond. skim, sweet. (30g)
130	cond. whole, sweet. (30g)
550	dried, skimmed (12g)
440	dried, whole (10g)
180	evap. whole, unsweet. (30g)
44	flavoured (230g)
50	fresh, skimmed (230g)
50	fresh, whole (230g)
50	longlife, UHT (230g)
40	goat's (230g)
10	human (100g)
–	Milkshake, flavoured (340g)
40	Yoghurt, flavoured (200g)
64	fruit, low-fat (200g)
76	natural, low-fat (200g)
40	plain (200g)

NUTS

6	Almonds (10=15g)
2	Brazil nuts (5=20g)
15	Cashews, roast (10=20g)
10	Chestnuts (4=20g)
30	Coconut, desiccated (15g)
1	Hazel nuts (10=15g)
–	Macadamia nuts (8=20g)
4	Peanuts, raw, in shells (5=25g)
440	roasted, salted (30=25g)
–	Pistachio nuts, shelled (25=15g)
3	Walnuts (5=20g)

SAUCES & CONDIMENTS

815	Barbecue sauce (10g)
–	Chilli sauce (–)

2	Peach, stewed, no sugar (120g)
1	Pear (inc. skin, core 120g)
1	canned (120g)
3	stewed, no sugar (120g)
2	Pineapple (80g)
1	canned (80g)
1	juice, canned (120g)
2	Plums (inc. stones 3 = 100g)
2	stewed, no sugar (inc. stones 100g)
10	Prunes (inc. stones 8=80g)
6	stewed, no sugar (inc. stones 120g)
3	Quince, raw (100g)
50	Raisins, dried (20g)
3	Raspberries (100g)
4	canned (100g)
3	stewed, no sugar (100g)
2	Rhubarb, stewed, no sugar (120g)
2	Strawberries (10=100g)
7	canned (100g)
50	Sultanas, dried (15g)
2	Watermelon (260g)

MEAT AND MEAT PRODUCTS

1870	Bacon rashers, middle, fried (2=40g)
2000	grilled (40g)
950	Beef, corned, canned (90g)
85	fillet steak, grilled (130g)
320	mince, stewed (120g)
50	rump steak, fried (150g)
60	grilled (150g)
910	silverside, salted, boiled (120g)
55	sirloin, roast (120g)
360	stewing steak, stewed (120g)
50	topside, roast (120g)
880	Beefburger, frozen, fried (60g)
400	Beef stew (250g)
440	Bolognese sauce (100g)
80	Chicken, boiled (100g)
640	crumbed, no bone (140g)
70	roast (130g)
50	leg quarter (inc. bone 130g)
40	wing quarter (inc. bone 130g)
240	Chicken livers, fried (130g)
80	Duck, roast (100g)

Food	Sodium (mg)
Gelatin (–)	–
Ham, canned (90g)	1250
Hamburger (170g)	660
with cheese (190g)	760
Irish stew (250g)	330
Lamb, brain, boiled (150g)	210
chops, loin, grilled (inc. bone 120g)	60
cutlets, grilled (inc. bone 100g)	50
heart, roast (140g)	150
kidney, fried (100g)	270
leg, roast (120g)	70
liver, fried (130g)	190
shoulder, roast (120g)	60
tongue, stewed (100g)	80
Luncheon meat, canned (90g)	1050
Meat pie (180g)	600
Moussaka (200g)	320
Pastie (160g)	590
Pork, chop, loin, grilled (100g)	70
leg, roast (120g)	80
sweet and sour (250g)	390
Pork pie (180g)	720
Rabbit, stewed (inc. bone 170g)	20
Salami, slices (3=90g)	1850
Sausage, liver (60g)	860
Sausage roll (100g)	650
Sausages, beef, fried (2=120g)	1090
grilled (2=120g)	1100
frankfurter (2=100g)	980
pork, fried (2=120g)	1050
grilled (2=120g)	1000
saveloy, large (2=150g)	890
Spring roll, fried (200g)	600
Steak and kidney pie (180g)	510
Stewed steak in gravy, canned (100g)	380
Tongue, canned (100g)	1050
Tripe, stewed (100g)	70
Turkey, roast (120g)	50
Veal, cutlet, fried (110g)	110
fillet, roast (100g)	100
schnitzel (140g)	260

MILK & MILK PRODUCTS

Food	Sodium (mg)
Cheese, camembert (25g)	1410
cheddar (25g)	610

Food	Sodium (mg)
Chutney, tomato (20g)	130
Curry powder (–)	450
French dressing (15g)	960
Ginger (ground) (–)	35
Mayonnaise (20g)	360
Mustard powder (–)	5
Oxo cubes (–)	10300
Pepper (–)	7
Pickles, mustard (20g)	1200
sweet (20g)	1700
Salad cream (25g)	840
Salt, table (–)	38850
Sesame seeds (–)	60
Soy sauce (–)	7325
Tartare sauce (20g)	705
Tomato sauce (25g)	340
Vinegar (–)	20
Worcestershire sauce (–)	–

SOUPS (as served)

Food	Sodium (mg)
Chicken, condensed (230g)	350
Chicken noodle, dried (230g)	370
Minestrone, dried (230g)	430
Mushroom, canned (230g)	470
Tomato, condensed (230g)	410
Tomato, dried (230g)	390
Vegetable, canned (230g)	500

SUGARS, JAMS AND SPREADS

Food	Sodium (mg)
Fish paste (5g)	600
Honey (30g)	10
Jam, fruit, edible seeds (30g)	20
Jam, stone fruit (30g)	10
Marmalade (30g)	20
Meat paste (5g)	740
Peanut butter (20g)	350
Sugar, white (–)	Tr
Syrup, golden (30g)	270
Topping, flavoured (40g)	–
Treacle, black (30g)	100
Vegemite (3g)	4160

SWEETS

Food	Sodium (mg)
Boiled sweet (5g)	30
Butterscotch (5g)	65
Caramel (5g)	225

Food	Sodium
Carob bar (75g)	80
Chocolate square, milk (5g)	120
Fruit and honey bar (50g)	45
Jelly bean (5g)	25
Liquorice allsort (7g)	80
Pastille (5g)	80
Peppermint (4g)	9
Popcorn, plain unsalted (15g)	1
Sesame bar (50g)	30
Toffee, mixed (5g)	320

VEGETABLES

Food	Sodium
Artichoke, globe, boiled (100g)	6
Asparagus, boiled (5=100g)	1
Bamboo shoots (50g)	–
Beans, French, boiled (100g)	3
baked, in tomato sauce (125g)	480
broad, boiled (100g)	20
kidney (and haricot), boiled (100g)	20
mung, cooked dahl (100g)	820
soya-, boiled (100g)	2
Beetroot, slices, boiled (2=30g)	60
canned (2=30g)	235
Broccoli, boiled (100g)	6
Brussels sprouts, boiled (7=70g)	2
Cabbage, raw (50g)	20
boiled (100g)	8
Carrots, raw (50g)	100
boiled (50g)	50
young, canned (50g)	280
Cauliflower, raw (50g)	8
boiled (100g)	4
Celeriac, boiled (3=60g)	30
Celery, raw (50g)	140
boiled (50g)	70
Chickpeas, cooked dahl (60g)	850
Cucumber, slices (5=30g)	10
Egg plant, baked (½=100g)	5
Endive, raw leaves (3=15g)	10
Leeks, boiled (4=100g)	6
Lentils, split, boiled (100g)	10
Lettuce, raw leaves (2=20g)	9
Marrow, boiled (100g)	1
Mushrooms, raw (3=30g)	9
fried (6=60g)	10
Onions, raw (¼=20g)	10
boiled (100g)	7
fried (70g)	20
spring (4=20g)	10
Parsley, sprigs (2=5g)	30
Parsnip, boiled (½=60g)	4
Peas, canned (60g)	230
canned, processed (60g)	330
fresh, boiled (60g)	Tr
frozen, boiled (60g)	2
split, boiled (60g)	10
Peppers, green, raw (¼=15g)	2
boiled (50g)	2
Potato, baked (inc. skin 120g)	6
boiled (120g)	3
chips, fresh, fried (12=120g)	10
chips, frozen, fried (8-14=120g)	30
crisps (10=25g)	550
mashed (100g)	20
instant, cooked (100g)	260
new, boiled (2=100g)	40
new, canned (2=100g)	260
roast (120g)	9
Pumpkin (100g)	1
Radishes (2=20g)	60
Spinach, leaves, boiled (3=60g)	120
Swede, boiled (80g)	10
Sweetcorn, on cob, boiled (150g)	1
canned kernels (80g)	310
Sweet potato, boiled (100g)	20
Tomato, raw (120g)	3
canned (120g)	30
fried (120g)	3
juice, canned (120g)	230
Turnip, boiled (80g)	30
Yam, boiled (100g)	20

☆ Yeast, dried, brewers (–) contains 130 milligram

26
POTASSIUM

Potassium, like sodium, is essential for normal body function. Potassium is necessary for muscle function, the transmission of nerve impulses and for carbohydrate and protein metabolism.

It is unlikely that we would have a dietary deficiency of potassium as it is present in a large number of foods. Deficiency can occur when there are large losses resulting from excessive urination or from prolonged vomiting and diarrhoea.

Although sodium is an important dietary factor in high blood pressure for some people, variations in the ratio of sodium and potassium will also affect blood pressure under certain circumstances. An increase in potassium intake appears to partly offset the adverse effect of sodium on blood pressure. If you are prone to high blood pressure it would be beneficial to decrease sodium intake and increase your *dietary* intake of potassium, by eating more foods that have low amounts of sodium and significant amounts of potassium, such as fruits and vegetables.

The use of potassium salts as substitutes for common salt (sodium chloride) is potentially dangerous, and overuse can be fatal. Excessive potassium intake can cause heart irregularities and can cause the heart to stop beating (cardiac arrest). Potassium supplements and bulk substitutes should not be used without medical advice. High potassium intake can be particularly dangerous for children.

POTASSIUM INTAKE

Recommended safe and adequate daily intake of potassium (Australia):

Adults:	2.5-5 grams
Infants:	0.4-1.4 grams
Children:	1-5.5 grams

milligrams per 100 grams

BEVERAGES

Beer (240g)	40
Cider, dry, alcoholic (180g)	70
sweet, alcoholic (180g)	70
sweet, non-alcoholic (220g)	100
Cocoa powder (5g)	1500
Coffee, percolated (230g)	70
Cola-type drinks (240g)	1
Cordial, diluted 1:4 (240g)	–
Drinking chocolate (10g)	410
Lemonade, carbonated drinks (240g)	1
Milo (10g)	700
Ovaltine (10g)	150
Port (60g)	100
Sherry, dry (60g)	60
medium (60g)	90
sweet (60g)	110
Spirits, e.g. whisky (30g)	Tr
Tea, infusion (230g)	20
Wine, red (100g)	130
white, dry (100g)	60
medium (100g)	90
sparkling (100g)	60
sweet (100g)	110

CEREALS, BISCUITS, CAKES, DESSERTS

Barley, pearl, boiled (–)	40
Biscuit, chocolate (20g)	230
cream-filled (20g)	–
crispbread, rye (20g)	500
wheat, starch-red. (11g)	210
gingernut (15g)	220
semi-sweet (15g)	140
short-sweet (15g)	110
Bran, wheat (8g)	1160
Bread, brown, slice (25g)	200
Lebanese (pita) (¼=25g)	100
white, slice (25g)	90
wholemeal, slice (25g)	200
roll, brown (35g)	240
starch-reduced (35g)	130
white (35g)	120
Cake, fruit (60g)	390
plain (60g)	120

FRUIT

Apple (inc. skin, core 100g)	90
baked, no sugar (inc. skin 110g)	100
stewed, no sugar (110g)	100
Apricots (inc. stones 3=100g)	290

Egg, fried (60g)	180
omelette (100g)	120
poached (55g)	120
raw (55g)	140
scrambled (70g)	130
Macaroni cheese (180g)	120
Quiche Lorraine (150g)	190

FATS AND OILS

Butter, salted (10g)	20
Dripping, beef (–)	4
Lard (–)	1
Margarine (10g)	20
Vegetable oils (–)	Tr

FISH AND OTHER SEAFOODS

Bream, steamed (100g)	280
Cod, baked (100g)	350
fried in batter (100g)	370
poached (100g)	330
steamed (100g)	360
Crab, boiled (150g)	270
canned (90g)	100
Fish cakes, fried (4=100g)	260
fingers, fried (5=100g)	260
in batter, fried (120g)	180
Flounder, baked (100g)	585
Haddock, fried (100g)	350
steamed (100g)	320
Lobster, boiled (120g)	260
Mussels, boiled (12=120g)	90
Oysters, raw (12=120g)	260
Prawns, boiled (6=120g)	260
Roe, cod, fried (100g)	260
Salmon, canned (100g)	300
Sardines, canned (60g)	360
Scallops, steamed (10=100g)	480
Tuna, canned in oil (120g)	280
Whiting, crumbed, fried (100g)	320
steamed (100g)	300

Food	Potassium
Apricots, canned (100g)	260
dried (25g)	1880
stewed, no sugar (inc. stones 110g)	250
Avocado pear (½=150g)	400
Banana (100g)	350
Blackberries (100g)	210
stewed, no sugar (100g)	180
Cantaloup (inc. skin 120g)	200
Cherries (inc. stones 20=100g)	240
stewed, no sugar (inc. stones 100g)	220
Currants, black (90g)	370
dried (15g)	710
red (90g)	280
Dates, dried (6=35g)	750
Figs (2=75g)	270
dried (2=40g)	1010
Fruit salad, canned (120g)	120
Grapes, black (20=100g)	270
white (20=100g)	240
Grapefruit, whole (200g)	110
canned (100g)	80
juice, canned (120g)	110
Guavas, canned (100g)	120
Lemon, slices (2=15g)	160
juice (15g)	140
Loganberries (100g)	260
canned (100g)	100
stewed, no sugar (100g)	240
Lychees, canned (100g)	80
Mandarins (2=100g)	170
canned (50g)	90
Mango (100g)	190
canned (100g)	100
Nectarines (inc. stones 3=100g)	250
Olives, in brine (5=20g)	70
Orange, whole (130g)	150
juice, fresh (120g)	180
canned (120g)	180
Passionfruit, whole (30g)	150
Papaw (100g)	235
canned (100g)	110
Peach (inc. stones 120g)	230
canned (120g)	150
dried (25g)	1100

Food	Potassium
Cake, sponge (60g)	80
Chapati (60g)	160
Cheesecake (120g)	120
Cornflakes (30g)	125
Crumpet (50g)	–
Custard (70g)	170
Custard tart (120g)	130
Doughnut (40g)	110
Eclair (50g)	90
Flour, corn- (–)	7
plain (–)	90
self-raising (–)	90
soya, full-fat (–)	1660
low-fat (–)	2030
wholemeal (–)	370
Fruit pie (150g)	120
Jam tart (35g)	110
Jelly, made with water (100g)	6
Lamington (60g)	160
Lemon meringue pie (120g)	80
Meringue (15g)	90
Milk pudding (e.g. sago) (160g)	160
Muesli (30g)	370
Noodles (chow mein) (250g)	90
Pancake (75g)	140
Pasta, macaroni, boiled (150g)	70
spaghetti, boiled (120g)	50
canned in tomato sauce (120g)	130
Pastry, flaky (–)	90
short crust (–)	110
Pizza, cheese and tomato (150g)	180
Porridge (30g)	40
Rice, boiled (160g)	40
fried (120g)	35
puffed (25g)	140
Scone (30g)	140
Sponge pudding, steamed (100g)	90
Trifle (100g)	150
Wheat, breakfast biscuit (35g)	350
Yeast, dried, baker's (–)	2000

EGG AND CHEESE DISHES

Food	Potassium
Cauliflower cheese (100g)	250
Cheese soufflé (100g)	150
Egg, boiled (55g)	140

Food	Potassium
cheese spread (10g)	150
cottage (25g)	50
cream cheese (15g)	160
Danish blue (25g)	190
edam (25g)	160
parmesan (10g)	150
processed (25g)	80
stilton (25g)	160
Swiss (25g)	100
Cream, 35% fat (30g)	230
sterilized, canned (15g)	120
Ice-cream (60g)	180
non-dairy (60g)	150
Milk, cow's, cond. skim, sweet. (30g)	390
cond. whole, sweet. (30g)	500
dried, skimmed (12g)	1650
dried, whole (10g)	1270
evap. whole, unsweet. (30g)	390
flavoured (230g)	145
fresh, skimmed (230g)	150
fresh, whole (230g)	150
longlife, UHT (230g)	140
goat's (230g)	180
human (100g)	60
Milkshake, flavoured (340g)	–
Yoghurt, flavoured (200g)	115
fruit, low-fat (200g)	220
natural, low-fat (200g)	240
plain (200g)	175

NUTS

Food	Potassium
Almonds (10 = 15g)	860
Brazil nuts (5 = 20g)	760
Cashews, roast (10 = 20g)	510
Chestnuts (4 = 20g)	500
Coconut, desiccated (15g)	750
Hazel nuts (10 = 15g)	350
Macadamia nuts (8 = 20g)	265
Peanuts, raw, in shells (5 = 25g)	470
roasted, salted (30 = 25g)	680
Pistachio nuts, shelled (25 = 15g)	970
Walnuts (5 = 20g)	690

SAUCES & CONDIMENTS

Food	Potassium
Barbecue sauce (10g)	175
Chilli sauce (–)	–

Food	Potassium
Peach, stewed, no sugar (120g)	410
Pear (inc. skin, core 120g)	90
canned (120g)	90
stewed, no sugar (120g)	90
Pineapple (80g)	250
canned (80g)	90
juice, canned (120g)	140
Plums (inc. stones 3 = 100g)	260
stewed, no sugar (inc. stones 100g)	220
Prunes (inc. stones 8 = 80g)	720
stewed, no sugar (inc. stones 120g)	400
Quince, raw (100g)	200
Raisins, dried (20g)	860
Raspberries (100g)	220
canned (100g)	100
stewed, no sugar (100g)	230
Rhubarb, stewed, no sugar (120g)	400
Strawberries (10 = 100g)	160
canned (100g)	100
Sultanas, dried (15g)	860
Watermelon (260g)	60

MEAT AND MEAT PRODUCTS

Food	Potassium
Bacon rashers, middle, fried (2 = 40g)	300
grilled (40g)	290
Beef, corned, canned (90g)	140
fillet steak, grilled (130g)	470
mince, stewed (120g)	290
rump steak, fried (150g)	360
grilled (150g)	380
silverside, salted, boiled (120g)	200
sirloin, roast (120g)	300
stewing steak, stewed (120g)	230
topside, roast (120g)	350
Beefburger, frozen, fried (60g)	340
Beef stew (250g)	200
Bolognese sauce (100g)	310
Chicken, boiled (100g)	300
crumbed, no bone (140g)	160
roast (130g)	270
leg quarter (inc. bone 130g)	190
wing quarter (inc. bone 130g)	160
Chicken livers, fried (130g)	290
Duck, roast (100g)	210

Food	Potassium
Chutney, tomato (20g)	310
Curry powder (–)	1840
French dressing (15g)	20
Ginger (ground) (–)	910
Mayonnaise (20g)	20
Mustard powder (–)	945
Oxo cubes (–)	730
Pepper (–)	40
Pickles, mustard (20g)	60
sweet (20g)	110
Salad cream (25g)	80
Salt, table (–)	Tr
Sesame seeds (–)	725
Soy sauce (–)	365
Tartare sauce (20g)	80
Tomato sauce (25g)	320
Vinegar (–)	90
Worcestershire sauce (–)	–

SOUPS (as served)

Food	Potassium
Chicken, condensed (230g)	30
Chicken noodle, dried (230g)	20
Minestrone, dried (230g)	60
Mushroom, canned (230g)	60
Tomato, condensed (230g)	180
Tomato, dried (230g)	90
Vegetable, canned (230g)	140

SUGARS, JAMS AND SPREADS

Food	Potassium
Fish paste (5g)	300
Honey (30g)	50
Jam, fruit, edible seeds (30g)	110
Jam, stone fruit (30g)	100
Marmalade (30g)	40
Meat paste (5g)	160
Peanut butter (20g)	700
Sugar, white (–)	2
Syrup, golden (30g)	240
Topping, flavoured (40g)	–
Treacle, black (30g)	1470
Vegemite (3g)	–

SWEETS

Food	Potassium
Boiled sweet (5g)	8
Butterscotch (5g)	2
Caramel (5g)	190

Food	Potassium
Gelatin (–)	–
Ham, canned (90g)	280
Hamburger (170g)	190
with cheese (190g)	210
Irish stew (250g)	310
Lamb, brain, boiled (150g)	190
chops, loin, grilled (inc. bone 120g)	250
cutlets, grilled (inc. bone 100g)	210
heart, roast (140g)	370
kidney, fried (100g)	340
leg, roast (120g)	310
liver, fried (130g)	300
shoulder, roast (120g)	260
tongue, stewed (100g)	110
Luncheon meat, canned (90g)	140
Meat pie (180g)	120
Moussaka (200g)	350
Pastie (160g)	190
Pork, chop, loin, grilled (100g)	300
leg, roast (120g)	350
sweet and sour (250g)	110
Pork pie (180g)	150
Rabbit, stewed (inc. bone 170g)	110
Salami, slices (3=90g)	160
Sausage, liver (60g)	170
Sausage roll (100g)	90
Sausages, beef, fried (2=120g)	180
grilled (2=120g)	190
frankfurter (2=100g)	100
pork, fried (2=120g)	200
grilled (2=120g)	200
saveloy, large (2=150g)	160
Spring roll, fried (200g)	600
Steak and kidney pie (180g)	140
Stewed steak in gravy, canned (100g)	240
Tongue, canned (100g)	100
Tripe, stewed (100g)	100
Turkey, roast (120g)	280
Veal, cutlet, fried (110g)	420
fillet, roast (100g)	430
schnitzel (140g)	350

MILK & MILK PRODUCTS

Food	Potassium
Cheese, camembert (25g)	110
cheddar (25g)	120

Food	Potassium (mg)
Carob bar (75g)	220
Chocolate square, milk (5g)	420
Fruit and honey bar (50g)	140
Jelly bean (5g)	5
Liquorice allsort (7g)	220
Pastille (5g)	40
Peppermint (4g)	Tr
Popcorn, plain unsalted (15g)	–
Sesame bar (50g)	140
Toffee, mixed (5g)	210

VEGETABLES

Food	Potassium (mg)
Artichoke, globe, boiled (100g)	140
Asparagus, boiled (5=100g)	120
Bamboo shoots (50g)	535
Beans, French, boiled (100g)	100
baked, in tomato sauce (125g)	300
broad, boiled (100g)	230
kidney (and haricot), boiled (100g)	320
mung, cooked dahl (100g)	270
soya-, boiled (100g)	540
Beetroot, slices, boiled (2=30g)	350
canned (2=30g)	160
Broccoli, boiled (100g)	220
Brussels sprouts, boiled (7=70g)	240
Cabbage, raw (50g)	260
boiled (100g)	120
Carrots, raw (50g)	220
boiled (50g)	90
young, canned (50g)	80
Cauliflower, raw (50g)	350
boiled (100g)	180
Celeriac, boiled (3=60g)	400
Celery, raw (50g)	280
boiled (50g)	130
Chickpeas, cooked dahl (60g)	400
Cucumber, slices (5=30g)	140
Egg plant, baked (½=100g)	190
Endive, raw leaves (3=15g)	380
Leeks, boiled (4=100g)	280
Lentils, split, boiled (100g)	210
Lettuce, raw leaves (2=20g)	240
Marrow, boiled (100g)	80
Mushrooms, raw (3=30g)	470
fried (6=60g)	570
Onions, raw (¼=20g)	140
boiled (100g)	80
fried (70g)	270
spring (4=20g)	230
Parsley, sprigs (2=5g)	1080
Parsnip, boiled (½=60g)	290
Peas, canned (60g)	130
canned, processed (60g)	170
fresh, boiled (60g)	170
frozen, boiled (60g)	130
split, boiled (60g)	270
Peppers, green, raw (¼=15g)	210
boiled (50g)	170
Potato, baked (inc. skin 120g)	550
boiled (120g)	330
chips, fresh, fried (12=120g)	680
chips, frozen, fried (8-14=120g)	560
crisps (10=25g)	1190
mashed (100g)	300
instant, cooked (100g)	340
new, boiled (2=100g)	330
new, canned (2=100g)	230
roast (120g)	750
Pumpkin (100g)	310
Radishes (2=20g)	240
Spinach, leaves, boiled (3=60g)	490
Swede, boiled (80g)	100
Sweetcorn, on cob, boiled (150g)	280
canned kernels (80g)	200
Sweet potato, boiled (100g)	300
Tomato, raw (120g)	290
canned (120g)	270
fried (120g)	340
juice, canned (120g)	260
Turnip, boiled (80g)	160
Yam, boiled (100g)	300

CALCIUM

Calcium, in combination with phosphorus and other elements, is necessary to give strength to bones and teeth. When our dietary intake of calcium is greater than our bodies' requirements some of the excess calcium is stored in our bones. When our day-to-day intake of calcium does not meet requirements, the calcium stored in bone becomes available to meet this shortfall.

Calcium has other important roles. It is essential for normal clotting of blood and is a vital link in transmission of nerve impulses. It is also an essential element in enzyme regulation, in the secretion of insulin in adults, and in regulation of muscle function.

During periods of growth the demand for calcium is greater than usual, although some calcium is incorporated into bone at certain other stages of life. Thus children, adolescents and pregnant and lactating women need additional calcium. Adults continually need to replace calcium that is lost from the body in urine and faeces and to a lesser extent in sweat.

Our bodies' utilization of the calcium in food can be adversely affected by the presence of two chemicals called phytic acid and oxalic acid. Phytic acid is found in the bran portion of cereals, and oxalic acid is present in significant quantities in spinach and rhubarb. The magnitude of the effect depends on the amount of these acids we consume and a higher intake of calcium may be necessary if large quantities of foods containing oxalic and/or phytic acids are eaten. Diets high in protein and also high in salt also increase the requirement for calcium.

Osteoporosis, a decrease in the density of the bone, is a disease that becomes especially evident in women after the menopause, and is responsible for many serious bone fractures that occur in this group. It is associated with a decrease of calcium in the bones and may be due to an imbalance between calcium and phosphorus earlier in life. Obtaining adequate calcium and avoiding factors that adversely affect calcium balance throughout life may be helpful in preventing the development of this disease. In old age it may be difficult to replace lost bone calcium.

Contrary to popular belief, fingernail changes are not an indicator of inadequate calcium intake.

CALCIUM INTAKE

Recommended daily dietary intake of calcium (Australia):

Children:	400-1400 milligrams
Adults:	400-800 milligrams
Pregnancy:	900-1300 milligrams
Lactation:	900-1300 milligrams

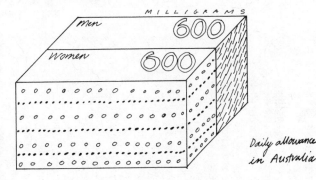

Daily allowance in Australia

milligrams per 100 grams

BEVERAGES

Food	mg
Beer (240g)	8
Cider, dry, alcoholic (180g)	8
sweet, alcoholic (180g)	8
sweet, non-alcoholic (220g)	6
Cocoa powder (5g)	130
Coffee, percolated (230g)	2
Cola-type drinks (240g)	4
Cordial, diluted 1:4 (240g)	3
Drinking chocolate (10g)	30
Lemonade, carbonated drinks (240g)	5
Milo (10g)	465
Ovaltine (10g)	270
Port (60g)	4
Sherry, dry (60g)	7
medium (60g)	9
sweet (60g)	7
Spirits, e.g. whisky (30g)	Tr
Tea, infusion (230g)	Tr
Wine, red (100g)	7
white, dry (100g)	9
medium (100g)	10
sparkling (100g)	3
sweet (100g)	10

CEREALS, BISCUITS, CAKES, DESSERTS

Food	mg
Barley, pearl, boiled (–)	3
Biscuit, chocolate (20g)	110
cream-filled (20g)	–
crispbread, rye (20g)	50
wheat, starch-red. (11g)	60
gingernut (15g)	130
semi-sweet (15g)	120
short-sweet (15g)	90
Bran, wheat (8g)	110
Bread, brown, slice (25g)	30
Lebanese (pita) (¼=25g)	20
white, slice (25g)	20
wholemeal, slice (25g)	30
roll, brown (35g)	30
starch-reduced (35g)	50
white (35g)	20
Cake, fruit (60g)	70
plain (60g)	40

Food	mg
Egg, fried (60g)	60
omelette (100g)	50
poached (55g)	50
raw (55g)	50
scrambled (70g)	60
Macaroni cheese (180g)	180
Quiche Lorraine (150g)	260

FATS AND OILS

Food	mg
Butter, salted (10g)	17
Dripping, beef (–)	1
Lard (–)	1
Margarine (10g)	20
Vegetable oils (–)	Tr

FISH AND OTHER SEAFOODS

Food	mg
Bream, steamed (100g)	35
Cod, baked (100g)	20
fried in batter (100g)	80
poached (100g)	30
steamed (100g)	20
Crab, boiled (150g)	30
canned (90g)	120
Fish cakes, fried (4=100g)	70
fingers, fried (5=100g)	40
in batter, fried (120g)	25
Flounder, baked (100g)	70
Haddock, fried (100g)	110
steamed (100g)	60
Lobster, boiled (120g)	60
Mussels, boiled (12=120g)	200
Oysters, raw (12=120g)	190
Prawns, boiled (6=120g)	150
Roe, cod, fried (100g)	20
Salmon, canned (100g)	90
Sardines, canned (60g)	460
Scallops, steamed (10=100g)	120
Tuna, canned in oil (120g)	7
Whiting, crumbed, fried (100g)	50
steamed (100g)	40

FRUIT

Food	mg
Apple (inc. skin, core 100g)	3
baked, no sugar (inc. skin 110g)	3
stewed, no sugar (110g)	3
Apricots (inc. stones 3=100g)	20

Calcium (mg)	Food
10	Apricots, canned (100g)
90	dried (25g)
10	stewed, no sugar (inc. stones 110g)
20	Avocado pear (½ = 150g)
7	Banana (100g)
60	Blackberries (100g)
50	stewed, no sugar (100g)
10	Cantaloup (inc. skin 120g)
10	Cherries (inc. stones 20 = 100g)
20	stewed, no sugar (inc. stones 100g)
60	Currants, black (90g)
100	dried (15g)
40	red (90g)
70	Dates, dried (6 = 35g)
30	Figs (2 = 75g)
280	dried (2 = 40g)
8	Fruit salad, canned (120g)
4	Grapes, black (20 = 100g)
20	white (20 = 100g)
8	Grapefruit, whole (200g)
20	canned (100g)
9	juice, canned (120g)
8	Guavas, canned (100g)
110	Lemon, slices (2 = 15g)
8	juice (15g)
40	Loganberries (100g)
20	canned (100g)
30	stewed, no sugar (100g)
4	Lychees, canned (100g)
35	Mandarins (2 = 100g)
20	canned (50g)
10	Mango (100g)
10	canned (100g)
4	Nectarines (inc. stones 3 = 100g)
50	Olives, in brine (5 = 20g)
30	Orange, whole (130g)
10	juice, fresh (120g)
9	canned (120g)
7	Passionfruit, whole (30g)
20	Papaw (100g)
20	canned (100g)
4	Peach (inc. stones 120g)
4	canned (120g)
40	dried (25g)

Calcium (mg)	Food
140	Cake, sponge (60g)
70	Chapati (60g)
70	Cheesecake (120g)
5	Cornflakes (30g)
–	Crumpet (50g)
140	Custard (70g)
110	Custard tart (120g)
70	Doughnut (40g)
50	Eclair (50g)
20	Flour, corn- (–)
20	plain (–)
90	self-raising (–)
210	soya, full-fat (–)
240	low-fat (–)
40	wholemeal (–)
50	Fruit pie (150g)
60	Jam tart (35g)
7	Jelly, made with water (100g)
30	Lamington (60g)
50	Lemon meringue pie (120g)
4	Meringue (15g)
130	Milk pudding (e.g. sago) (160g)
60	Muesli (30g)
10	Noodles (chow mein) (250g)
120	Pancake (75g)
8	Pasta, macaroni, boiled (150g)
7	spaghetti, boiled (120g)
20	canned in tomato sauce (120g)
90	Pastry, flaky (–)
110	short crust (–)
240	Pizza, cheese and tomato (150g)
6	Porridge (30g)
1	Rice, boiled (160g)
10	fried (120g)
30	puffed (25g)
620	Scone (30g)
210	Sponge pudding, steamed (100g)
80	Trifle (100g)
50	Wheat, breakfast biscuit (35g)
80	Yeast, dried, baker's (–)

EGG AND CHEESE DISHES

Calcium (mg)	Food
160	Cauliflower cheese (100g)
230	Cheese soufflé (100g)
50	Egg, boiled (55g)

Value	Food
510	cheese spread (10g)
60	cottage (25g)
100	cream cheese (15g)
580	Danish blue (25g)
740	edam (25g)
1220	parmesan (10g)
700	processed (25g)
360	stilton (25g)
950	Swiss (25g)
80	Cream, 35% fat (30g)
80	sterilized, canned (15g)
140	Ice-cream (60g)
120	non-dairy (60g)
380	Milk, cow's, cond. skim, sweet. (30g)
280	cond. whole, sweet. (30g)
1190	dried, skimmed (12g)
1020	dried, whole (10g)
280	evap. whole, unsweet. (30g)
110	flavoured (230g)
130	fresh, skimmed (230g)
120	fresh, whole (230g)
120	longlife, UHT (230g)
130	goat's (230g)
30	human (100g)
110	Milkshake, flavoured (340g)
130	Yoghurt, flavoured (200g)
160	fruit, low-fat (200g)
180	natural, low-fat (200g)
145	plain (200g)

NUTS

Value	Food
250	Almonds (10=15g)
180	Brazil nuts (5=20g)
45	Cashews, roast (10=20g)
50	Chestnuts (4=20g)
20	Coconut, desiccated (15g)
40	Hazel nuts (10=15g)
50	Macadamia nuts (8=20g)
40	Peanuts, raw, in shells (5=25g)
60	roasted, salted (30=25g)
130	Pistachio nuts, shelled (25=15g)
60	Walnuts (5=20g)

SAUCES & CONDIMENTS

Value	Food
20	Barbecue sauce (10g)
10	Chilli sauce (–)

Value	Food
10	Peach, stewed, no sugar (120g)
6	Pear (inc. skin, core 120g)
5	canned (120g)
6	stewed, no sugar (120g)
10	Pineapple (80g)
10	canned (80g)
10	juice, canned (120g)
20	Plums (inc. stones 3=100g)
20	stewed, no sugar (inc. stones 100g)
30	Prunes (inc. stones 8=80g)
20	stewed, no sugar (inc. stones 120g)
10	Quince, raw (100g)
60	Raisins, dried (20g)
40	Raspberries (100g)
10	canned (100g)
40	stewed, no sugar (100g)
90	Rhubarb, stewed, no sugar (120g)
20	Strawberries (10=100g)
10	canned (100g)
50	Sultanas, dried (15g)
3	Watermelon (260g)

MEAT AND MEAT PRODUCTS

Value	Food
15	Bacon rashers, middle, fried (2=40g)
10	grilled (40g)
10	Beef, corned, canned (90g)
15	fillet steak, grilled (130g)
20	mince, stewed (120g)
7	rump steak, fried (150g)
7	grilled (150g)
10	silverside, salted, boiled (120g)
10	sirloin, roast (120g)
20	stewing steak, stewed (120g)
6	topside, roast (120g)
30	Beefburger, frozen, fried (60g)
20	Beef stew (250g)
30	Bolognese sauce (100g)
10	Chicken, boiled (100g)
65	crumbed, no bone (140g)
9	roast (130g)
6	leg quarter (inc. bone 130g)
5	wing quarter (inc. bone 130g)
20	Chicken livers, fried (130g)
10	Duck, roast (100g)

Value	Food
30	Chutney, tomato (20g)
645	Curry powder (-)
5	French dressing (15g)
95	Ginger (ground) (-)
20	Mayonnaise (20g)
335	Mustard powder (-)
180	Oxo cubes (-)
130	Pepper (-)
20	Pickles, mustard (20g)
20	sweet (20g)
30	Salad cream (25g)
30	Salt, table (-)
1160	Sesame seeds (-)
80	Soy sauce (-)
20	Tartare sauce (20g)
30	Tomato sauce (25g)
20	Vinegar (-)
100	Worcestershire sauce (-)

SOUPS (as served)

Value	Food
20	Chicken, condensed (230g)
3	Chicken noodle, dried (230g)
9	Minestrone, dried (230g)
30	Mushroom, canned (230g)
20	Tomato, condensed (230g)
10	Tomato, dried (230g)
20	Vegetable, canned (230g)

SUGARS, JAMS AND SPREADS

Value	Food
280	Fish paste (5g)
5	Honey (30g)
20	Jam, fruit, edible seeds (30g)
10	Jam, stone fruit (30g)
40	Marmalade (30g)
90	Meat paste (5g)
40	Peanut butter (20g)
2	Sugar, white (-)
30	Syrup, golden (30g)
10	Topping, flavoured (40g)
500	Treacle, black (30g)
90	Vegemite (3g)

SWEETS

Value	Food
5	Boiled sweet (5g)
15	Butterscotch (5g)
140	Caramel (5g)

Value	Food
-	Gelatin (-)
10	Ham, canned (90g)
20	Hamburger (170g)
80	with cheese (190g)
10	Irish stew (250g)
10	Lamb, brain, boiled (150g)
7	chops, loin, grilled (inc. bone 120g)
6	cutlets, grilled (inc. bone 100g)
10	heart, roast (140g)
10	kidney, fried (100g)
8	leg, roast (120g)
10	liver, fried (130g)
9	shoulder, roast (120g)
10	tongue, stewed (100g)
20	Luncheon meat, canned (90g)
10	Meat pie (180g)
90	Moussaka (200g)
60	Pastie (160g)
9	Pork, chop, loin, grilled (100g)
10	leg, roast (120g)
15	sweet and sour (250g)
50	Pork pie (180g)
6	Rabbit, stewed (inc. bone 170g)
10	Salami, slices (3=90g)
30	Sausage, liver (60g)
20	Sausage roll (100g)
60	Sausages, beef, fried (2=120g)
70	grilled (2=120g)
30	frankfurter (2=100g)
60	pork, fried (2=120g)
50	grilled (2=120g)
20	saveloy, large (2=150g)
20	Spring roll, fried (200g)
50	Steak and kidney pie (180g)
10	Stewed steak in gravy, canned (100g)
30	Tongue, canned (100g)
150	Tripe, stewed (100g)
9	Turkey, roast (120g)
10	Veal, cutlet, fried (110g)
10	fillet, roast (100g)
25	schnitzel (140g)

MILK & MILK PRODUCTS

Value	Food
380	Cheese, camembert (25g)
800	cheddar (25g)

Calcium (mg)	Food
160	Carob bar (75g)
220	Chocolate square, milk (5g)
70	Fruit and honey bar (50g)
10	Jelly bean (5g)
60	Liquorice allsort (7g)
40	Pastille (5g)
7	Peppermint (4g)
5	Popcorn, plain unsalted (15g)
90	Sesame bar (50g)
100	Toffee, mixed (5g)

VEGETABLES

Calcium (mg)	Food
20	Artichoke, globe, boiled (100g)
10	Asparagus, boiled (5=100g)
15	Bamboo shoots (50g)
40	Beans, French, boiled (100g)
30	baked, in tomato sauce (125g)
20	broad, boiled (100g)
70	kidney (and haricot), boiled (100g)
30	mung, cooked dahl (100g)
75	soya-, boiled (100g)
30	Beetroot, slices, boiled (2=30g)
15	canned (2=30g)
80	Broccoli, boiled (100g)
30	Brussels sprouts, boiled (7=70g)
80	Cabbage, raw (50g)
50	boiled (100g)
50	Carrots, raw (50g)
40	boiled (50g)
30	young, canned (50g)
20	Cauliflower, raw (50g)
20	boiled (100g)
50	Celeriac, boiled (3=60g)
50	Celery, raw (50g)
50	boiled (50g)
60	Chickpeas, cooked dahl (60g)
20	Cucumber, slices (5=30g)
10	Egg plant, baked (½=100g)
40	Endive, raw leaves (3=15g)
60	Leeks, boiled (4=100g)
10	Lentils, split, boiled (100g)
20	Lettuce, raw leaves (2=20g)
10	Marrow, boiled (100g)
3	Mushrooms, raw (3=30g)
4	fried (6=60g)
30	Onions, raw (¼=20g)
20	boiled (100g)
60	fried (70g)
140	spring (4=20g)
330	Parsley, sprigs (2=5g)
40	Parsnip, boiled (½=60g)
20	Peas, canned (60g)
30	canned, processed (60g)
10	fresh, boiled (60g)
30	frozen, boiled (60g)
10	split, boiled (60g)
9	Peppers, green, raw (¼=15g)
9	boiled (50g)
8	Potato, baked (inc. skin 120g)
4	boiled (120g)
10	chips, fresh, fried (12=120g)
10	chips, frozen, fried (8-14=120g)
40	crisps (10=25g)
10	mashed (100g)
20	instant, cooked (100g)
5	new, boiled (2=100g)
10	new, canned (2=100g)
10	roast (120g)
40	Pumpkin (100g)
40	Radishes (2=20g)
600	Spinach, leaves, boiled (3=60g)
40	Swede, boiled (80g)
4	Sweetcorn, on cob, boiled (150g)
3	canned kernels (80g)
20	Sweet potato, boiled (100g)
10	Tomato, raw (120g)
9	canned (120g)
20	fried (120g)
10	juice, canned (120g)
60	Turnip, boiled (80g)
9	Yam, boiled (100g)

2 8
MAGNESIUM

Many enzyme (natural substances required for chemical reactions in the body) systems that are needed for the transfer of· energy within our bodies must have a supply of magnesium. Magnesium also plays a part in the normal functioning of muscles and nerves.

Magnesium occurs widely in foods, and cereals and vegetables are particularly good sources. An inadequate supply of magnesium in the diet is rare. However, deficiency can occur as a result of prolonged vomiting, diarrhoea and other gastrointestinal disorders. Chronic alcoholics frequently suffer from magnesium deficiency, which may be due to low intake and large losses in urine.

MAGNESIUM INTAKE

There is no recommended dietary intake for magnesium in Australia.

However, in the U.S.A. the recommended daily dietary intake is:

Adult men:	350 milligrams
Adult women:	300 milligrams
Pregnant and lactating women:	450 milligrams

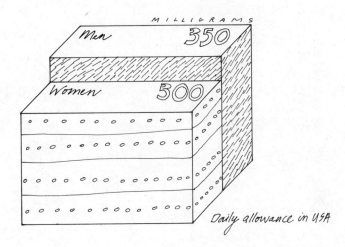

Daily allowance in USA

milligrams per 100 grams

BEVERAGES

Item	mg
Beer (240g)	7
Cider, dry, alcoholic (180g)	3
sweet, alcoholic (180g)	3
sweet, non-alcoholic (220g)	–
Cocoa powder (5g)	520
Coffee, percolated (230g)	6
Cola-type drinks (240g)	1
Cordial, diluted 1:4 (240g)	–
Drinking chocolate (10g)	150
Lemonade, carbonated drinks (240g)	Tr
Milo (10g)	210
Ovaltine (10g)	–
Port (60g)	10
Sherry, dry (60g)	10
medium (60g)	8
sweet (60g)	10
Spirits, e.g. whisky (30g)	Tr
Tea, infusion (230g)	1
Wine, red (100g)	10
white, dry (100g)	8
medium (100g)	9
sparkling (100g)	6
sweet (100g)	10

CEREALS, BISCUITS, CAKES, DESSERTS

Item	mg
Barley, pearl, boiled (–)	7
Biscuit, chocolate (20g)	40
cream-filled (20g)	–
crispbread, rye (20g)	100
wheat, starch-red. (11g)	60
gingernut (15g)	25
semi-sweet (15g)	20
short-sweet (15g)	15
Bran, wheat (8g)	520
Bread, brown, slice (25g)	80
Lebanese (pita) (¼ = 25g)	–
white, slice (25g)	30
wholemeal, slice (25g)	90
roll, brown (35g)	90
starch-reduced (35g)	60
white (35g)	30
Cake, fruit (60g)	25
plain (60g)	12

Item	mg
Egg, fried (60g)	10
omelette (100g)	20
poached (55g)	10
raw (55g)	10
scrambled (70g)	20
Macaroni cheese (180g)	20
Quiche Lorraine (150g)	20

FATS AND OILS

Item	mg
Butter, salted (10g)	–
Dripping, beef (–)	Tr
Lard (–)	1
Margarine (10g)	–
Vegetable oils (–)	Tr

FISH AND OTHER SEAFOODS

Item	mg
Bream, steamed (100g)	–
Cod, baked (100g)	30
fried in batter (100g)	20
poached (100g)	30
steamed (100g)	20
Crab, boiled (150g)	50
canned (90g)	30
Fish cakes, fried (4 = 100g)	20
fingers, fried (5 = 100g)	20
in batter, fried (120g)	25
Flounder, baked (100g)	–
Haddock, fried (100g)	30
steamed (100g)	30
Lobster, boiled (120g)	30
Mussels, boiled (12 = 120g)	30
Oysters, raw (12 = 120g)	40
Prawns, boiled (6 = 120g)	40
Roe, cod, fried (100g)	10
Salmon, canned (100g)	30
Sardines, canned (60g)	40
Scallops, steamed (10 = 100g)	40
Tuna, canned in oil (120g)	30
Whiting, crumbed, fried (100g)	30
steamed (100g)	20

FRUIT

Item	mg
Apple (inc. skin, core 100g)	4
baked, no sugar (inc. skin 110g)	2
stewed, no sugar (110g)	3
Apricots (inc. stones 3 = 100g)	10

	Value	Food
■	10	Cake, sponge (60g)
▬▬	40	Chapati (60g)
■	10	Cheesecake (120g)
–	–	Cornflakes (30g)
–	–	Crumpet (50g)
■	10	Custard (70g)
▬	20	Custard tart (120g)
▬	20	Doughnut (40g)
▬	20	Eclair (50g)
–	–	Flour, corn- (–)
▬	20	plain (–)
▬▬	40	self-raising (–)
▬▬▬▬▬▬	240	soya, full-fat (–)
▬▬▬▬▬▬▬	290	low-fat (–)
▬▬▬	140	wholemeal (–)
■	10	Fruit pie (150g)
■	10	Jam tart (35g)
ı	1	Jelly, made with water (100g)
–	–	Lamington (60g)
■	9	Lemon meringue pie (120g)
■	6	Meringue (15g)
■	10	Milk pudding (e.g. sago) (160g)
–	–	Muesli (30g)
■	10	Noodles (chow mein) (250g)
■	10	Pancake (75g)
▬	20	Pasta, macaroni, boiled (150g)
■	10	spaghetti, boiled (120g)
■	10	canned in tomato sauce (120g)
▬	20	Pastry, flaky (–)
▬	20	short crust (–)
▬	20	Pizza, cheese and tomato (150g)
■	10	Porridge (30g)
ı	4	Rice, boiled (160g)
■	10	fried (120g)
–	–	puffed (25g)
▬	20	Scone (30g)
■	10	Sponge pudding, steamed (100g)
■	10	Trifle (100g)
–	–	Wheat, breakfast biscuit (35g)
▬▬▬▬▬▬	230	Yeast, dried, baker's (–)

EGG AND CHEESE DISHES

	Value	Food
▬	20	Cauliflower cheese (100g)
▬	20	Cheese soufflé (100g)
■	10	Egg, boiled (55g)

	Value	Food
■	7	Apricots, canned (100g)
▬▬▬	70	dried (25g)
■	9	stewed, no sugar (inc. stones 110g)
▬	30	Avocado pear (½=150g)
▬▬	40	Banana (100g)
▬	30	Blackberries (100g)
▬	30	stewed, no sugar (100g)
■	10	Cantaloup (inc. skin 120g)
■	8	Cherries (inc. stones 20=100g)
■	9	stewed, no sugar (inc. stones 100g)
▬	20	Currants, black (90g)
▬▬	40	dried (15g)
■	10	red (90g)
▬▬	60	Dates, dried (6=35g)
▬	20	Figs (2=75g)
▬▬▬	90	dried (2=40g)
■	8	Fruit salad, canned (120g)
ı	3	Grapes, black (20=100g)
■	6	white (20=100g)
■	5	Grapefruit, whole (200g)
■	7	canned (100g)
■	8	juice, canned (120g)
■	6	Guavas, canned (100g)
■	10	Lemon, slices (2=15g)
■	7	juice (15g)
▬▬	30	Loganberries (100g)
■	10	canned (100g)
▬	20	stewed, no sugar (100g)
■	6	Lychees, canned (100g)
–	–	Mandarins (2=100g)
■	9	canned (50g)
▬	20	Mango (100g)
■	7	canned (100g)
■	10	Nectarines (inc. stones 3=100g)
▬	20	Olives, in brine (5=20g)
■	10	Orange, whole (130g)
■	10	juice, fresh (120g)
■	9	canned (120g)
▬	20	Passionfruit, whole (30g)
–	–	Papaw (100g)
■	8	canned (100g)
■	7	Peach (inc. stones 120g)
■	6	canned (120g)
▬▬	50	dried (25g)

Food	Magnesium (mg)
cheese spread (10g)	30
cottage (25g)	6
cream cheese (15g)	10
Danish blue (25g)	20
edam (25g)	30
parmesan (10g)	50
processed (25g)	20
stilton (25g)	30
Swiss (25g)	–
Cream, 35% fat (30g)	–
sterilized, canned (15g)	6
Ice-cream (60g)	10
non-dairy (60g)	11
Milk, cow's, cond. skim, sweet. (30g)	40
cond. whole, sweet. (30g)	10
dried, skimmed (12g)	120
dried, whole (10g)	80
evap. whole, unsweet. (30g)	30
flavoured (230g)	–
fresh, skimmed (230g)	10
fresh, whole (230g)	10
longlife, UHT (230g)	10
goat's (230g)	20
human (100g)	3
Milkshake, flavoured (340g)	–
Yoghurt, flavoured (200g)	–
fruit, low-fat (200g)	20
natural, low-fat (200g)	20
plain (200g)	–

NUTS

Food	Magnesium (mg)
Almonds (10=15g)	260
Brazil nuts (5=20g)	410
Cashews, roast (10=20g)	–
Chestnuts (4=20g)	30
Coconut, desiccated (15g)	90
Hazel nuts (10=15g)	60
Macadamia nuts (8=20g)	–
Peanuts, raw, in shells (5=25g)	130
roasted, salted (30=25g)	180
Pistachio nuts, shelled (25=15g)	–
Walnuts (5=20g)	130

SAUCES & CONDIMENTS

Food	Magnesium (mg)
Barbecue sauce (10g)	–
Chilli sauce (–)	–

Food	Magnesium (mg)
Peach, stewed, no sugar (120g)	20
Pear (inc. skin, core 120g)	5
canned (120g)	6
stewed, no sugar (120g)	3
Pineapple (80g)	20
canned (80g)	8
juice, canned (120g)	10
Plums (inc. stones 3=100g)	10
stewed, no sugar (inc. stones 100g)	9
Prunes (inc. stones 8=80g)	70
stewed, no sugar (inc. stones 120g)	40
Quince, raw (100g)	20
Raisins, dried (20g)	30
Raspberries (100g)	30
canned (100g)	10
stewed, no sugar (100g)	30
Rhubarb, stewed, no sugar (120g)	20
Strawberries (10=100g)	20
canned (100g)	20
Sultanas, dried (15g)	35
Watermelon (260g)	6

MEAT AND MEAT PRODUCTS

Food	Magnesium (mg)
Bacon rashers, middle, fried (2=40g)	20
grilled (40g)	15
Beef, corned, canned (90g)	20
fillet steak, grilled (130g)	–
mince, stewed (120g)	20
rump steak, fried (150g)	20
grilled (150g)	30
silverside, salted, boiled (120g)	20
sirloin, roast (120g)	20
stewing steak, stewed (120g)	20
topside, roast (120g)	20
Beefburger, frozen, fried (60g)	20
Beef stew (250g)	10
Bolognese sauce (100g)	20
Chicken, boiled (100g)	30
crumbed, no bone (140g)	25
roast (130g)	20
leg quarter (inc. bone 130g)	20
wing quarter (inc. bone 130g)	10
Chicken livers, fried (130g)	20
Duck, roast (100g)	20

Gelatin (–)	–
Ham, canned (90g)	20
Hamburger (170g)	–
with cheese (190g)	–
Irish stew (250g)	20
Lamb, brain, boiled (150g)	20
chops, loin, grilled (inc. bone 120g)	20
cutlets, grilled (inc. bone 100g)	20
heart, roast (140g)	40
kidney, fried (100g)	30
leg, roast (120g)	30
liver, fried (130g)	20
shoulder, roast (120g)	20
tongue, stewed (100g)	10
Luncheon meat, canned (90g)	10
Meat pie (180g)	–
Moussaka (200g)	20
Pastie (160g)	20
Pork, chop, loin, grilled (100g)	20
leg, roast (120g)	20
sweet and sour (250g)	10
Pork pie (180g)	20
Rabbit, stewed (inc. bone 170g)	10
Salami, slices (3=90g)	10
Sausage, liver (60g)	10
Sausage roll (100g)	–
Sausages, beef, fried (2=120g)	20
grilled (2=120g)	20
frankfurter (2=100g)	10
pork, fried (2=120g)	20
grilled (2=120g)	20
saveloy, large (2=150g)	10
Spring roll, fried (200g)	–
Steak and kidney pie (180g)	20
Stewed steak in gravy, canned (100g)	10
Tongue, canned (100g)	10
Tripe, stewed (100g)	20
Turkey, roast (120g)	20
Veal, cutlet, fried (110g)	30
fillet, roast (100g)	30
schnitzel (140g)	–

MILK & MILK PRODUCTS

Cheese, camembert (25g)	20
cheddar (25g)	30

Chutney, tomato (20g)	20
Curry powder (–)	–
French dressing (15g)	10
Ginger (ground) (–)	–
Mayonnaise (20g)	7
Mustard powder (–)	–
Oxo cubes (–)	60
Pepper (–)	50
Pickles, mustard (20g)	10
sweet (20g)	10
Salad cream (25g)	20
Salt, table (–)	290
Sesame seeds (–)	–
Soy sauce (–)	–
Tartare sauce (20g)	–
Tomato sauce (25g)	10
Vinegar (–)	20
Worcestershire sauce (–)	–

SOUPS (as served)

Chicken, condensed (230g)	4
Chicken noodle, dried (230g)	3
Minestrone, dried (230g)	7
Mushroom, canned (230g)	4
Tomato, condensed (230g)	8
Tomato, dried (230g)	4
Vegetable, canned (230g)	10

SUGARS, JAMS AND SPREADS

Fish paste (5g)	30
Honey (30g)	2
Jam, fruit, edible seeds (30g)	10
Jam, stone fruit (30g)	5
Marmalade (30g)	4
Meat paste (5g)	20
Peanut butter (20g)	180
Sugar, white (–)	Tr
Syrup, golden (30g)	10
Topping, flavoured (40g)	–
Treacle, black (30g)	140
Vegemite (3g)	–

SWEETS

Boiled sweet (5g)	2
Butterscotch (5g)	–
Caramel (5g)	–

Carob bar (75g)	30
Chocolate square, milk (5g)	60
Fruit and honey bar (50g)	200
Jelly bean (5g)	–
Liquorice allsort (7g)	40
Pastille (5g)	10
Peppermint (4g)	3
Popcorn, plain unsalted (15g)	1
Sesame bar (50g)	140
Toffee, mixed (5g)	30

VEGETABLES

Artichoke, globe, boiled (100g)	10
Asparagus, boiled (5=100g)	5
Bamboo shoots (50g)	–
Beans, French, boiled (100g)	10
baked, in tomato sauce (125g)	30
broad, boiled (100g)	30
kidney (and haricot), boiled (100g)	50
mung, cooked dahl (100g)	50
soya-, boiled (100g)	–
Beetroot, slices, boiled (2=30g)	20
canned (2=30g)	–
Broccoli, boiled (100g)	10
Brussels sprouts, boiled (7=70g)	10
Cabbage, raw (50g)	20
boiled (100g)	7
Carrots, raw (50g)	10
boiled (50g)	6
young, canned (50g)	5
Cauliflower, raw (50g)	10
boiled (100g)	8
Celeriac, boiled (3=60g)	10
Celery, raw (50g)	10
boiled (50g)	9
Chickpeas, cooked dahl (60g)	70
Cucumber, slices (5=30g)	9
Egg plant, baked (½=100g)	–
Endive, raw leaves (3=15g)	10
Leeks, boiled (4=100g)	10
Lentils, split, boiled (100g)	30
Lettuce, raw leaves (2=20g)	8
Marrow, boiled (100g)	7
Mushrooms, raw (3=30g)	10
fried (6=60g)	20
Onions, raw (¼=20g)	8
boiled (100g)	5
fried (70g)	20
spring (4=20g)	10
Parsley, sprigs (2=5g)	50
Parsnip, boiled (½=60g)	10
Peas, canned (60g)	20
canned, processed (60g)	20
fresh, boiled (60g)	20
frozen, boiled (60g)	20
split, boiled (60g)	30
Peppers, green, raw (¼=15g)	10
boiled (50g)	10
Potato, baked (inc. skin 120g)	20
boiled (120g)	20
chips, fresh, fried (12=120g)	40
chips, frozen, fried (8-14=120g)	30
crisps (10=25g)	60
mashed (100g)	10
instant, cooked (100g)	20
new, boiled (2=100g)	20
new, canned (2=100g)	10
roast (120g)	30
Pumpkin (100g)	8
Radishes (2=20g)	10
Spinach, leaves, boiled (3=60g)	60
Swede, boiled (80g)	7
Sweetcorn, on cob, boiled (150g)	50
canned kernels (80g)	20
Sweet potato, boiled (100g)	10
Tomato, raw (120g)	10
canned (120g)	10
fried (120g)	10
juice, canned (120g)	10
Turnip, boiled (80g)	7
Yam, boiled (100g)	10

I R O N

Iron is an essential element in the diet. It is a component of body systems that are involved in the utilization of oxygen. It forms part of haemoglobin, the red pigment in blood, which allows oxygen to be carried from the lungs to the tissues.

We cannot use all food sources of iron with equal efficiency. This means that not all of the iron consumed is available to our bodies.

Animal sources of iron are more readily utilized than those from plant foods. The recommended dietary intake for iron takes into account the varying availability of the iron from food. The presence of vitamin C in the meal can enhance the availability of iron.

Iron deficiency is the most commonly occurring nutrient deficiency. In healthy people, iron deficiency can occur in infancy, during periods of rapid growth, from menstruation, and in pregnancy. Additional amounts of iron are needed during these periods. Blood loss and disorders of the gastrointestinal tract can also lead to deficiency. Severe iron deficiency can result in anaemia.

IRON INTAKE

Recommended daily dietary intake of iron (Australia):

Infants:	4-8 milligrams
Children:	5-12 milligrams
Adult men:	10 milligrams
Adult women:	12 milligrams
Pregnancy:	15 milligrams
Lactation:	15 milligrams

TOXIC LEVEL OF INTAKE

Excessive body levels of iron can result in poisoning, although, for healthy individuals, daily intakes of 25 to 75 milligrams should not cause untoward effects. Poisoning has occurred in children who have eaten adults' iron supplements.

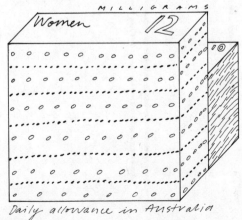

Daily allowance in Australia

milligrams per 100 grams

BEVERAGES

.01	Beer (240g)
.5	Cider, dry, alcoholic (180g)
.5	sweet, alcoholic (180g)
.5	sweet, non-alcoholic (220g)
11	Cocoa powder (5g)
Tr	Coffee, percolated (230g)
Tr	Cola-type drinks (240g)
–	Cordial, diluted 1:4 (240g)
2	Drinking chocolate (10g)
Tr	Lemonade, carbonated drinks (240g)
20	Milo (10g)
18	Ovaltine (10g)
.4	Port (60g)
.4	Sherry, dry (60g)
.5	medium (60g)
.4	sweet (60g)
Tr	Spirits, e.g. whisky (30g)
Tr	Tea, infusion (230g)
.9	Wine, red (100g)
.5	white, dry (100g)
1	medium (100g)
.5	sparkling (100g)
.6	sweet (100g)

CEREALS, BISCUITS, CAKES, DESSERTS

.2	Barley, pearl, boiled (–)
2	Biscuit, chocolate (20g)
–	cream-filled (20g)
4	crispbread, rye (20g)
5	wheat, starch-red. (11g)
4	gingernut (15g)
2	semi-sweet (15g)
2	short-sweet (15g)
13	Bran, wheat (8g)
3	Bread, brown, slice (25g)
2	Lebanese (pita) (¼=25g)
2	white, slice (25g)
3	wholemeal, slice (25g)
3	roll, brown (35g)
4	starch-reduced (35g)
2	white (35g)
2	Cake, fruit (60g)
1	plain (60g)

3	Egg, fried (60g)
2	omelette (100g)
2	poached (55g)
2	raw (55g)
2	scrambled (70g)
.4	Macaroni cheese (180g)
1	Quiche Lorraine (150g)

FATS AND OILS

–	Butter, salted (10g)
.2	Dripping, beef (–)
.1	Lard (–)
0	Margarine (10g)
Tr	Vegetable oils (–)

FISH AND OTHER SEAFOODS

.6	Bream, steamed (100g)
.4	Cod, baked (100g)
.5	fried in batter (100g)
.3	poached (100g)
.5	steamed (100g)
1	Crab, boiled (150g)
3	canned (90g)
1	Fish cakes, fried (4=100g)
.7	fingers, fried (5=100g)
.7	in batter, fried (120g)
1	Flounder, baked (100g)
1	Haddock, fried (100g)
.7	steamed (100g)
1	Lobster, boiled (120g)
8	Mussels, boiled (12=120g)
6	Oysters, raw (12=120g)
1	Prawns, boiled (6=120g)
2	Roe, cod, fried (100g)
1	Salmon, canned (100g)
2	Sardines, canned (60g)
3	Scallops, steamed (10=100g)
1	Tuna, canned in oil (120g)
.7	Whiting, crumbed, fried (100g)
1	steamed (100g)

FRUIT

.2	Apple (inc. skin, core 100g)
.2	baked, no sugar (inc. skin 110g)
.2	stewed, no sugar (110g)
.3	Apricots (inc. stones 3=100g)

Food	Iron
Apricots, canned (100g)	.7
dried (25g)	4
stewed, no sugar (inc. stones 110g)	.3
Avocado pear (½=150g)	2
Banana (100g)	.4
Blackberries (100g)	.9
stewed, no sugar (100g)	.8
Cantaloup (inc. skin 120g)	.5
Cherries (inc. stones 20 = 100g)	.3
stewed, no sugar (inc. stones 100g)	.3
Currants, black (90g)	1
dried (15g)	2
red (90g)	1
Dates, dried (6=35g)	2
Figs (2=75g)	.4
dried (2=40g)	4
Fruit salad, canned (120g)	1
Grapes, black (20=100g)	.3
white (20=100g)	.3
Grapefruit, whole (200g)	.1
canned (100g)	.7
juice, canned (120g)	.3
Guavas, canned (100g)	.5
Lemon, slices (2=15g)	.4
juice (15g)	.1
Loganberries (100g)	1
canned (100g)	1
stewed, no sugar (100g)	1
Lychees, canned (100g)	.7
Mandarins (2=100g)	.4
canned (50g)	.4
Mango (100g)	.5
Nectarines (inc. stones 3=100g)	.4
Olives, in brine (5=20g)	.8
Orange, whole (130g)	.3
juice, fresh (120g)	.3
canned (120g)	.5
Passionfruit, whole (30g)	.5
Papaw (100g)	.3
canned (100g)	.4
Peach (inc. stones 120g)	.3
canned (120g)	.4
dried (25g)	7

Food	Iron
Cake, sponge (60g)	1
Chapati (60g)	2
Cheesecake (120g)	.7
Cornflakes (30g)	9
Crumpet (50g)	-
Custard (70g)	.1
Custard tart (120g)	1
Doughnut (40g)	2
Eclair (50g)	1
Flour, corn- (-)	.5
plain (-)	1
self-raising (-)	1
soya, full-fat (-)	7
low-fat (-)	9
wholemeal (-)	3
Fruit pie (150g)	1
Jam tart (35g)	2
Jelly, made with water (100g)	.4
Lamington (60g)	2
Lemon meringue pie (120g)	1
Meringue (15g)	.1
Milk pudding (e.g. sago) (160g)	.1
Muesli (30g)	11
Noodles (chow mein) (250g)	.9
Pancake (75g)	.9
Pasta, macaroni, boiled (150g)	.5
spaghetti, boiled (120g)	.4
canned in tomato sauce (120g)	.4
Pastry, flaky (-)	2
short crust (-)	2
Pizza, cheese and tomato (150g)	1
Porridge (30g)	.5
Rice, boiled (160g)	.2
fried (120g)	.9
puffed (25g)	8
Scone (30g)	2
Sponge pudding, steamed (100g)	1
Trifle (100g)	.7
Wheat, breakfast biscuit (35g)	4
Yeast, dried, baker's (-)	20

EGG AND CHEESE DISHES

Food	Iron
Cauliflower cheese (100g)	.4
Cheese soufflé (100g)	1
Egg, boiled (55g)	2

Food	Iron
cheese spread (10g)	.7
cottage (25g)	.1
cream cheese (15g)	.1
Danish blue (25g)	.2
edam (25g)	.2
parmesan (10g)	.4
processed (25g)	.5
stilton (25g)	.5
Swiss (25g)	.9
Cream, 35% fat (30g)	–
sterilized, canned (15g)	.3
Ice-cream (60g)	.2
non-dairy (60g)	.3
Milk, cow's, cond. skim, sweet. (30g)	.3
cond. whole, sweet. (30g)	.2
dried, skimmed (12g)	.4
dried, whole (10g)	.4
evap. whole, unsweet. (30g)	.2
flavoured (230g)	.2
fresh, skimmed (230g)	.1
fresh, whole (230g)	.1
longlife, UHT (230g)	.1
goat's (230g)	.04
human (100g)	.1
Milkshake, flavoured (340g)	.3
Yoghurt, flavoured (200g)	Tr
fruit, low-fat (200g)	.2
natural, low-fat (200g)	.1
plain (200g)	Tr

NUTS

Food	Iron
Almonds (10=15g)	4
Brazil nuts (5=20g)	3
Cashews, roast (10=20g)	5
Chestnuts (4=20g)	.9
Coconut, desiccated (15g)	4
Hazel nuts (10=15g)	1
Macadamia nuts (8=20g)	2
Peanuts, raw, in shells (5=25g)	1
roasted, salted (30=25g)	2
Pistachio nuts, shelled (25=15g)	7
Walnuts (5=20g)	2

SAUCES & CONDIMENTS

Food	Iron
Barbecue sauce (10g)	.8
Chilli sauce (–)	.5

Food	Iron
Peach, stewed, no sugar (120g)	3
Pear (inc. skin, core 120g)	.1
canned (120g)	.3
stewed, no sugar (120g)	.2
Pineapple (80g)	.4
canned (80g)	.4
juice, canned (120g)	.7
Plums (inc. stones 3=100g)	.4
stewed, no sugar (inc. stones 100g)	.3
Prunes (inc. stones 8=80g)	2
stewed, no sugar (inc. stones 120g)	1
Quince, raw (100g)	.3
Raisins, dried (20g)	2
Raspberries (100g)	1
canned (100g)	2
stewed, no sugar (100g)	1
Rhubarb, stewed, no sugar (120g)	.4
Strawberries (10=100g)	.7
canned (100g)	.9
Sultanas, dried (15g)	2
Watermelon (260g)	.2

MEAT AND MEAT PRODUCTS

Food	Iron
Bacon rashers, middle, fried (2=40g)	1
grilled (40g)	2
Beef, corned, canned (90g)	3
fillet steak, grilled (130g)	4
mince, stewed (120g)	3
rump steak, fried (150g)	3
grilled (150g)	3
silverside, salted, boiled (120g)	3
sirloin, roast (120g)	2
stewing steak, stewed (120g)	3
topside, roast (120g)	3
Beefburger, frozen, fried (60g)	3
Beef stew (250g)	1
Bolognese sauce (100g)	2
Chicken, boiled (100g)	1
crumbed, no bone (140g)	1
roast (130g)	.8
leg quarter (inc. bone 130g)	.5
wing quarter (inc. bone 130g)	.4
Chicken livers, fried (130g)	9
Duck, roast (100g)	3

Food	Iron
Gelatin (–)	–
Ham, canned (90g)	1
Hamburger (170g)	2
with cheese (190g)	2
Irish stew (250g)	–
Lamb, brain, boiled (150g)	1
chops, loin, grilled (inc. bone 120g)	2
cutlets, grilled (inc. bone 100g)	1
heart, roast (140g)	8
kidney, fried (100g)	12
leg, roast (120g)	3
liver, fried (130g)	10
shoulder, roast (120g)	2
tongue, stewed (100g)	3
Luncheon meat, canned (90g)	1
Meat pie (180g)	1
Moussaka (200g)	1
Pastie (160g)	2
Pork, chop, loin, grilled (100g)	.9
leg, roast (120g)	1
sweet and sour (250g)	3
Pork pie (180g)	1
Rabbit, stewed (inc. bone 170g)	1
Salami, slices (3=90g)	1
Sausage, liver (60g)	6
Sausage roll (100g)	1
Sausages, beef, fried (2=120g)	2
grilled (2=120g)	2
frankfurter (2=100g)	2
pork, fried (2=120g)	2
grilled (2=120g)	2
saveloy, large (2=150g)	2
Spring roll, fried (200g)	.9
Steak and kidney pie (180g)	3
Stewed steak in gravy, canned (100g)	2
Tongue, canned (100g)	3
Tripe, stewed (100g)	1
Turkey, roast (120g)	.9
Veal, cutlet, fried (110g)	2
fillet, roast (100g)	2
schnitzel (140g)	3

MILK & MILK PRODUCTS

Food	Iron
Cheese, camembert (25g)	.8
cheddar (25g)	.4

Food	Iron
Chutney, tomato (20g)	1
Curry powder (–)	75
French dressing (15g)	.1
Ginger (ground) (–)	17
Mayonnaise (20g)	.7
Mustard powder (–)	11
Oxo cubes (–)	25
Pepper (–)	10
Pickles, mustard (20g)	.9
sweet (20g)	2
Salad cream (25g)	.8
Salt, table (–)	.2
Sesame seeds (–)	11
Soy sauce (–)	5
Tartare sauce (20g)	.9
Tomato sauce (25g)	.7
Vinegar (–)	.5
Worcestershire sauce (–)	6

SOUPS (as served)

Food	Iron
Chicken, condensed (230g)	.3
Chicken noodle, dried (230g)	.2
Minestrone, dried (230g)	.2
Mushroom, canned (230g)	.3
Tomato, condensed (230g)	.3
Tomato, dried (230g)	.2
Vegetable, canned (230g)	.6

SUGARS, JAMS AND SPREADS

Food	Iron
Fish paste (5g)	9
Honey (30g)	.4
Jam, fruit, edible seeds (30g)	2
Jam, stone fruit (30g)	1
Marmalade (30g)	1
Meat paste (5g)	2
Peanut butter (20g)	2
Sugar, white (–)	Tr
Syrup, golden (30g)	2
Topping, flavoured (40g)	Tr
Treacle, black (30g)	9
Vegemite (3g)	–

SWEETS

Food	Iron
Boiled sweet (5g)	.4
Butterscotch (5g)	1
Caramel (5g)	2

7	Carob bar (75g)
2	Chocolate square, milk (5g)
4	Fruit and honey bar (50g)
1	Jelly bean (5g)
8	Liquorice allsort (7g)
1	Pastille (5g)
.2	Peppermint (4g)
–	Popcorn, plain unsalted (15g)
3	Sesame bar (50g)
2	Toffee, mixed (5g)

VEGETABLES

.2	Artichoke, globe, boiled (100g)
1	Asparagus, boiled (5=100g)
.5	Bamboo shoots (50g)
1	Beans, French, boiled (100g)
1	baked, in tomato sauce (125g)
1	broad, boiled (100g)
3	kidney (and haricot), boiled (100g)
3	mung, cooked dahl (100g)
3	soya-, boiled (100g)
.4	Beetroot, slices, boiled (2=30g)
.6	canned (2=30g)
1	Broccoli, boiled (100g)
.5	Brussels sprouts, boiled (7=70g)
.9	Cabbage, raw (50g)
.7	boiled (100g)
.6	Carrots, raw (50g)
.4	boiled (50g)
1	young, canned (50g)
.5	Cauliflower, raw (50g)
.4	boiled (100g)
.8	Celeriac, boiled (3=60g)
.6	Celery, raw (50g)
.4	boiled (50g)
3	Chickpeas, cooked dahl (60g)
.3	Cucumber, slices (5=30g)
.3	Egg plant, baked (½=100g)
3	Endive, raw leaves (3=15g)
2	Leeks, boiled (4=100g)
2	Lentils, split, boiled (100g)
.9	Lettuce, raw leaves (2=20g)
.2	Marrow, boiled (100g)
1	Mushrooms, raw (3=30g)
1	fried (6=60g)

.3	Onions, raw (¼=20g)
.3	boiled (100g)
.6	fried (70g)
1	spring (4=20g)
8	Parsley, sprigs (2=5g)
.5	Parsnip, boiled (½=60g)
2	Peas, canned (60g)
2	canned, processed (60g)
1	fresh, boiled (60g)
1	frozen, boiled (60g)
2	split, boiled (60g)
.4	Peppers, green, raw (¼=15g)
.4	boiled (50g)
.6	Potato, baked (inc. skin 120g)
.3	boiled (120g)
.9	chips, fresh, fried (12=120g)
1	chips, frozen, fried (8-14=120g)
2	crisps (10=25g)
.3	mashed (100g)
.5	instant, cooked (100g)
.4	new, boiled (2=100g)
.7	new, canned (2=100g)
.7	roast (120g)
.4	Pumpkin (100g)
2	Radishes (2=20g)
4	Spinach, leaves, boiled (3=60g)
.3	Swede, boiled (80g)
.9	Sweetcorn, on cob, boiled (150g)
.6	canned kernels (80g)
.6	Sweet potato, boiled (100g)
.4	Tomato, raw (120g)
.9	canned (120g)
.5	fried (120g)
.5	juice, canned (120g)
.4	Turnip, boiled (80g)
.3	Yam, boiled (100g)

P H O S P H O R U S

Phosphorus is an important element for many essential processes in the body. In combination with calcium it is necessary for the formation of bones and teeth. Phosphorus is also involved in the metabolism of fat, carbohydrate and protein, and in the effective utilization of many of the B-group vitamins, and in energy metabolism.

Phosphorus is very widely distributed in both plant and animal foods. Because of its widespread occurrence, it is unlikely that you will have any dietary deficiency. But you could become deficient if you used large amounts of antacids for a long time. Also, people with faulty kidneys could have a deficiency of phosphorus.

PHOSPHORUS INTAKE

There is no recommended intake for phosphorus in Australia.

In the U.S.A. the allowance for adults is 800 milligrams per day. Pregnant and lactating women, and children during years of rapid growth (10 to 18 years) should have a higher intake of 1200 milligrams per day.

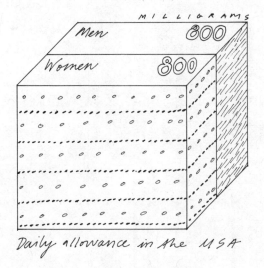

Daily allowance in the USA

milligrams per 100 grams

BEVERAGES

Beer (240g)	10
Cider, dry, alcoholic (180g)	3
sweet, alcoholic (180g)	3
sweet, non-alcoholic (220g)	9
Cocoa powder (5g)	660
Coffee, percolated (230g)	2
Cola-type drinks (240g)	Tr
Cordial, diluted 1:4 (240g)	–
Drinking chocolate (10g)	190
Lemonade, carbonated drinks (240g)	Tr
Milo (10g)	625
Ovaltine (10g)	400
Port (60g)	10
Sherry, dry (60g)	10
medium (60g)	7
sweet (60g)	10
Spirits, e.g. whisky (30g)	Tr
Tea, infusion (230g)	1
Wine, red (100g)	10
white, dry (100g)	6
medium (100g)	8
sparkling (100g)	7
sweet (100g)	10

CEREALS, BISCUITS, CAKES, DESSERTS

Barley, pearl, boiled (–)	70
Biscuit, chocolate (20g)	130
cream-filled (20g)	–
crispbread, rye (20g)	310
wheat, starch-red. (11g)	220
gingernut (15g)	90
semi-sweet (15g)	85
short-sweet (15g)	85
Bran, wheat (8g)	1200
Bread, brown, slice (25g)	160
Lebanese (pita) (¼=25g)	–
white, slice (25g)	70
wholemeal, slice (25g)	200
roll, brown (35g)	160
starch-reduced (35g)	190
white (35g)	70
Cake, fruit (60g)	110
plain (60g)	120

Egg, fried (60g)	260
omelette (100g)	190
poached (55g)	240
raw (55g)	220
scrambled (70g)	190
Macaroni cheese (180g)	140
Quiche Lorraine (150g)	240

FATS AND OILS

Butter, salted (10g)	–
Dripping, beef (–)	10
Lard (–)	3
Margarine (10g)	20
Vegetable oils (–)	Tr

FISH AND OTHER SEAFOODS

Bream, steamed (100g)	240
Cod, baked (100g)	190
fried in batter (100g)	200
poached (100g)	180
steamed (100g)	240
Crab, boiled (150g)	350
canned (90g)	140
Fish cakes, fried (4=100g)	110
fingers, fried (5=100g)	220
in batter, fried (120g)	–
Flounder, baked (100g)	245
Haddock, fried (100g)	250
steamed (100g)	230
Lobster, boiled (120g)	280
Mussels, boiled (12=120g)	330
Oysters, raw (12=120g)	270
Prawns, boiled (6=120g)	350
Roe, cod, fried (100g)	500
Salmon, canned (100g)	240
Sardines, canned (60g)	430
Scallops, steamed (10=100g)	340
Tuna, canned in oil (120g)	190
Whiting, crumbed, fried (100g)	260
steamed (100g)	190

FRUIT

Apple (inc. skin, core 100g)	6
baked, no sugar (inc. skin 110g)	10
stewed, no sugar (110g)	10
Apricots (inc. stones 3=100g)	20

Value	Food
150	Cake, sponge (60g)
130	Chapati (60g)
90	Cheesecake (120g)
60	Cornflakes (30g)
–	Crumpet (50g)
110	Custard (70g)
100	Custard tart (120g)
60	Doughnut (40g)
70	Eclair (50g)
30	Flour, corn- (–)
90	plain (–)
480	self-raising (–)
600	soya, full-fat (–)
640	low-fat (–)
370	wholemeal (–)
60	Fruit pie (150g)
50	Jam tart (35g)
2	Jelly, made with water (100g)
140	Lamington (60g)
70	Lemon meringue pie (120g)
20	Meringue (15g)
110	Milk pudding (e.g. sago) (160g)
–	Muesli (30g)
–	Noodles (chow mein) (250g)
120	Pancake (75g)
50	Pasta, macaroni, boiled (150g)
40	spaghetti, boiled (120g)
30	canned in tomato sauce (120g)
70	Pastry, flaky (–)
80	short crust (–)
170	Pizza, cheese and tomato (150g)
40	Porridge (30g)
35	Rice, boiled (160g)
–	fried (120g)
260	puffed (25g)
470	Scone (30g)
190	Sponge pudding, steamed (100g)
90	Trifle (100g)
–	Wheat, breakfast biscuit (35g)
1290	Yeast, dried, baker's (–)

EGG AND CHEESE DISHES

Value	Food
120	Cauliflower cheese (100g)
230	Cheese soufflé (100g)
220	Egg, boiled (55g)

Value	Food
10	Apricots, canned (100g)
120	dried (25g)
20	stewed, no sugar (inc. stones 110g)
30	Avocado pear (½=150g)
30	Banana (100g)
20	Blackberries (100g)
20	stewed, no sugar (100g)
20	Cantaloup (inc. skin 120g)
20	Cherries (inc. stones 20=100g)
20	stewed, no sugar (inc. stones 100g)
40	Currants, black (90g)
40	dried (15g)
30	red (90g)
60	Dates, dried (6=35g)
30	Figs (2=75g)
90	dried (2=40g)
10	Fruit salad, canned (120g)
10	Grapes, black (20=100g)
20	white (20=100g)
8	Grapefruit, whole (200g)
10	canned (100g)
10	juice, canned (120g)
10	Guavas, canned (100g)
20	Lemon, slices (2=15g)
10	juice (15g)
20	Loganberries (100g)
20	canned (100g)
20	stewed, no sugar (100g)
10	Lychees, canned (100g)
20	Mandarins (2=100g)
10	canned (50g)
10	Mango (100g)
10	canned (100g)
20	Nectarines (inc. stones 3=100g)
10	Olives, in brine (5=20g)
20	Orange, whole (130g)
20	juice, fresh (120g)
20	canned (120g)
20	Passionfruit, whole (30g)
15	Papaw (100g)
6	canned (100g)
20	Peach (inc. stones 120g)
10	canned (120g)
120	dried (25g)

440	cheese spread (10g)
140	cottage (25g)
100	cream cheese (15g)
430	Danish blue (25g)
520	edam (25g)
770	parmesan (10g)
490	processed (25g)
300	stilton (25g)
605	Swiss (25g)
–	Cream, 35% fat (30g)
40	sterilized, canned (15g)
100	Ice-cream (60g)
90	non-dairy (60g)
270	Milk, cow's, cond. skim, sweet. (30g)
220	cond. whole, sweet. (30g)
950	dried, skimmed (12g)
740	dried, whole (10g)
250	evap. whole, unsweet. (30g)
95	flavoured (230g)
100	fresh, skimmed (230g)
100	fresh, whole (230g)
100	longlife, UHT (230g)
110	goat's (230g)
10	human (100g)
95	Milkshake, flavoured (340g)
95	Yoghurt, flavoured (200g)
140	fruit, low-fat (200g)
140	natural, low-fat (200g)
100	plain (200g)

NUTS

440	Almonds (10 = 15g)
590	Brazil nuts (5 = 20g)
400	Cashews, roast (10 = 20g)
70	Chestnuts (4 = 20g)
160	Coconut, desiccated (15g)
230	Hazel nuts (10 = 15g)
200	Macadamia nuts (8 = 20g)
250	Peanuts, raw, in shells (5 = 25g)
370	roasted, salted (30 = 25g)
500	Pistachio nuts, shelled (25 = 15g)
510	Walnuts (5 = 20g)

SAUCES & CONDIMENTS

20	Barbecue sauce (10g)
15	Chilli sauce (–)

40	Peach, stewed, no sugar (120g)
7	Pear (inc. skin, core 120g)
5	canned (120g)
10	stewed, no sugar (120g)
8	Pineapple (80g)
5	canned (80g)
10	juice, canned (120g)
20	Plums (inc. stones 3 = 100g)
10	stewed, no sugar (inc. stones 100g)
70	Prunes (inc. stones 8 = 80g)
40	stewed, no sugar (inc. stones 120g)
20	Quince, raw (100g)
30	Raisins, dried (20g)
30	Raspberries (100g)
10	canned (100g)
30	stewed, no sugar (100g)
20	Rhubarb, stewed, no sugar (120g)
20	Strawberries (10 = 100g)
20	canned (100g)
100	Sultanas, dried (15g)
4	Watermelon (260g)

MEAT AND MEAT PRODUCTS

170	Bacon rashers, middle, fried (2 = 40g)
160	grilled (40g)
120	Beef, corned, canned (90g)
265	fillet steak, grilled (130g)
170	mince, stewed (120g)
220	rump steak, fried (150g)
220	grilled (150g)
140	silverside, salted, boiled (120g)
170	sirloin, roast (120g)
160	stewing steak, stewed (120g)
200	topside, roast (120g)
250	Beefburger, frozen, fried (60g)
70	Beef stew (250g)
80	Bolognese sauce (100g)
190	Chicken, boiled (100g)
–	crumbed, no bone (140g)
170	roast (130g)
130	leg quarter (inc. bone 130g)
110	wing quarter (inc. bone 130g)
350	Chicken livers, fried (130g)
150	Duck, roast (100g)

Food	Phosphorus (mg)
Gelatin (–)	–
Ham, canned (90g)	280
Hamburger (170g)	–
with cheese (190g)	–
Irish stew (250g)	60
Lamb, brain, boiled (150g)	320
chops, loin, grilled (inc. bone 120g)	160
cutlets, grilled (inc. bone 100g)	130
heart, roast (140g)	390
kidney, fried (100g)	360
leg, roast (120g)	200
liver, fried (130g)	400
shoulder, roast (120g)	150
tongue, stewed (100g)	200
Luncheon meat, canned (90g)	200
Meat pie (180g)	–
Moussaka (200g)	130
Pastie (160g)	110
Pork, chop, loin, grilled (100g)	180
leg, roast (120g)	200
sweet and sour (250g)	–
Pork pie (180g)	120
Rabbit, stewed (inc. bone 170g)	100
Salami, slices (3=90g)	160
Sausage, liver (60g)	230
Sausage roll (100g)	–
Sausages, beef, fried (2=120g)	210
grilled (2=120g)	210
frankfurter (2=100g)	130
pork, fried (2=120g)	210
grilled (2=120g)	210
saveloy, large (2=150g)	210
Spring roll, fried (200g)	–
Steak and kidney pie (180g)	110
Stewed steak in gravy, canned (100g)	100
Tongue, canned (100g)	140
Tripe, stewed (100g)	90
Turkey, roast (120g)	200
Veal, cutlet, fried (110g)	280
fillet, roast (100g)	360
schnitzel (140g)	225

MILK & MILK PRODUCTS

Food	Phosphorus (mg)
Cheese, camembert (25g)	290
cheddar (25g)	520

Food	Phosphorus (mg)
Chutney, tomato (20g)	40
Curry powder (–)	260
French dressing (15g)	8
Ginger (ground) (–)	135
Mayonnaise (20g)	60
Mustard powder (–)	175
Oxo cubes (–)	360
Pepper (–)	130
Pickles, mustard (20g)	20
sweet (20g)	10
Salad cream (25g)	90
Salt, table (–)	8
Sesame seeds (–)	615
Soy sauce (–)	105
Tartare sauce (20g)	40
Tomato sauce (25g)	40
Vinegar (–)	30
Worcestershire sauce (–)	60

SOUPS (as served)

Food	Phosphorus (mg)
Chicken, condensed (230g)	20
Chicken noodle, dried (230g)	10
Minestrone, dried (230g)	10
Mushroom, canned (230g)	30
Tomato, canned (230g)	20
Tomato, dried (230g)	10
Vegetable, canned (230g)	30

SUGARS, JAMS AND SPREADS

Food	Phosphorus (mg)
Fish paste (5g)	310
Honey (30g)	20
Jam, fruit, edible seeds (30g)	20
Jam, stone fruit (30g)	20
Marmalade (30g)	10
Meat paste (5g)	170
Peanut butter (20g)	330
Sugar, white (–)	Tr
Syrup, golden (30g)	20
Topping, flavoured (40g)	–
Treacle, black (30g)	30
Vegemite (3g)	1080

SWEETS

Food	Phosphorus (mg)
Boiled sweet (5g)	10
Butterscotch (5g)	5
Caramel (5g)	105

Food	Phosphorus
Carob bar (75g)	-
Chocolate square, milk (5g)	240
Fruit and honey bar (50g)	-
Jelly bean (5g)	2
Liquorice allsort (7g)	30
Pastille (5g)	Tr
Peppermint (4g)	Tr
Popcorn, plain unsalted (15g)	135
Sesame bar (50g)	-
Toffee, mixed (5g)	60

VEGETABLES

Food	Phosphorus
Artichoke, globe, boiled (100g)	20
Asparagus, boiled (5=100g)	40
Bamboo shoots (50g)	60
Beans, French, boiled (100g)	20
baked, in tomato sauce (125g)	90
broad, boiled (100g)	100
kidney (and haricot), boiled (100g)	120
mung, cooked dahl (100g)	100
soya-, boiled (100g)	180
Beetroot, slices, boiled (2=30g)	40
canned (2=30g)	20
Broccoli, boiled (100g)	60
Brussels sprouts, boiled (7=70g)	50
Cabbage, raw (50g)	70
boiled (100g)	30
Carrots, raw (50g)	20
boiled (50g)	20
young, canned (50g)	20
Cauliflower, raw (50g)	50
boiled (100g)	30
Celeriac, boiled (3=60g)	70
Celery, raw (50g)	30
boiled (50g)	20
Chickpeas, cooked dahl (60g)	130
Cucumber, slices (5=30g)	70
Egg plant, baked (½=100g)	25
Endive, raw leaves (3=15g)	70
Leeks, boiled (4=100g)	30
Lentils, split, boiled (100g)	80
Lettuce, raw leaves (2=20g)	30
Marrow, boiled (100g)	10
Mushrooms, raw (3=30g)	140
fried (6=60g)	170
Onions, raw (¼=20g)	30
boiled (100g)	20
fried (70g)	60
spring (4=20g)	25
Parsley, sprigs (2=5g)	130
Parsnip, boiled (½=60g)	30
Peas, canned (60g)	70
canned, processed (60g)	90
fresh, boiled (60g)	80
frozen, boiled (60g)	80
split, boiled (60g)	120
Peppers, green, raw (¼=15g)	30
boiled (50g)	20
Potato, baked (inc. skin 120g)	40
boiled (120g)	30
chips, fresh, fried (12=120g)	70
chips, frozen, fried (8-14=120g)	80
crisps (10=25g)	130
mashed (100g)	30
instant, cooked (100g)	50
new, boiled (2=100g)	30
new, canned (2=100g)	30
roast (120g)	50
Pumpkin (100g)	20
Radishes (2=20g)	30
Spinach, leaves, boiled (3=60g)	90
Swede, boiled (80g)	20
Sweetcorn, on cob, boiled (150g)	120
canned kernels (80g)	70
Sweet potato, boiled (100g)	40
Tomato, raw (120g)	20
canned (120g)	20
fried (120g)	30
juice, canned (120g)	20
Turnip, boiled (80g)	20
Yam, boiled (100g)	30

3 1
S U L P H U R

We obtain most of our sulphur from proteins in the
diet. The essential amino acid methionine (see page
67) is one of several sulphur-containing components
of protein. The proteins are broken down into their
constituent amino acids, and the sulphur-containing
amino acids are reused for the formation of body proteins needed for growth, tissue maintenance and
enzyme production. New sulphur-containing compounds are also made by our bodies from the protein
components. Some of these have metabolic function,
and some are used to remove potentially toxic substances, including certain drugs, from the body.

SULPHUR INTAKE

There is no recommended dietary intake for sulphur.
The sulphur that is essential for the functions
described above is provided by protein and is
included in the recommended dietary intake for protein.

milligrams per 100 grams

BEVERAGES

Beer (240g)	–
Cider, dry, alcoholic (180g)	–
sweet, alcoholic (180g)	–
sweet, non-alcoholic (220g)	–
Cocoa powder (5g)	–
Coffee, percolated (230g)	–
Cola-type drinks (240g)	–
Cordial, diluted 1:4 (240g)	–
Drinking chocolate (10g)	–
Lemonade, carbonated drinks (240g)	–
Milo (10g)	–
Ovaltine (10g)	–
Port (60g)	–
Sherry, dry (60g)	–
medium (60g)	–
sweet (60g)	–
Spirits, e.g. whisky (30g)	Tr
Tea, infusion (230g)	–
Wine, red (100g)	–
white, dry (100g)	–
medium (100g)	–
sparkling (100g)	–
sweet (100g)	–

CEREALS, BISCUITS, CAKES, DESSERTS

Barley, pearl, boiled (–)	35
Biscuit, chocolate (20g)	–
cream-filled (20g)	–
crispbread, rye (20g)	–
wheat, starch-red. (11g)	–
gingernut (15g)	–
semi-sweet (15g)	–
short-sweet (15g)	–
Bran, wheat (8g)	65
Bread, brown, slice (25g)	90
Lebanese (pita) (¼=25g)	–
white, slice (25g)	80
wholemeal, slice (25g)	80
roll, brown (35g)	170
starch-reduced (35g)	–
white (35g)	150
Cake, fruit (60g)	–
plain (60g)	–

Egg, fried (60g)	210
omelette (100g)	160
poached (55g)	180
raw (55g)	180
scrambled (70g)	150
Macaroni cheese (180g)	–
Quiche Lorraine (150g)	–

FATS AND OILS

Butter, salted (10g)	–
Dripping, beef (–)	10
Lard (–)	30
Margarine (10g)	–
Vegetable oils (–)	Tr

FISH AND OTHER SEAFOODS

Bream, steamed (100g)	–
Cod, baked (100g)	230
fried in batter (100g)	–
poached (100g)	250
steamed (100g)	210
Crab, boiled (150g)	470
canned (90g)	–
Fish cakes, fried (4=100g)	–
fingers, fried (5=100g)	–
in batter, fried (120g)	–
Flounder, baked (100g)	–
Haddock, fried (100g)	290
steamed (100g)	300
Lobster, boiled (120g)	510
Mussels, boiled (12=120g)	350
Oysters, raw (12=120g)	250
Prawns, boiled (6=120g)	370
Roe, cod, fried (100g)	240
Salmon, canned (100g)	220
Sardines, canned (60g)	260
Scallops, steamed (10=100g)	570
Tuna, canned in oil (120g)	–
Whiting, crumbed, fried (100g)	270
steamed (100g)	310

FRUIT

Apple (inc. skin, core 100g)	5
baked, no sugar (inc. skin 110g)	2
stewed, no sugar (110g)	3
Apricots (inc. stones 3=100g)	6

Apricots, canned (100g)	1
dried (25g)	160
stewed, no sugar (inc. stones 110g)	5
Avocado pear (½=150g)	20
Banana (100g)	10
Blackberries (100g)	10
stewed, no sugar (100g)	10
Cantaloup (inc. skin 120g)	7
Cherries (inc. stones 20=100g)	6
stewed, no sugar (inc. stones 100g)	10
Currants, black (90g)	30
dried (15g)	30
red (90g)	30
Dates, dried (6=35g)	50
Figs (2=75g)	10
dried (2=40g)	80
Fruit salad, canned (120g)	2
Grapes, black (20=100g)	6
white (20=100g)	10
Grapefruit, whole (200g)	3
canned (100g)	–
juice, canned (120g)	–
Guavas, canned (100g)	–
Lemon, slices (2=15g)	10
juice (15g)	2
Loganberries (100g)	20
canned (100g)	3
stewed, no sugar (100g)	20
Lychees, canned (100g)	–
Mandarins (2=100g)	–
canned (50g)	–
Mango (100g)	–
canned (100g)	–
Nectarines (inc. stones 3=100g)	10
Olives, in brine (5=20g)	30
Orange, whole (130g)	7
juice, fresh (120g)	5
canned (120g)	–
Passionfruit, whole (30g)	8
Papaw (100g)	–
canned (100g)	–
Peach (inc. stones 120g)	5
canned (120g)	1
dried (25g)	240

Cake, sponge (60g)	–
Chapati (60g)	–
Cheesecake (120g)	–
Cornflakes (30g)	–
Crumpet (50g)	–
Custard (70g)	40
Custard tart (120g)	–
Doughnut (40g)	60
Eclair (50g)	–
Flour, corn- (–)	–
plain (–)	–
self-raising (–)	–
soya, full-fat (–)	–
low-fat (–)	–
wholemeal (–)	–
Fruit pie (150g)	–
Jam tart (35g)	–
Jelly, made with water (100g)	10
Lamington (60g)	–
Lemon meringue pie (120g)	–
Meringue (15g)	110
Milk pudding (e.g. sago) (160g)	40
Muesli (30g)	–
Noodles (chow mein) (250g)	–
Pancake (75g)	–
Pasta, macaroni, boiled (150g)	30
spaghetti, boiled (120g)	30
canned in tomato sauce (120g)	–
Pastry, flaky (–)	–
short crust (–)	–
Pizza, cheese and tomato (150g)	–
Porridge (30g)	20
Rice, boiled (160g)	30
fried (120g)	–
puffed (25g)	–
Scone (30g)	–
Sponge pudding, steamed (100g)	–
Trifle (100g)	–
Wheat, breakfast biscuit (35g)	–
Yeast, dried, baker's (–)	–

EGG AND CHEESE DISHES

Cauliflower cheese (100g)	–
Cheese soufflé (100g)	–
Egg, boiled (55g)	180

	Food
90	Peach, stewed, no sugar (120g)
4	Pear (inc. skin, core 120g)
1	canned (120g)
3	stewed, no sugar (120g)
3	Pineapple (80g)
3	canned (80g)
–	juice, canned (120g)
6	Plums (inc. stones 3=100g)
5	stewed, no sugar (inc. stones 100g)
20	Prunes (inc. stones 8=80g)
10	stewed, no sugar (inc. stones 120g)
5	Quince, raw (100g)
20	Raisins, dried (20g)
20	Raspberries (100g)
–	canned (100g)
20	stewed, no sugar (100g)
7	Rhubarb, stewed, no sugar (120g)
10	Strawberries (10=100g)
–	canned (100g)
40	Sultanas, dried (15g)
–	Watermelon (260g)

MEAT AND MEAT PRODUCTS

	Food
–	Bacon rashers, middle, fried (2=40g)
–	grilled (40g)
240	Beef, corned, canned (90g)
–	fillet steak, grilled (130g)
220	mince, stewed (120g)
–	rump steak, fried (150g)
–	grilled (150g)
–	silverside, salted, boiled (120g)
–	sirloin, roast (120g)
–	stewing steak, stewed (120g)
–	topside, roast (120g)
220	Beefburger, frozen, fried (60g)
–	Beef stew (250g)
80	Bolognese sauce (100g)
300	Chicken, boiled (100g)
–	crumbed, no bone (140g)
–	roast (130g)
160	leg quarter (inc. bone 130g)
130	wing quarter (inc. bone 130g)
250	Chicken livers, fried (130g)
–	Duck, roast (100g)

	Food
–	cheese spread (10g)
–	cottage (25g)
–	cream cheese (15g)
–	Danish blue (25g)
–	edam (25g)
250	parmesan (10g)
–	processed (25g)
230	stilton (25g)
–	Swiss (25g)
–	Cream, 35% fat (30g)
–	sterilized, canned (15g)
–	Ice-cream (60g)
–	non-dairy (60g)
90	Milk, cow's, cond. skim, sweet. (30g)
80	cond. whole, sweet. (30g)
320	dried, skimmed (12g)
240	dried, whole (10g)
80	evap. whole, unsweet. (30g)
–	flavoured (230g)
30	fresh, skimmed (230g)
30	fresh, whole (230g)
30	longlife, UHT (230g)
–	goat's (230g)
–	human (100g)
–	Milkshake, flavoured (340g)
–	Yoghurt, flavoured (200g)
–	fruit, low-fat (200g)
–	natural, low-fat (200g)
–	plain (200g)

NUTS

	Food
150	Almonds (10=15g)
290	Brazil nuts (5=20g)
–	Cashews, roast (10=20g)
30	Chestnuts (4=20g)
80	Coconut, desiccated (15g)
80	Hazel nuts (10=15g)
–	Macadamia nuts (8=20g)
260	Peanuts, raw, in shells (5=25g)
380	roasted, salted (30=25g)
–	Pistachio nuts, shelled (25=15g)
100	Walnuts (5=20g)

SAUCES & CONDIMENTS

	Food
–	Barbecue sauce (10g)
–	Chilli sauce (–)

Gelatin (–)	–
Ham, canned (90g)	180
Hamburger (170g)	–
with cheese (190g)	–
Irish stew (250g)	–
Lamb, brain, boiled (150g)	–
chops, loin, grilled (inc. bone 120g)	–
cutlets, grilled (inc. bone 100g)	–
heart, roast (140g)	300
kidney, fried (100g)	290
leg, roast (120g)	–
liver, fried (130g)	270
shoulder, roast (120g)	–
tongue, stewed (100g)	190
Luncheon meat, canned (90g)	120
Meat pie (180g)	–
Moussaka (200g)	100
Pastie (160g)	100
Pork, chop, loin, grilled (100g)	–
leg, roast (120g)	–
sweet and sour (250g)	–
Pork pie (180g)	100
Rabbit, stewed (inc. bone 170g)	130
Salami, slices (3 = 90g)	190
Sausage, liver (60g)	130
Sausage roll (100g)	–
Sausages, beef, fried (2 = 120g)	140
grilled (2 = 120g)	140
frankfurter (2 = 100g)	90
pork, fried (2 = 120g)	160
grilled (2 = 120g)	160
saveloy, large (2 = 150g)	90
Spring roll, fried (200g)	–
Steak and kidney pie (180g)	–
Stewed steak in gravy, canned (100g)	130
Tongue, canned (100g)	210
Tripe, stewed (100g)	140
Turkey, roast (120g)	–
Veal, cutlet, fried (110g)	330
fillet, roast (100g)	330
schnitzel (140g)	–

MILK & MILK PRODUCTS

Cheese, camembert (25g)	–
cheddar (25g)	230
Chutney, tomato (20g)	30
Curry powder (–)	–
French dressing (15g)	6
Ginger (ground) (–)	–
Mayonnaise (20g)	20
Mustard powder (–)	–
Oxo cubes (–)	–
Pepper (–)	100
Pickles, mustard (20g)	–
sweet (20g)	–
Salad cream (25g)	–
Salt, table (–)	20
Sesame seeds (–)	–
Soy sauce (–)	–
Tartare sauce (20g)	–
Tomato sauce (25g)	–
Vinegar (–)	20
Worcestershire sauce (–)	–

SOUPS (as served)

Chicken, condensed (230g)	–
Chicken noodle, dried (230g)	–
Minestrone, dried (230g)	–
Mushroom, canned (230g)	–
Tomato, canned (230g)	–
Tomato, condensed (230g)	–
Tomato, dried (230g)	–
Vegetable, canned (230g)	–

SUGARS, JAMS AND SPREADS

Fish paste (5g)	–
Honey (30g)	1
Jam, fruit, edible seeds (30g)	7
Jam, stone fruit (30g)	3
Marmalade (30g)	2
Meat paste (5g)	150
Peanut butter (20g)	–
Sugar, white (–)	Tr
Syrup, golden (30g)	50
Topping, flavoured (40g)	–
Treacle, black (30g)	70
Vegemite (3g)	–

SWEETS

Boiled sweet (5g)	–
Butterscotch (5g)	–
Caramel (5g)	–

Carob bar (75g)	–
Chocolate square, milk (5g)	–
Fruit and honey bar (50g)	–
Jelly bean (5g)	–
Liquorice allsort (7g)	–
Pastille (5g)	–
Peppermint (4g)	–
Popcorn, plain unsalted (15g)	–
Sesame bar (50g)	–
Toffee, mixed (5g)	–

VEGETABLES

Artichoke, globe, boiled (100g)	10
Asparagus, boiled (5=100g)	20
Bamboo shoots (50g)	–
Beans, French, boiled (100g)	10
baked, in tomato sauce (125g)	40
broad, boiled (100g)	30
kidney (and haricot), boiled (100g)	50
mung, cooked dahl (100g)	60
soya-, boiled (100g)	–
Beetroot, slices, boiled (2=30g)	20
canned (2=30g)	–
Broccoli, boiled (100g)	–
Brussels sprouts, boiled (7=70g)	80
Cabbage, raw (50g)	90
boiled (100g)	30
Carrots, raw (50g)	10
boiled (50g)	10
young, canned (50g)	–
Cauliflower, raw (50g)	–
boiled (100g)	–
Celeriac, boiled (3=60g)	10
Celery, raw (50g)	20
boiled (50g)	10
Chickpeas, cooked dahl (60g)	80
Cucumber, slices (5=30g)	10
Egg plant, baked (½=100g)	–
Endive, raw leaves (3=15g)	30
Leeks, boiled (4=100g)	50
Lentils, split, boiled (100g)	40
Lettuce, raw leaves (2=20g)	–
Marrow, boiled (100g)	10
Mushrooms, raw (3=30g)	30
fried (6=60g)	70
Onions, raw (¼=20g)	50
boiled (100g)	20
fried (70g)	90
spring (4=20g)	50
Parsley, sprigs (2=5g)	–
Parsnip, boiled (½=60g)	20
Peas, canned (60g)	–
canned, processed (60g)	–
fresh, boiled (60g)	40
frozen, boiled (60g)	–
split, boiled (60g)	50
Peppers, green, raw (¼=15g)	–
boiled (50g)	–
Potato, baked (inc. skin 120g)	30
boiled (120g)	20
chips, fresh, fried (12=120g)	50
chips, frozen, fried (8-14=120g)	–
crisps (10=25g)	–
mashed (100g)	20
instant, cooked (100g)	–
new, boiled (2=100g)	20
new, canned (2=100g)	–
roast (120g)	60
Pumpkin (100g)	10
Radishes (2=20g)	40
Spinach, leaves, boiled (3=60g)	90
Swede, boiled (80g)	30
Sweetcorn, on cob, boiled (150g)	–
canned kernels (80g)	–
Sweet potato, boiled (100g)	20
Tomato, raw (120g)	10
canned (120g)	–
fried (120g)	10
juice, canned (120g)	–
Turnip, boiled (80g)	20
Yam, boiled (100g)	–

32
CHLORINE

Chlorine is present in food and our body almost entirely in the form of chloride. Chloride is important in maintaining water balance, and is an essential component of gastric juice. We get our supplies of chlorine from food mainly in the form of sodium chloride (salt).

Dietary deficiency of chlorine is rare and is only likely to occur if you have excessive losses from your body. This can result from prolonged vomiting, diarrhoea or profuse sweating. If you are on a severe sodium-restricted diet it may be necessary to obtain chlorine from other sources.

CHLORINE INTAKE

There is no recommended dietary intake for chlorine in Australia. For the average adult an estimated safe and adequate amount of chlorine is closely related to that for sodium and is in the range of 1700 to 5100 milligrams of chlorine per day. To keep to this level, most of us would need to reduce the amount of salt used in cooking or added at the table. Additionally, highly salted foods should be avoided.

milligrams per 100 grams

BEVERAGES

Food	Cl (mg)
Beer (240g)	–
Cider, dry, alcoholic (180g)	6
sweet, alcoholic (180g)	6
sweet, non-alcoholic (220g)	–
Cocoa powder (5g)	460
Coffee, percolated (230g)	Tr
Cola-type drinks (240g)	10
Cordial, diluted 1:4 (240g)	–
Drinking chocolate (10g)	130
Lemonade, carbonated drinks (240g)	Tr
Milo (10g)	–
Ovaltine (10g)	–
Port (60g)	8
Sherry, dry (60g)	10
medium (60g)	7
sweet (60g)	10
Spirits, e.g. whisky (30g)	Tr
Tea, infusion (230g)	Tr
Wine, red (100g)	20
white, dry (100g)	10
medium (100g)	4
sparkling (100g)	7
sweet (100g)	7

CEREALS, BISCUITS, CAKES, DESSERTS

Food	Cl (mg)
Barley, pearl, boiled (–)	35
Biscuit, chocolate (20g)	250
cream-filled (20g)	–
crispbread, rye (20g)	370
wheat, starch-red. (11g)	980
gingernut (15g)	320
semi-sweet (15g)	520
short-sweet (15g)	490
Bran, wheat (8g)	150
Bread, brown, slice (25g)	880
Lebanese (pita) (¼=25g)	–
white, slice (25g)	890
wholemeal, slice (25g)	860
roll, brown (35g)	1030
starch-reduced (35g)	980
white (35g)	1040
Cake, fruit (60g)	320
plain (60g)	500

Food	Cl (mg)
Egg, fried (60g)	200
omelette (100g)	1540
poached (55g)	160
raw (55g)	160
scrambled (70g)	1580
Macaroni cheese (180g)	480
Quiche Lorraine (150g)	970

FATS AND OILS

Food	Cl (mg)
Butter, salted (10g)	1300
Dripping, beef (–)	2
Lard (–)	4
Margarine (10g)	–
Vegetable oils (–)	Tr

FISH AND OTHER SEAFOODS

Food	Cl (mg)
Bream, steamed (100g)	–
Cod, baked (100g)	520
fried in batter (100g)	150
poached (100g)	150
steamed (100g)	120
Crab, boiled (150g)	570
canned (90g)	830
Fish cakes, fried (4=100g)	730
fingers, fried (5=100g)	400
in batter, fried (120g)	–
Flounder, baked (100g)	–
Haddock, fried (100g)	180
steamed (100g)	140
Lobster, boiled (120g)	530
Mussels, boiled (12=120g)	320
Oysters, raw (12=120g)	820
Prawns, boiled (6=120g)	2550
Roe, cod, fried (100g)	190
Salmon, canned (100g)	880
Sardines, canned (60g)	830
Scallops, steamed (10=100g)	410
Tuna, canned in oil (120g)	690
Whiting, crumbed, fried (100g)	190
steamed (100g)	90

FRUIT

Food	Cl (mg)
Apple (inc. skin, core 100g)	1
baked, no sugar (inc. skin 110g)	4
stewed, no sugar (110g)	4
Apricots (inc. stones 3=100g)	Tr

Chlorine (mg)	Food
2	Apricots, canned (100g)
40	dried (25g)
Tr	stewed, no sugar (inc. stones 110g)
6	Avocado pear (½=150g)
80	Banana (100g)
20	Blackberries (100g)
20	stewed, no sugar (100g)
30	Cantaloup (inc. skin 120g)
Tr	Cherries (inc. stones 20=100g)
Tr	stewed, no sugar (inc. stones 100g)
20	Currants, black (90g)
20	dried (15g)
10	red (90g)
290	Dates, dried (6=35g)
20	Figs (2=75g)
170	dried (2=40g)
3	Fruit salad, canned (120g)
Tr	Grapes, black (20=100g)
Tr	white (20=100g)
1	Grapefruit, whole (200g)
5	canned (100g)
10	juice, canned (120g)
10	Guavas, canned (100g)
5	Lemon, slices (2=15g)
3	juice (15g)
20	Loganberries (100g)
5	canned (100g)
20	stewed, no sugar (100g)
5	Lychees, canned (100g)
–	Mandarins (2=100g)
2	canned (50g)
–	Mango (100g)
5	canned (100g)
4	Nectarines (inc. stones 3=100g)
3000	Olives, in brine (5=20g)
2	Orange, whole (130g)
1	juice, fresh (120g)
10	canned (120g)
20	Passionfruit, whole (30g)
–	Papaw (100g)
40	canned (100g)
Tr	Peach (inc. stones 120g)
4	canned (120g)
10	dried (25g)

Chlorine (mg)	Food
400	Cake, sponge (60g)
250	Chapati (60g)
360	Cheesecake (120g)
–	Cornflakes (30g)
–	Crumpet (50g)
140	Custard (70g)
390	Custard tart (120g)
90	Doughnut (40g)
250	Eclair (50g)
–	Flour, corn- (–)
45	plain (–)
45	self-raising (–)
–	soya, full-fat (–)
–	low-fat (–)
40	wholemeal (–)
260	Fruit pie (150g)
360	Jam tart (35g)
5	Jelly, made with water (100g)
–	Lamington (60g)
310	Lemon meringue pie (120g)
100	Meringue (15g)
110	Milk pudding (e.g. sago) (160g)
–	Muesli (30g)
–	Noodles (chow mein) (250g)
90	Pancake (75g)
10	Pasta, macaroni, boiled (150g)
20	spaghetti, boiled (120g)
800	canned in tomato sauce (120g)
740	Pastry, flaky (–)
760	short crust (–)
570	Pizza, cheese and tomato (150g)
890	Porridge (30g)
10	Rice, boiled (160g)
–	fried (120g)
–	puffed (25g)
480	Scone (30g)
260	Sponge pudding, steamed (100g)
90	Trifle (100g)
–	Wheat, breakfast biscuit (35g)
–	Yeast, dried, baker's (–)

EGG AND CHEESE DISHES

Chlorine (mg)	Food
410	Cauliflower cheese (100g)
670	Cheese soufflé (100g)
160	Egg, boiled (55g)

Food	Chlorine (mg)
cheese spread (10g)	760
cottage (25g)	670
cream cheese (15g)	480
Danish blue (25g)	2390
edam (25g)	1640
parmesan (10g)	1110
processed (25g)	1020
stilton (25g)	1720
Swiss (25g)	–
Cream, 35% fat (30g)	–
sterilized, canned (15g)	140
Ice-cream (60g)	140
non-dairy (60g)	140
Milk, cow's, cond. skim, sweet. (30g)	310
cond. whole, sweet. (30g)	260
dried, skimmed (12g)	1100
dried, whole (10g)	810
evap. whole, unsweet. (30g)	350
flavoured (230g)	–
fresh, skimmed (230g)	100
fresh, whole (230g)	100
longlife, UHT (230g)	100
goat's (230g)	130
human (100g)	40
Milkshake, flavoured (340g)	–
Yoghurt, flavoured (200g)	–
fruit, low-fat (200g)	150
natural, low-fat (200g)	180
plain (200g)	–

NUTS

Food	Chlorine (mg)
Almonds (10=15g)	2
Brazil nuts (5=20g)	60
Cashews, roast (10=20g)	–
Chestnuts (4=20g)	15
Coconut, desiccated (15g)	200
Hazel nuts (10=15g)	6
Macadamia nuts (8=20g)	–
Peanuts, raw, in shells (5=25g)	5
roasted, salted (30=25g)	660
Pistachio nuts, shelled (25=15g)	–
Walnuts (5=20g)	25

SAUCES & CONDIMENTS

Food	Chlorine (mg)
Barbecue sauce (10g)	–
Chilli sauce (–)	–

Food	Chlorine (mg)
Peach, stewed, no sugar (120g)	4
Pear (inc. skin, core 120g)	Tr
canned (120g)	3
stewed, no sugar (120g)	2
Pineapple (80g)	30
canned (80g)	4
juice, canned (120g)	40
Plums (inc. stones 3=100g)	Tr
stewed, no sugar (inc. stones 100g)	Tr
Prunes (inc. stones 8=80g)	2
stewed, no sugar (inc. stones 120g)	1
Quince, raw (100g)	2
Raisins, dried (20g)	9
Raspberries (100g)	20
canned (100g)	5
stewed, no sugar (100g)	20
Rhubarb, stewed, no sugar (120g)	80
Strawberries (10=100g)	20
canned (100g)	5
Sultanas, dried (15g)	20
Watermelon (260g)	–

MEAT AND MEAT PRODUCTS

Food	Chlorine (mg)
Bacon rashers, middle, fried (2=40g)	2910
grilled (40g)	2940
Beef, corned, canned (90g)	1430
fillet steak, grilled (130g)	–
mince, stewed (120g)	470
rump steak, fried (150g)	60
grilled (150g)	60
silverside, salted, boiled (120g)	1420
sirloin, roast (120g)	60
stewing steak, stewed (120g)	550
topside, roast (120g)	50
Beefburger, frozen, fried (60g)	1120
Beef stew (250g)	590
Bolognese sauce (100g)	670
Chicken, boiled (100g)	90
crumbed, no bone (140g)	–
roast (130g)	80
leg quarter (inc. bone 130g)	50
wing quarter (inc. bone 130g)	40
Chicken livers, fried (130g)	350
Duck, roast (100g)	80

Food	Chlorine
Gelatin (–)	–
Ham, canned (90g)	1670
Hamburger (170g)	–
with cheese (190g)	–
Irish stew (250g)	520
Lamb, brain, boiled (150g)	250
chops, loin, grilled (inc. bone 120g)	70
cutlets, grilled (inc. bone 100g)	50
heart, roast (140g)	130
kidney, fried (100g)	330
leg, roast (120g)	60
liver, fried (130g)	250
shoulder, roast (120g)	60
tongue, stewed (100g)	80
Luncheon meat, canned (90g)	1290
Meat pie (180g)	–
Moussaka (200g)	510
Pastie (160g)	860
Pork, chop, loin, grilled (100g)	60
leg, roast (120g)	80
sweet and sour (250g)	–
Pork pie (180g)	1030
Rabbit, stewed (inc. bone 170g)	20
Salami, slices (3=90g)	2460
Sausage, liver (60g)	1140
Sausage roll (100g)	–
Sausages, beef, fried (2=120g)	1470
grilled (2=120g)	1490
frankfurter (2=100g)	1280
pork, fried (2=120g)	1440
grilled (2=120g)	1340
saveloy, large (2=150g)	1030
Spring roll, fried (200g)	–
Steak and kidney pie (180g)	720
Stewed steak in gravy, canned (100g)	550
Tongue, canned (100g)	1430
Tripe, stewed (100g)	60
Turkey, roast (120g)	50
Veal, cutlet, fried (110g)	120
fillet, roast (100g)	110
schnitzel (140g)	–

MILK & MILK PRODUCTS

Food	Chlorine
Cheese, camembert (25g)	2320
cheddar (25g)	1060

Food	Chlorine
Chutney, tomato (20g)	230
Curry powder (–)	–
French dressing (15g)	1480
Ginger (ground) (–)	–
Mayonnaise (20g)	570
Mustard powder (–)	–
Oxo cubes (–)	16000
Pepper (–)	60
Pickles, mustard (20g)	1700
sweet (20g)	2600
Salad cream (25g)	1300
Salt, table (–)	59900
Sesame seeds (–)	–
Soy sauce (–)	–
Tartare sauce (20g)	–
Tomato sauce (25g)	560
Vinegar (–)	50
Worcestershire sauce (–)	–

SOUPS (as served)

Food	Chlorine
Chicken, condensed (230g)	530
Chicken noodle, dried (230g)	550
Minestrone, dried (230g)	590
Mushroom, canned (230g)	750
Tomato, condensed (230g)	660
Tomato, dried (230g)	640
Vegetable, canned (230g)	750

SUGARS, JAMS AND SPREADS

Food	Chlorine
Fish paste (5g)	940
Honey (30g)	20
Jam, fruit, edible seeds (30g)	9
Jam, stone fruit (30g)	4
Marmalade (30g)	7
Meat paste (5g)	1060
Peanut butter (20g)	500
Sugar, white (–)	Tr
Syrup, golden (30g)	40
Topping, flavoured (40g)	–
Treacle, black (30g)	820
Vegemite (3g)	–

SWEETS

Food	Chlorine
Boiled sweet (5g)	70
Butterscotch (5g)	–
Caramel (5g)	–

Food	Chlorine (mg)
Carob bar (75g)	–
Chocolate square, milk (5g)	270
Fruit and honey bar (50g)	–
Jelly bean (5g)	–
Liquorice allsort (7g)	120
Pastille (5g)	120
Peppermint (4g)	20
Popcorn, plain unsalted (15g)	–
Sesame bar (50g)	–
Toffee, mixed (5g)	480

VEGETABLES

Food	Chlorine (mg)
Artichoke, globe, boiled (100g)	40
Asparagus, boiled (5=100g)	20
Bamboo shoots (50g)	–
Beans, French, boiled (100g)	10
baked, in tomato sauce (125g)	800
broad, boiled (100g)	10
kidney (and haricot), boiled (100g)	1
mung, cooked dahl (100g)	1260
soya-, boiled (100g)	–
Beetroot, slices, boiled (2=30g)	80
canned (2=30g)	–
Broccoli, boiled (100g)	40
Brussels sprouts, boiled (7=70g)	20
Cabbage, raw (50g)	20
boiled (100g)	9
Carrots, raw (50g)	70
boiled (50g)	30
young, canned (50g)	450
Cauliflower, raw (50g)	30
boiled (100g)	10
Celeriac, boiled (3=60g)	20
Celery, raw (50g)	180
boiled (50g)	100
Chickpeas, cooked dahl (60g)	310
Cucumber, slices (5=30g)	30
Egg plant, baked (½=100g)	–
Endive, raw leaves (3=15g)	70
Leeks, boiled (4=100g)	40
Lentils, split, boiled (100g)	20
Lettuce, raw leaves (2=20g)	50
Marrow, boiled (100g)	10
Mushrooms, raw (3=30g)	90
fried (6=60g)	100
Onions, raw (¼=20g)	20
boiled (100g)	5
fried (70g)	40
spring (4=20g)	40
Parsley, sprigs (2=5g)	160
Parsnip, boiled (½=60g)	30
Peas, canned (60g)	350
canned, processed (60g)	510
fresh, boiled (60g)	8
frozen, boiled (60g)	10
split, boiled (60g)	10
Peppers, green, raw (¼=15g)	20
boiled (50g)	20
Potato, baked (inc. skin 120g)	80
boiled (120g)	40
chips, fresh, fried (12=120g)	140
chips, frozen, fried (8-14=120g)	70
crisps (10=25g)	890
mashed (100g)	70
instant, cooked (100g)	380
new, boiled (2=100g)	50
new, canned (2=100g)	440
roast (120g)	100
Pumpkin (100g)	40
Radishes (2=20g)	20
Spinach, leaves, boiled (3=60g)	60
Swede, boiled (80g)	9
Sweetcorn, on cob, boiled (150g)	10
canned kernels (80g)	460
Sweet potato, boiled (100g)	60
Tomato, raw (120g)	50
canned (120g)	80
fried (120g)	60
juice, canned (120g)	4
Turnip, boiled (80g)	30
Yam, boiled (100g)	40

33
COPPER

Copper is an essential part of several body enzymes (natural substances required for chemical reactions in the body). It is necessary for iron metabolism, for the formation of the brown pigment, melanin, in hair and skin, and in the functioning of the body's central nervous system.

Copper deficiency due to inadequate dietary intake is rare. However, a deficiency may arise due to an inherited metabolic abnormality. Sources of copper include shellfish, liver, kidney and nuts. The amount of copper in household water supplies depends on the type of pipe and the hardness of the water. More copper is present in water from the hot tap than from the cold. For preparing hot drinks it is probably safer to heat cold water rather than use water from the hot tap, particularly for children.

COPPER INTAKE

There is no recommended dietary intake for copper in Australia.

In the U.S.A. an intake of 2 to 3 milligrams per day for adults is considered to be safe and adequate. (It is assumed that up to an occasional 10 milligrams per day is safe for adults.)

milligrams per 100 grams

BEVERAGES

Tr	Beer (240g)
.04	Cider, dry, alcoholic (180g)
.04	sweet, alcoholic (180g)
–	sweet, non-alcoholic (220g)
4	Cocoa powder (5g)
Tr	Coffee, percolated (230g)
.03	Cola-type drinks (240g)
–	Cordial, diluted 1:4 (240g)
1.1	Drinking chocolate (10g)
.01	Lemonade, carbonated drinks (240g)
–	Milo (10g)
–	Ovaltine (10g)
.1	Port (60g)
.03	Sherry, dry (60g)
.1	medium (60g)
.1	sweet (60g)
Tr	Spirits, e.g. whisky (30g)
Tr	Tea, infusion (230g)
.1	Wine, red (100g)
.01	white, dry (100g)
.01	medium (100g)
.01	sparkling (100g)
.05	sweet (100g)

CEREALS, BISCUITS, CAKES, DESSERTS

.04	Barley, pearl, boiled (–)
.3	Biscuit, chocolate (20g)
–	cream-filled (20g)
.4	crispbread, rye (20g)
.5	wheat, starch-red. (11g)
.2	gingernut (15g)
.08	semi-sweet (15g)
.1	short-sweet (15g)
1.3	Bran, wheat (8g)
.2	Bread, brown, slice (25g)
–	Lebanese (pita) (¼=25g)
.2	white, slice (25g)
.3	wholemeal, slice (25g)
.3	roll, brown (35g)
.5	starch-reduced (35g)
.2	white (35g)
.3	Cake, fruit (60g)
.1	plain (60g)

.1	Egg, fried (60g)
.09	omelette (100g)
.1	poached (55g)
.1	raw (55g)
.09	scrambled (70g)
.03	Macaroni cheese (180g)
.1	Quiche Lorraine (150g)

FATS AND OILS

–	Butter, salted (10g)
–	Dripping, beef (–)
.02	Lard (–)
–	Margarine (10g)
Tr	Vegetable oils (–)

FISH AND OTHER SEAFOODS

–	Bream, steamed (100g)
.05	Cod, baked (100g)
.05	fried in batter (100g)
.1	poached (100g)
.1	steamed (100g)
4.8	Crab, boiled (150g)
.4	canned (90g)
.1	Fish cakes, fried (4=100g)
.1	fingers, fried (5=100g)
–	in batter, fried (120g)
–	Flounder, baked (100g)
–	Haddock, fried (100g)
.1	steamed (100g)
1.7	Lobster, boiled (120g)
.5	Mussels, boiled (12=120g)
7.6	Oysters, raw (12=120g)
.7	Prawns, boiled (6=120g)
.1	Roe, cod, fried (100g)
.1	Salmon, canned (100g)
.2	Sardines, canned (60g)
–	Scallops, steamed (10=100g)
.1	Tuna, canned in oil (120g)
–	Whiting, crumbed, fried (100g)
–	steamed (100g)

FRUIT

.03	Apple (inc. skin, core 100g)
.1	baked, no sugar (inc. skin 110g)
.1	stewed, no sugar (110g)
.1	Apricots (inc. stones 3 = 100g)

	Copper (mg)
Apricots, canned (100g)	.1
dried (25g)	.3
stewed, no sugar (inc. stones 110g)	.1
Avocado pear (½ = 150g)	.2
Banana (100g)	.2
Blackberries (100g)	.1
stewed, no sugar (100g)	.1
Cantaloup (inc. skin 120g)	.03
Cherries (inc. stones 20 = 100g)	.1
stewed, no sugar (inc. stones 100g)	.1
Currants, black (90g)	.1
dried (15g)	.5
red (90g)	.1
Dates, dried (6 = 35g)	.2
Figs (2 = 75g)	.1
dried (2 = 40g)	.2
Fruit salad, canned (120g)	.03
Grapes, black (20 = 100g)	.1
white (20 = 100g)	.1
Grapefruit, whole (200g)	.03
canned (100g)	.03
juice, canned (120g)	.03
Guavas, canned (100g)	.1
Lemon, slices (2 = 15g)	.3
juice (15g)	.1
Loganberries (100g)	.1
canned (100g)	.04
stewed, no sugar (100g)	.1
Lychees, canned (100g)	.1
Mandarins (2 = 100g)	–
canned (50g)	.1
Mango (100g)	.1
canned (100g)	.1
Nectarines (inc. stones 3 = 100g)	.1
Olives, in brine (5 = 20g)	.2
Orange, whole (130g)	.1
juice, fresh (120g)	.1
canned (120g)	.03
Passionfruit, whole (30g)	.1
Papaw (100g)	–
canned (100g)	.1
Peach (inc. stones 120g)	.04
canned (120g)	.1
dried (25g)	.6

	Copper (mg)
Cake, sponge (60g)	.1
Chapati (60g)	.2
Cheesecake (120g)	.1
Cornflakes (30g)	–
Crumpet (50g)	–
Custard (70g)	.03
Custard tart (120g)	.08
Doughnut (40g)	.1
Eclair (50g)	.2
Flour, corn- (–)	–
plain (–)	.2
self-raising (–)	.2
soya, full-fat (–)	–
low-fat (–)	–
wholemeal (–)	.4
Fruit pie (150g)	.1
Jam tart (35g)	.2
Jelly, made with water (100g)	.04
Lamington (60g)	–
Lemon meringue pie (120g)	.09
Meringue (15g)	.05
Milk pudding (e.g. sago) (160g)	.03
Muesli (30g)	–
Noodles (chow mein) (250g)	–
Pancake (75g)	.07
Pasta, macaroni, boiled (150g)	.02
spaghetti, boiled (120g)	.08
canned in tomato sauce (120g)	.1
Pastry, flaky (–)	.1
short crust (–)	.1
Pizza, cheese and tomato (150g)	.1
Porridge (30g)	.03
Rice, boiled (160g)	.02
fried (120g)	–
puffed (25g)	–
Scone (30g)	.1
Sponge pudding, steamed (100g)	.09
Trifle (100g)	.09
Wheat, breakfast biscuit (35g)	–
Yeast, dried, baker's (–)	5

EGG AND CHEESE DISHES

	Copper (mg)
Cauliflower cheese (100g)	.03
Cheese soufflé (100g)	.07
Egg, boiled (55g)	.1

Food	Copper
cheese spread (10g)	.1
cottage (25g)	.02
cream cheese (15g)	.04
Danish blue (25g)	.1
edam (25g)	.03
parmesan (10g)	–
processed (25g)	.5
stilton (25g)	.1
Swiss (25g)	–
Cream, 35% fat (30g)	–
sterilized, canned (15g)	.2
Ice-cream (60g)	.03
non-dairy (60g)	.03
Milk, cow's, cond. skim, sweet. (30g)	.03
cond. whole, sweet. (30g)	.04
dried, skimmed (12g)	.2
dried, whole (10g)	.1
evap. whole, unsweet. (30g)	.04
flavoured (230g)	–
fresh, skimmed (230g)	.02
fresh, whole (230g)	.02
longlife, UHT (230g)	.02
goat's (230g)	.1
human (100g)	.04
Milkshake, flavoured (340g)	–
Yoghurt, flavoured (200g)	–
fruit, low-fat (200g)	.1
natural, low-fat (200g)	.04
plain (200g)	–

NUTS

Food	Copper
Almonds (10=15g)	.1
Brazil nuts (5=20g)	1.1
Cashews, roast (10=20g)	–
Chestnuts (4=20g)	.2
Coconut, desiccated (15g)	.6
Hazel nuts (10=15g)	.2
Macadamia nuts (8=20g)	–
Peanuts, raw, in shells (5=25g)	.2
roasted, salted (30=25g)	.3
Pistachio nuts, shelled (25=15g)	–
Walnuts (5=20g)	.3

SAUCES & CONDIMENTS

Food	Copper
Barbecue sauce (10g)	–
Chilli sauce (–)	–

Food	Copper
Peach, stewed, no sugar (120g)	.2
Pear (inc. skin, core 120g)	.1
canned (120g)	.04
stewed, no sugar (120g)	.1
Pineapple (80g)	.1
canned (80g)	.1
juice, canned (120g)	.1
Plums (inc. stones 3=100g)	.1
stewed, no sugar (inc. stones 100g)	.1
Prunes (inc. stones 8=80g)	.1
stewed, no sugar (inc. stones 120g)	.1
Quince, raw (100g)	.1
Raisins, dried (20g)	.2
Raspberries (100g)	.2
canned (100g)	.1
stewed, no sugar (100g)	.2
Rhubarb, stewed, no sugar (120g)	.1
Strawberries (10=100g)	.1
canned (100g)	.03
Sultanas, dried (15g)	.4
Watermelon (260g)	.02

MEAT AND MEAT PRODUCTS

Food	Copper
Bacon rashers, middle, fried (2=40g)	.1
grilled (40g)	.2
Beef, corned, canned (90g)	.2
fillet steak, grilled (130g)	–
mince, stewed (120g)	.2
rump steak, fried (150g)	.2
grilled (150g)	.2
silverside, salted, boiled (120g)	.3
sirloin, roast (120g)	.2
stewing steak, stewed (120g)	.3
topside, roast (120g)	.1
Beefburger, frozen, fried (60g)	.3
Beef stew (250g)	.1
Bolognese sauce (100g)	.1
Chicken, boiled (100g)	.2
crumbed, no bone (140g)	–
roast (130g)	.1
leg quarter (inc. bone 130g)	.1
wing quarter (inc. bone 130g)	.1
Chicken livers, fried (130g)	.5
Duck, roast (100g)	.3

Gelatin (–)	–
Ham, canned (90g)	.2
Hamburger (170g)	–
with cheese (190g)	–
Irish stew (250g)	.1
Lamb, brain, boiled (150g)	.2
chops, loin, grilled (inc. bone 120g)	.1
cutlets, grilled (inc. bone 100g)	.1
heart, roast (140g)	–
kidney, fried (100g)	.7
leg, roast (120g)	.3
liver, fried (130g)	9.9
shoulder, roast (120g)	.2
tongue, stewed (100g)	–
Luncheon meat, canned (90g)	.2
Meat pie (180g)	–
Moussaka (200g)	.1
Pastie (160g)	.4
Pork, chop, loin, grilled (100g)	.1
leg, roast (120g)	.3
sweet and sour (250g)	–
Pork pie (180g)	.3
Rabbit, stewed (inc. bone 170g)	–
Salami, slices (3=90g)	.2
Sausage, liver (60g)	.6
Sausage roll (100g)	–
Sausages, beef, fried (2=120g)	.4
grilled (2=120g)	.3
frankfurter (2=100g)	.2
pork, fried (2=120g)	.4
grilled (2=120g)	.3
saveloy, large (2=150g)	.3
Spring roll, fried (200g)	–
Steak and kidney pie (180g)	.1
Stewed steak in gravy, canned (100g)	.2
Tongue, canned (100g)	.3
Tripe, stewed (100g)	.1
Turkey, roast (120g)	.1
Veal, cutlet, fried (110g)	–
fillet, roast (100g)	–
schnitzel (140g)	–

MILK & MILK PRODUCTS

Cheese, camembert (25g)	.1
cheddar (25g)	.03

Chutney, tomato (20g)	.1
Curry powder (–)	–
French dressing (15g)	.01
Ginger (ground) (–)	–
Mayonnaise (20g)	.03
Mustard powder (–)	–
Oxo cubes (–)	.7
Pepper (–)	1.1
Pickles, mustard (20g)	.1
sweet (20g)	.1
Salad cream (25g)	.1
Salt, table (–)	.1
Sesame seeds (–)	–
Soy sauce (–)	–
Tartare sauce (20g)	–
Tomato sauce (25g)	.1
Vinegar (–)	.04
Worcestershire sauce (–)	–

SOUPS (as served)

Chicken, condensed (230g)	.02
Chicken noodle, dried (230g)	.02
Minestrone, dried (230g)	.02
Mushroom, canned (230g)	.04
Tomato, canned (230g)	.1
Tomato, condensed (230g)	.1
Tomato, dried (230g)	.03
Vegetable, canned (230g)	.1

SUGARS, JAMS AND SPREADS

Fish paste (5g)	.4
Honey (30g)	.05
Jam, fruit, edible seeds (30g)	.2
Jam, stone fruit (30g)	.1
Marmalade (30g)	.1
Meat paste (5g)	.3
Peanut butter (20g)	.7
Sugar, white (–)	.02
Syrup, golden (30g)	.1
Topping, flavoured (40g)	–
Treacle, black (30g)	.4
Vegemite (3g)	–

SWEETS

Boiled sweet (5g)	.1
Butterscotch (5g)	–
Caramel (5g)	–

Food	Copper (mg)
Carob bar (75g)	—
Chocolate square, milk (5g)	.3
Fruit and honey bar (50g)	—
Jelly bean (5g)	—
Liquorice allsort (7g)	.4
Pastille (5g)	.3
Peppermint (4g)	.04
Popcorn, plain unsalted (15g)	—
Sesame bar (50g)	—
Toffee, mixed (5g)	.4

VEGETABLES

Food	Copper (mg)
Artichoke, globe, boiled (100g)	.04
Asparagus, boiled (5=100g)	.1
Bamboo shoots (50g)	—
Beans, French, boiled (100g)	.1
baked, in tomato sauce (125g)	.2
broad, boiled (100g)	.4
kidney (and haricot), boiled (100g)	.1
mung, cooked dahl (100g)	.3
soya-, boiled (100g)	—
Beetroot, slices, boiled (2=30g)	.1
canned (2=30g)	—
Broccoli, boiled (100g)	.1
Brussels sprouts, boiled (7=70g)	.1
Cabbage, raw (50g)	.1
boiled (100g)	.1
Carrots, raw (50g)	.1
boiled (50g)	.1
young, canned (50g)	.04
Cauliflower, raw (50g)	.03
boiled (100g)	.03
Celeriac, boiled (3=60g)	.1
Celery, raw (50g)	.1
boiled (50g)	.1
Chickpeas, cooked dahl (60g)	.3
Cucumber, slices (5=30g)	.1
Egg plant, baked (½=100g)	—
Endive, raw leaves (3=15g)	.1
Leeks, boiled (4=100g)	.1
Lentils, split, boiled (100g)	.2
Lettuce, raw leaves (2=20g)	.03
Marrow, boiled (100g)	.03
Mushrooms, raw (3=30g)	.6
fried (6=60g)	.8
Onions, raw (¼=20g)	.1
boiled (100g)	.1
fried (70g)	.2
spring (4=20g)	.1
Parsley, sprigs (2=5g)	.5
Parsnip, boiled (½=60g)	.1
Peas, canned (60g)	.2
canned, processed (60g)	.2
fresh, boiled (60g)	.2
frozen, boiled (60g)	.2
split, boiled (60g)	.3
Peppers, green, raw (¼=15g)	.1
boiled (50g)	.1
Potato, baked (inc. skin 120g)	.2
boiled (120g)	.1
chips, fresh, fried (12=120g)	.3
chips, frozen, fried (8-14=120g)	.2
crisps (10=25g)	.2
mashed (100g)	.1
instant, cooked (100g)	.1
new, boiled (2=100g)	.2
new, canned (2=100g)	.1
roast (120g)	.2
Pumpkin (100g)	.1
Radishes (2=20g)	.1
Spinach, leaves, boiled (3=60g)	.3
Swede, boiled (80g)	.04
Sweetcorn, on cob, boiled (150g)	.2
canned kernels (80g)	.1
Sweet potato, boiled (100g)	.2
Tomato, raw (120g)	.1
canned (120g)	.1
fried (120g)	.1
juice, canned (120g)	.05
Turnip, boiled (80g)	.04
Yam, boiled (100g)	.2

34

ZINC

Our bodies need zinc for many different functions, which include protein and carbohydrate metabolism, wound healing, growth and vision.

Several groups of people are at risk of developing dietary zinc deficiency. If you restrict your food to vegetables, and particularly wholegrain cereals, you could become deficient in zinc. Although zinc is present in these foods, it is not utilized by the body as efficiently as the zinc in other sources, such as meat, eggs and liver. Alcoholics also develop zinc deficiency, due to an inadequate diet and to large losses of zinc in their urine. Zinc deficiency also appears to be a problem in some disease states. Inadequate zinc intake can result in retarded growth, delayed wound healing, loss of taste sensation and dermatitis.

ZINC INTAKE

The dietary requirement for zinc must take into account the different degree of availability of zinc in different foods. Animal products are more efficient sources compared with cereals. The recommended dietary intake for zinc assumes that the zinc comes from mixed animal and plant sources. For people who do not eat animal products a higher intake may be necessary.

Recommended daily dietary intake of zinc (Australia):

Infants:	4.5-6.0 milligrams
Children:	4.5-18.0 milligrams
Adults:	12-16 milligrams

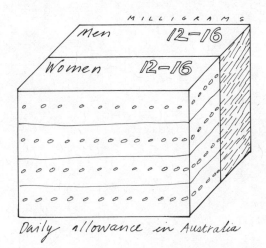

Daily allowance in Australia

milligrams per 100 grams

BEVERAGES

Food	mg
Beer (240g)	Tr
Cider, dry, alcoholic (180g)	–
sweet, alcoholic (180g)	–
sweet, non-alcoholic (220g)	–
Cocoa powder (5g)	7
Coffee, percolated (230g)	–
Cola-type drinks (240g)	Tr
Cordial, diluted 1:4 (240g)	–
Drinking chocolate (10g)	2
Lemonade, carbonated drinks (240g)	–
Milo (10g)	–
Ovaltine (10g)	–
Port (60g)	–
Sherry, dry (60g)	–
medium (60g)	.3
sweet (60g)	–
Spirits, e.g. whisky (30g)	Tr
Tea, infusion (230g)	Tr
Wine, red (100g)	–
white, dry (100g)	.01
medium (100g)	–
sparkling (100g)	–
sweet (100g)	–

CEREALS, BISCUITS, CAKES, DESSERTS

Food	mg
Barley, pearl, boiled (–)	–
Biscuit, chocolate (20g)	.8
cream-filled (20g)	–
crispbread, rye (20g)	3
wheat, starch-red. (11g)	3
gingernut (15g)	.5
semi-sweet (15g)	.6
short-sweet (15g)	.6
Bran, wheat (8g)	16
Bread, brown, slice (25g)	2
Lebanese (pita) (¼=25g)	–
white, slice (25g)	.8
wholemeal, slice (25g)	2
roll, brown (35g)	2
starch-reduced (35g)	–
white (35g)	1
Cake, fruit (60g)	.5
plain (60g)	.5

Food	mg
Egg, fried (60g)	2
omelette (100g)	1
poached (55g)	2
raw (55g)	2
scrambled (70g)	1
Macaroni cheese (180g)	.9
Quiche Lorraine (150g)	2

FATS AND OILS

Food	mg
Butter, salted (10g)	–
Dripping, beef (–)	–
Lard (–)	–
Margarine (10g)	–
Vegetable oils (–)	Tr

FISH AND OTHER SEAFOODS

Food	mg
Bream, steamed (100g)	–
Cod, baked (100g)	.5
fried in batter (100g)	–
poached (100g)	.5
steamed (100g)	.5
Crab, boiled (150g)	6
canned (90g)	5
Fish cakes, fried (4=100g)	.4
fingers, fried (5=100g)	.4
in batter, fried (120g)	.5
Flounder, baked (100g)	–
Haddock, fried (100g)	–
steamed (100g)	.4
Lobster, boiled (120g)	2
Mussels, boiled (12=120g)	2
Oysters, raw (12=120g)	45
Prawns, boiled (6=120g)	2
Roe, cod, fried (100g)	–
Salmon, canned (100g)	1
Sardines, canned (60g)	3
Scallops, steamed (10=100g)	–
Tuna, canned in oil (120g)	.8
Whiting, crumbed, fried (100g)	–
steamed (100g)	–

FRUIT

Food	mg
Apple (inc. skin, core 100g)	.1
baked, no sugar (inc. skin 110g)	.1
stewed, no sugar (110g)	.1
Apricots (inc. stones 3=100g)	.1

	Zinc (mg)
Apricots, canned (100g)	.1
dried (25g)	.2
stewed, no sugar (inc. stones 110g)	.1
Avocado pear (½=150g)	–
Banana (100g)	.2
Blackberries (100g)	–
stewed, no sugar (100g)	–
Cantaloup (inc. skin 120g)	.1
Cherries (inc. stones 20 = 100g)	.1
stewed, no sugar (inc. stones 100g)	.1
Currants, black (90g)	–
dried (15g)	.1
red (90g)	–
Dates, dried (6=35g)	.3
Figs (2=75g)	.3
dried (2=40g)	.9
Fruit salad, canned (120g)	–
Grapes, black (20 = 100g)	.1
white (20 = 100g)	.1
Grapefruit, whole (200g)	.1
canned (100g)	.4
juice, canned (120g)	.4
Guavas, canned (100g)	.4
Lemon, slices (2 = 15g)	.1
juice (15g)	Tr
Loganberries (100g)	–
canned (100g)	.1
stewed, no sugar (100g)	–
Lychees, canned (100g)	.2
Mandarins (2 = 100g)	–
canned (50g)	.4
Mango (100g)	–
canned (100g)	.3
Nectarines (inc. stones 3 = 100g)	.1
Olives, in brine (5 = 20g)	–
Orange, whole (130g)	.2
juice, fresh (120g)	.2
canned (120g)	.3
Passionfruit, whole (30g)	–
Papaw (100g)	–
canned (100g)	.3
Peach (inc. stones 120g)	.1
canned (120g)	–
dried (25g)	–

	Zinc (mg)
Cake, sponge (60g)	.6
Chapati (60g)	1
Cheesecake (120g)	.5
Cornflakes (30g)	–
Crumpet (50g)	–
Custard (70g)	.4
Custard tart (120g)	.5
Doughnut (40g)	–
Eclair (50g)	.4
Flour, corn– (–)	–
plain (–)	.7
self-raising (–)	.6
soya, full-fat (–)	–
low-fat (–)	–
wholemeal (–)	3
Fruit pie (150g)	.5
Jam tart (35g)	–
Jelly, made with water (100g)	–
Lamington (60g)	–
Lemon meringue pie (120g)	.4
Meringue (15g)	Tr
Milk pudding (e.g. sago) (160g)	–
Muesli (30g)	–
Noodles (chow mein) (250g)	.8
Pancake (75g)	.6
Pasta, macaroni, boiled (150g)	–
spaghetti, boiled (120g)	.3
canned in tomato sauce (120g)	–
Pastry, flaky (–)	.4
short crust (–)	.5
Pizza, cheese and tomato (150g)	1
Porridge (30g)	.3
Rice, boiled (160g)	.4
fried (120g)	1
puffed (25g)	–
Scone (30g)	.6
Sponge pudding, steamed (100g)	.5
Trifle (100g)	.4
Wheat, breakfast biscuit (35g)	–
Yeast, dried, baker's (–)	8

EGG AND CHEESE DISHES

	Zinc (mg)
Cauliflower cheese (100g)	.8
Cheese soufflé (100g)	1
Egg, boiled (55g)	2

Food	Zinc
cheese spread (10g)	—
cottage (25g)	.5
cream cheese (15g)	.5
Danish blue (25g)	—
edam (25g)	4
parmesan (10g)	4
processed (25g)	3
stilton (25g)	—
Swiss (25g)	—
Cream, 35% fat (30g)	—
sterilized, canned (15g)	.3
Ice-cream (60g)	.4
non-dairy (60g)	.4
Milk, cow's, cond. skim, sweet. (30g)	1
cond. whole, sweet. (30g)	1
dried, skimmed (12g)	4
dried, whole (10g)	3
evap. whole, unsweet. (30g)	1
flavoured (230g)	—
fresh, skimmed (230g)	.4
fresh, whole (230g)	.4
longlife, UHT (230g)	.4
goat's (230g)	.3
human (100g)	.3
Milkshake, flavoured (340g)	—
Yoghurt, flavoured (200g)	—
fruit, low-fat (200g)	.6
natural, low-fat (200g)	.6
plain (200g)	—

NUTS

Food	Zinc
Almonds (10=15g)	3
Brazil nuts (5=20g)	4
Cashews, roast (10=20g)	—
Chestnuts (4=20g)	—
Coconut, desiccated (15g)	—
Hazel nuts (10=15g)	2
Macadamia nuts (8=20g)	—
Peanuts, raw, in shells (5=25g)	2
roasted, salted (30=25g)	3
Pistachio nuts, shelled (25=15g)	—
Walnuts (5=20g)	3

SAUCES & CONDIMENTS

Food	Zinc
Barbecue sauce (10g)	—
Chilli sauce (—)	—

Food	Zinc
Peach, stewed, no sugar (120g)	—
Pear (inc. skin, core 120g)	.1
canned (120g)	—
stewed, no sugar (120g)	.1
Pineapple (80g)	.1
canned (80g)	—
juice, canned (120g)	—
Plums (inc. stones 3=100g)	.1
stewed, no sugar (inc. stones 100g)	.1
Prunes (inc. stones 8=80g)	—
stewed, no sugar (inc. stones 120g)	—
Quince, raw (100g)	—
Raisins, dried (20g)	.1
Raspberries (100g)	—
canned (100g)	—
stewed, no sugar (100g)	—
Rhubarb, stewed, no sugar (120g)	.1
Strawberries (10=100g)	.1
canned (100g)	.2
Sultanas, dried (15g)	.1
Watermelon (260g)	Tr

MEAT AND MEAT PRODUCTS

Food	Zinc
Bacon rashers, middle, fried (2=40g)	3
grilled (40g)	3
Beef, corned, canned (90g)	6
fillet steak, grilled (130g)	—
mince, stewed (120g)	6
rump steak, fried (150g)	5
grilled (150g)	5
silverside, salted, boiled (120g)	6
sirloin, roast (120g)	5
stewing steak, stewed (120g)	8
topside, roast (120g)	5
Beefburger, frozen, fried (60g)	4
Beef stew (250g)	2
Bolognese sauce (100g)	2
Chicken, boiled (100g)	2
crumbed, no bone (140g)	1
roast (130g)	1
leg quarter (inc. bone 130g)	.9
wing quarter (inc. bone 130g)	.8
Chicken livers, fried (130g)	3
Duck, roast (100g)	2

Zinc	Food
–	Gelatin (–)
2	Ham, canned (90g)
2	Hamburger (170g)
2	with cheese (190g)
1	Irish stew (250g)
1	Lamb, brain, boiled (150g)
3	chops, loin, grilled (inc. bone 120g)
2	cutlets, grilled (inc. bone 100g)
–	heart, roast (140g)
4	kidney, fried (100g)
5	leg, roast (120g)
4	liver, fried (130g)
4	shoulder, roast (120g)
–	tongue, stewed (100g)
2	Luncheon meat, canned (90g)
.8	Meat pie (180g)
2	Moussaka (200g)
1	Pastie (160g)
2	Pork, chop, loin, grilled (100g)
3	leg, roast (120g)
1	sweet and sour (250g)
1	Pork pie (180g)
–	Rabbit, stewed (inc. bone 170g)
2	Salami, slices (3=90g)
2	Sausage, liver (60g)
1	Sausage roll (100g)
2	Sausages, beef, fried (2=120g)
2	grilled (2=120g)
1	frankfurter (2=100g)
2	pork, fried (2=120g)
2	grilled (2=120g)
1	saveloy, large (2=150g)
–	Spring roll, fried (200g)
1	Steak and kidney pie (180g)
3	Stewed steak in gravy, canned (100g)
2	Tongue, canned (100g)
2	Tripe, stewed (100g)
2	Turkey, roast (120g)
–	Veal, cutlet, fried (110g)
–	fillet, roast (100g)
–	schnitzel (140g)

MILK & MILK PRODUCTS

Zinc	Food
3	Cheese, camembert (25g)
4	cheddar (25g)

Zinc	Food
.2	Chutney, tomato (20g)
–	Curry powder (–)
–	French dressing (15g)
–	Ginger (ground) (–)
.4	Mayonnaise (20g)
–	Mustard powder (–)
–	Oxo cubes (–)
2	Pepper (–)
.2	Pickles, mustard (20g)
1	sweet (20g)
–	Salad cream (25g)
–	Salt, table (–)
–	Sesame seeds (–)
–	Soy sauce (–)
–	Tartare sauce (20g)
.4	Tomato sauce (25g)
–	Vinegar (–)
–	Worcestershire sauce (–)

SOUPS (as served)

Zinc	Food
.3	Chicken, condensed (230g)
.1	Chicken noodle, dried (230g)
.1	Minestrone, dried (230g)
.3	Mushroom, canned (230g)
.2	Tomato, condensed (230g)
.1	Tomato, dried (230g)
.3	Vegetable, canned (230g)

SUGARS, JAMS AND SPREADS

Zinc	Food
1	Fish paste (5g)
–	Honey (30g)
–	Jam, fruit, edible seeds (30g)
–	Jam, stone fruit (30g)
–	Marmalade (30g)
2	Meat paste (5g)
3	Peanut butter (20g)
–	Sugar, white (–)
–	Syrup, golden (30g)
–	Topping, flavoured (40g)
–	Treacle, black (30g)
–	Vegemite (3g)

SWEETS

Zinc	Food
–	Boiled sweet (5g)
–	Butterscotch (5g)
–	Caramel (5g)

Food	Zinc
Carob bar (75g)	.8
Chocolate square, milk (5g)	.2
Fruit and honey bar (50g)	3
Jelly bean (5g)	-
Liquorice allsort (7g)	-
Pastille (5g)	-
Peppermint (4g)	-
Popcorn, plain unsalted (15g)	-
Sesame bar (50g)	2
Toffee, mixed (5g)	-

VEGETABLES

Food	Zinc
Artichoke, globe, boiled (100g)	-
Asparagus, boiled (5=100g)	.1
Bamboo shoots (50g)	-
Beans, French, boiled (100g)	.3
baked, in tomato sauce (125g)	1
broad, boiled (100g)	1
kidney (and haricot), boiled (100g)	1
mung, cooked dahl (100g)	-
soya-, boiled (100g)	.4
Beetroot, slices, boiled (2=30g)	-
canned (2=30g)	-
Broccoli, boiled (100g)	.4
Brussels sprouts, boiled (7=70g)	.4
Cabbage, raw (50g)	.3
boiled (100g)	.2
Carrots, raw (50g)	.4
boiled (50g)	.3
young, canned (50g)	.3
Cauliflower, raw (50g)	.3
boiled (100g)	.2
Celeriac, boiled (3=60g)	-
Celery, raw (50g)	.1
boiled (50g)	.1
Chickpeas, cooked dahl (60g)	-
Cucumber, slices (5=30g)	.1
Egg plant, baked (½=100g)	-
Endive, raw leaves (3=15g)	-
Leeks, boiled (4=100g)	.1
Lentils, split, boiled (100g)	1
Lettuce, raw leaves (2=20g)	.2
Marrow, boiled (100g)	.2
Mushrooms, raw (3=30g)	.1
fried (6=60g)	.1
Onions, raw (¼=20g)	.1
boiled (100g)	.1
fried (70g)	.1
spring (4=20g)	-
Parsley, sprigs (2=5g)	.9
Parsnip, boiled (½=60g)	.1
Peas, canned (60g)	.7
canned, processed (60g)	.8
fresh, boiled (60g)	.5
frozen, boiled (60g)	.7
split, boiled (60g)	1
Peppers, green, raw (¼=15g)	.2
boiled (50g)	.2
Potato, baked (inc. skin 120g)	.2
boiled (120g)	.2
chips, fresh, fried (12=120g)	.6
chips, frozen, fried (8-14=120g)	.4
crisps (10=25g)	.8
mashed (100g)	.3
instant, cooked (100g)	.2
new, boiled (2=100g)	.3
new, canned (2=100g)	.3
roast (120g)	.4
Pumpkin (100g)	.2
Radishes (2=20g)	.1
Spinach, leaves, boiled (3=60g)	.4
Swede, boiled (80g)	-
Sweetcorn, on cob, boiled (150g)	1
canned kernels (80g)	.6
Sweet potato, boiled (100g)	-
Tomato, raw (120g)	.2
canned (120g)	.3
fried (120g)	.2
juice, canned (120g)	.4
Turnip, boiled (80g)	-
Yam, boiled (100g)	.4

I O D I N E

Our bodies must have an adequate intake of iodine to form the hormones produced by the thyroid gland. These hormones regulate our bodies' metabolic rate. If the dietary level of iodine is inadequate, the gland, which is in the neck, swells and produces goitre. Unless treated, this condition can cause mental retardation and stunted growth in children, and hair loss, slowed reflexes, dry, coarse skin and other effects in adults. Foods produced in regions where soils are low in iodine, such as Tasmania in Australia, the Thames Valley in the U.K., and the north-west region of the U.S.A., are deficient in this element. Goitre caused by iodine deficiency can be prevented by supplementing the diet with added iodine. This is commonly done by adding sodium iodide to table salt to produce iodized salt. For some people, iodized salt can be an important source of iodine, and a change to a low-salt diet should make allowance for the decrease in iodine intake. Some foods, such as cabbage, sprouts and other brassicas contain natural anti-thyroid substances. In circumstances where both large quantities of these foods are eaten and the levels of dietary iodine are marginal, goitre could develop.

IODINE INTAKE

Excessive amounts of iodine can also lead to goitre. This has occurred where foods, such as seaweeds, which are rich in iodine, are commonly eaten. Although excessive iodine intake is not common, it should be noted that, in addition to food, many cough medicines and milk contaminated with an iodine-containing sanitizing agent also contribute to iodine intake. But it is unlikely that any harmful effects would occur with habitual intakes up to 300 micrograms per day.

Recommended daily dietary intake of iodine (Australia):

Infants:	50-60 micrograms
Children:	70-150 micrograms
Adult men:	150 micrograms
Adult women:	120 micrograms
Pregnancy:	150 micrograms
Lactation:	170 micrograms

FIGURE 52: IODINE CONTENT OF SOME FOODS

FOOD	IODINE CONTENT (micrograms per 100 grams of food)
Salt (iodized)	3000
Seafood	66
Vegetables	32
Meat	26
Eggs	26
Dairy products	13
Bread and cereals	10
Fruits	4

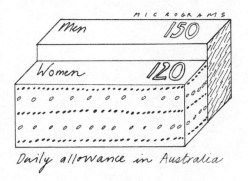

Daily allowance in Australia

The usual form of fluorine in our bodies is fluoride. Populations with a low intake of fluoride (about 1.2 milligrams per day for adults) have more dental decay (caries) than those with a higher intake (3.5 to 4.5 milligrams per day for adults). The fluoridation of public water supplies in low fluoride areas has significantly reduced decay in these areas. The fluoride content of a water supply is often described by the term 'parts per million' (ppm). 1 ppm = 0.1 milligram per 100 millilitres. About 1 ppm seems to be the optimal level of fluoride in the water supply; a litre of such water would provide 1 milligram of fluoride. At 2 ppm, mottling of tooth enamel may occur. The condition of 'fluorosis' or excessive deposition of fluoride in bones, with associated skeleton deformities, is only present after prolonged consumption of 20 to 80 milligrams of fluoride per day.

FLUORIDE INTAKE

The intake of fluoride, at the higher end of the safe range, has also been associated with reduced osteoporosis ('thinning of bones'), which is a fairly common condition in elderly people. Therefore, this also may be favourably affected by the fluoridation of water.

Safe and adequate daily intake of fluoride (U.S.A.):

Infants:	0.1-0.5 milligram
Children:	1-3 years: 0.5-1.5 milligrams
	4-6 years: 1.0-2.5 milligrams
	7+ years: 1.5-2.5 milligrams
Adults:	1.5-4.0 milligrams

FIGURE 53: FLUORIDE CONTENT OF SOME FOODS AND BEVERAGES

FOOD	FLUORIDE CONTENT (milligrams per 100 grams of food or beverage)
Crude sea salt	3.5-5.5
Fish and seafood	0.5-1
Fluoridated water	0.1
Tea	0.05-0.2

Note: 1 ml of beverage weighs approximately 1 gram.

Chromium is considered to be an essential element for humans. Those without it in their diets, such as hospital patients on artificial feeds, develop a diabetes-like condition, with high blood sugar (glucose) levels. The availability of chromium to the body may depend on the form in which it is present in food. For example, it is found in a form in association with other compounds in Brewer's Yeast and known as 'Glucose Tolerance Factor (GTF)'. Elderly people may be an at-risk group from chromium deficiency.

Relatively few foods have been analysed for chromium.

CHROMIUM INTAKE

Safe and adequate chromium intake (U.S.A.):

Infants:	0.01-0.06 milligram
Children:	1-3 years: 0.02-0.08 milligram
	4-6 years: 0.03-0.12 milligram
	7+ years: 0.05-0.2 milligram
Adults:	0.05-0.2 milligram

FIGURE 54: CHROMIUM CONTENT OF SOME FOODS

FOOD	CHROMIUM CONTENT (micrograms per 100 grams of food)
Egg yolk	183
Brewer's yeast	112
Beef	57
Cheese	56
Liver	55
Wine	45
Bread, wholemeal, wheat	42
Black pepper	35
Rye bread	30
Chilli, fresh	30
Apple peel	27
Potatoes, old	27
Oysters	26
Potatoes, new	21
Margarine	18
Spaghetti	15
Cornflakes	14
Spirits	14
Butter	13
Spinach	10
Egg white	8
Oranges	5
Beer	3-30
Apples, peeled	1

Although the element manganese forms a part of substances essential for body metabolism, known as enzymes, no definite deficiency has been recognized in humans. In animals, deficiency can lead to abnormalities of the developing skeleton, of balance, and of carbohydrate and fat metabolism. Manganese poisoning from food is very unlikely.

MANGANESE INTAKE

The safe and adequate range of intake for adults (U.S.A.) is 2500 to 5000 micrograms per day.

FIGURE 55: MANGANESE CONTENT OF SOME FOODS

FOOD	MANGANESE CONTENT (micrograms per 100 grams of food)
Nuts	1700
Wholegrain cereals	700
Vegetables	250
Fats and oils	180
Fruits	100
Meat	20
Poultry	20
Fish and seafood	5

Selenium is an element that forms part of an important body enzyme (substances essential for body metabolism), which has an antioxidant action in preventing, for example, breakdown of fats (lipids) to substances that can be damaging to the body. The enzyme probably takes care of what other antioxidants like vitamin E have failed to do because they were not present in sufficient amounts.

Selenium deficiency has been observed in patients receiving all their nutrition via the veins (parenteral nutrition), but with selenium-poor solutions. 'Keshan disease', a disease of heart muscle affecting children, is a selenium-deficiency disease seen in a selenium-poor area of North-Eastern China.

SELENIUM INTAKE

The safe and adequate range of intake for adults (U.S.A.) is 50 to 200 micrograms per day.

FIGURE 56: SELENIUM CONTENT OF SOME FOODS

FOOD	SELENIUM CONTENT (micrograms per 100 grams of food)
Seafood	100
Organ meats	20
Muscle meats	20
Cereals	20
Dairy products	6
Fruits	1
Vegetables	1
Brown sugar	1
White sugar	0.3

COBALT

MOLYBDENUM

Cobalt is essential for humans because it is a part of vitamin B-12. This form of cobalt is obtainable from micro-organisms or from animal sources. Vegetable sources of cobalt are more important to animals that are ruminants (sheep and cattle). Cobalt deficiency in humans is like vitamin B-12 deficiency, with anaemia and nervous system problems. As little as 0.1 microgram cobalt as vitamin B-12 per day is needed by adults. Total cobalt intake may be in a range from 10 to 1800 micrograms per day. Cobalt in a different chemical form (i.e. not as part of vitamin B-12) will stimulate blood formation, but this is probably not a normal action.

When cobalt was used to stabilize beer froth, it was found to have a toxic effect on the heart. Its toxicity, at cobalt intakes of about 8000 micrograms per day, probably arose from its interaction with alcohol itself, and other nutritional problems created by alcohol.

COBALT INTAKE

A safe and adequate range of intake has not been specified.

FIGURE 57: COBALT CONTENT OF SOME FOODS

FOOD	COBALT CONTENT (micrograms per 100 grams of food)
Green leafy vegetables	20-60
Organ meats	15-25
Muscle meats	7-12

Some cobalt is present as vitamin B-12 in foods of animal origin.

No definite disease due to deficient molybdenum intake in humans has been recognized. However, it is an element that is part of enzymes (natural substances essential for body metabolism) that are involved in the production of waste products prior to excretion.

The molybdenum content of foods depends on the soil where plant foods are grown.

MOLYBDENUM INTAKE

The safe and adequate range of intake for adults (U.S.A.) is 150 to 500 micrograms per day.

FIGURE 58: MOLYBDENUM CONTENT OF SOME FOODS

FOOD	MOLYBDENUM CONTENT (micrograms per 100 grams of food)
Potatoes	600
Cabbage	280
Carrots	200
Leguminous seeds	20-470
Cereal grains	10-110

NICKEL

Nickel is probably an essential element for humans, with several possible roles in maintenance and production of body cells.

Adequate amounts are probably obtained from most diets, provided that the gut is functioning properly.

There is some evidence that a few people may develop a skin sensitivity reaction to nickel. For these people, acid food cooked in stainless steel utensils and canned food may need to be avoided.

NICKEL INTAKE

The safe and adequate intake is not known.

FIGURE 59: NICKEL CONTENT OF SOME FOODS

FOOD	NICKEL CONTENT (micrograms per 100 grams of food)
Green leafy vegetables	150-300
Fruits	15-35
Tuberous vegetables	15-35
Grains	15-35
Muscle meat	very low
Milk	very low

TIN

Tin is an essential element for the growth of rats, but whether this applies to human growth is not known.

TIN INTAKE

The safe and adequate intake is not known.

FIGURE 60: TIN CONTENT OF SOME FOODS

FOOD	TIN CONTENT (micrograms per 100 grams of food)
Foods in contact with tin plate, not-resin coated (this tin is only poorly absorbed by food)	10000-15000
Cereals	100-800
Fresh meat	100
Fresh vegetables	100

SILICON

After oxygen, silicon is the most abundant element on earth. Its presence in our bodies might be thought of as that of an environmental contaminant. From the health point of view, most interest has centered on toxicity to the lungs from inhalation of silica dust. However, it has been shown in animals that silicon is essential for normal growth. Its action appears to be connected with bone mineralization and formation of connective tissue.

The best known form of silicon is silica or sand, but this is not the form that has been used to prevent growth abnormalities in animals. In a different chemical form, known as a 'salt' form, it appears to be more available to metabolic processes.

Good sources are wholegrain cereals and citrus fruits.

SILICON INTAKE

The safe and adequate intake is not known.

45
VANADIUM

46
CADMIUM

Vanadium is an essential element in the diets of chickens; deficiency affects bones, feathers and blood. It is not known whether it is essential for humans.

VANADIUM INTAKE

The safe and adequate intake is not known.

Toxicity has not been seen with intakes below 4500 micrograms per day.

FIGURE 61: VANADIUM CONTENT OF SOME FOODS

FOOD	VANADIUM CONTENT (micrograms per 100 grams of food)
Radishes	79
Dill	14
Wheat grains	0.6-2
Liver	0.2-1
Fish	0.2-1
Meat	0.2-1
Carrots	0.01
Peas	0.01
Pears	0.01

Most of the interest in the element cadmium derives from its potentially toxic effects on the lungs, and also on the kidneys, leading to high blood pressure and bone disease. However, the function of certain proteins may be dependent on the presence of cadmium.

Cadmium levels in our bodies progressively increase with age. Cigarettes also contribute additional cadmium.

CADMIUM INTAKE

The World Health Organisation has proposed a maximum tolerable weekly intake of 8.3 micrograms per kilogram of body weight.

FIGURE 62: CADMIUM CONTENT OF SOME FOODS

FOOD	CADMIUM CONTENT (micrograms per 100 grams of food)
Oysters	4-14
Wheat	5
Vegetables	1-8
Fruits	1-8
Nuts	1-4

OTHER CHEMICAL
ELEMENTS IN FOOD

ELEMENT	USUAL FOOD SOURCE	FUNCTION, IF ANY	HAZARD CAUSED BY EXCESS IN FOOD (IF KNOWN)
Aluminium	From cooking vessels, aluminium-containing medications, some fruits and vegetables	Poorly absorbed; no known function	Decreased phosphate absorption leading to bone diseases, altered mental function
Antimony	Foods stored in enamel vessels and cans	No known function	Very low toxicity
Arsenic	Crustaceans and fish, contaminated water, fruits and vegetables grown in contaminated areas or with spray residues	Possibly essential for growth in rodents, pigs and poultry	Gut, skin, brain and nerves affected
Barium	Brazil nuts, cereals grown in barium-rich soil	No known function; used for X-ray studies	Very low toxicity
Boron	Plant foods	Not essential for animals, although it is for some plants	Very low toxicity
Bromine	From fumigated grain and its products	Will replace chloride and so accumulate; will also be taken up by the thyroid gland instead of iodine	Adverse effects on brain and thyroid function
Gold	Information inadequate	No known function; gold injections are used in the treatment of rheumatoid arthritis.	Skin, gut and kidney damage
Lead	Variable content in food; more in produce grown near highways with vehicles using leaded petrol; more in food from metal cans than from glass or aluminium containers; some from reticulated water	Not essential	World Health Organisation suggests tolerable weekly intake of 50 micrograms per kilogram body weight for adults. Excess affects brain, blood, bone and kidneys.
Mercury	Inorganic mercury to which miners are exposed; mercurial fungicides contaminating food; organic mercury in fish from contaminated water, such as near paper mills; from shark, which is high up in the marine food chain with progressive concentration of mercury	Interacts with selenium	Brain damage, kidney damage
Rubidium	Soya beans, beef	Can act partly as a substitute for potassium	More toxic on low potassium diets, with effects on growth and reproduction
Silver	From food prepared in silver-plated vessels, contaminated by silver–lead solders or stored in silver foil	Not essential	Low toxicity
Strontium	Plant foods have more than animal foods, unless bone is a part. More in bran than the remainder of cereal grain.	Found in bone, and can be replaced by radioactive strontium from fall-out; interacts with calcium	May affect growth

48
LECITHIN

Lecithin belongs to a class of lipids (fats) known as phospholipids, because they contain phosphorus. Lecithin also contains choline, which can be used to make a brain chemical, acetylcholine, used to transmit information between some nerve cells, and also between nerve and muscle. Only in one rare disorder of movement, 'tardive dyskinesia', has dietary choline supplementation been shown to be of value. Lecithin also contains fatty acids, which may be saturated, monounsaturated or polyunsaturated. These same fatty acids can be obtained from lipids other than lecithin.

Lecithin is not an essential dietary item as the body can produce enough of its own. It is a component of bile, produced by the liver, which is used to aid the digestion of fat.

Lecithin is sometimes used as a food additive. It acts as an emulsifier and helps to disperse oils in water. It can be found in chocolate, salad dressings, frozen desserts and baked goods. The lecithin occurring naturally in eggs helps to perform the same function.

LECITHIN INTAKE

The safe and adequate intake of lecithin has not been specified.

FIGURE 63: TYPE OF FATTY ACID IN SOME LECITHIN-CONTAINING FOODS

FOOD	MAIN TYPE OF FATTY ACIDS PRESENT
Good source:	
Brains	Polyunsaturated
Egg yolks	Saturated
Kidney	Saturated
Liver	Saturated
Meat	Saturated
Soya beans	Polyunsaturated
Whole grains	Polyunsaturated
Milk	Saturated
Poor source:	
Fruits	Various
Vegetables	Various

49
CAFFEINE

Caffeine occurs naturally in a variety of plants. The main dietary sources of caffeine are coffee, tea, cocoa and cola-type beverages. In addition, some drugs contain caffeine. Undoubtedly the popularity of these beverages is due to the stimulant effect of caffeine. Individuals react differently to caffeine and, in addition to stimulation, caffeine can cause other effects, such as insomnia, frequent urination, stomach upsets, nervousness and irritability. Caffeine and coffee drinking have also been associated with heart disease and birth defects. Although there is no clear-cut evidence to support these studies, it would be prudent if you are pregnant to limit caffeine intake.

The amount of caffeine consumed in tea or coffee depends on factors such as the variety used, the length of brewing time, and the size of the cup. With decaffeinated coffee, over 95 per cent of the caffeine is removed prior to roasting. Cocoa contains only a small amount of caffeine, but has larger amounts of theobromine, a substance that has somewhat similar effects to those of caffeine.

FIGURE 64: CAFFEINE CONTENT OF SOME BEVERAGES

BEVERAGE	CAFFEINE CONTENT (milligrams per 150 millilitre cup)
Brewed coffee	85
Instant coffee	60
Decaffeinated coffee	3
Tea	50
Cocoa	5 (+ 250 milligrams of theobromine)
Cola-type soft drinks	35 (per can)

Gluten is a part of the protein found in wheat, and to a lesser extent in rye, barley and oats. Gluten is largely responsible for the ability of wheat flour to form 'elastic' batters and doughs. Without gluten in flour it would not be possible to produce light-baked products or the well-risen breads that are characteristic of wheat flour.

There are some people who have a condition in which the lining of the intestine is damaged by gluten; this is known as coeliac disease. This damage interferes with the normal absorption of nutrients from digested foods and can lead to an illness that resembles general malnutrition.

Coeliac disease is controlled by excluding gluten from the diet. This means avoiding foods containing wheat, rye, and barley. The position of oats is controversial but some people who suffer from coeliac disease also have a sensitivity to oats. If you have coeliac disease you must strictly adhere to the gluten-free diet, and it is usually necessary to continue for life. Good dietary guidance is essential, as wheat flour is 'hidden' in many convenience foods, in which it is used as a filler. There are gluten-free goods available, as well as specially prepared gluten-free products, such as bread, biscuits and cake.

For specific food advice, check with your doctor, dietitian or local Coeliac Society. In Australia, the Commonwealth Department of Health has compiled a *Dietary Guide for the Treatment of Coeliac Disease*, which is available from Australian Government bookshops.

General guidelines for gluten-free foods are shown in Figure 65. (Other foods labelled 'gluten-free' may also be used.)

FIGURE 65: GUIDELINES FOR A GLUTEN-FREE DIET

FOODS THAT CAN BE EATEN	FOODS TO AVOID
Butter	All canned and packaged foods
Cornflour.*	Bread/bread crumbs
Eggs	Bread seasonings
Fruit	Breakfast cereals containing wheat
Margarine	and oats
Meat	Sausages and luncheon sausage
Milk	meats
Potato flour	
Rice	
Rice flour	
Sago	
Soya bean flour	
Vegetables	

*Some 'cornflours' are made from wheat flour — check the label.

FURTHER READING

NUTRITION

Mark L. Wahlqvist (ed.), *Food and nutrition in Australia*, Methuen Australia, 1982.

Sir Stanley Davidson, R. Passmore, J. F. Brock, and A. S. Truswell, *Human nutrition and dietetics*, 7th edition, Churchill Livingstone, 1979.

FOOD COMPOSITION

Catherine Adams, *Nutritive value of American foods*, United States Department of Agriculture, Agriculture Handbook No. 456, Washington, D.C., 1975.

A. A. Paul and D. A. T. Southgate, *The composition of foods*, 4th revised edition, Elsevier/North Holland Biomedical Press, 1978.

Sucy Thomas and Margaret Corden, *Metric tables of composition of Australian food*, Australian Government Publishing Service, Canberra, 1977.

NUTRIENT ALLOWANCES

Nutrition Committee, *Dietary allowances for use in Australia*, Australian Government Publishing Service, Canberra, 1979.

Department of Health and Social Security, *Recommended intakes of nutrients for the United Kingdom*, Her Majesty's Stationery Office, London, 1973.

Food and Nutrition Board, *Recommended dietary allowances*, 9th revised edition, National Academy of Sciences, Washington, D.C., 1980.

ORGANIZATIONS THAT CAN PROVIDE NUTRITION INFORMATION

Australian Nutrition Foundation (ANF), c/o CSIRO Division of Human Nutrition, Kintore Avenue, Adelaide, S.A. 5000. (See also Capital City telephone directory.)

National Heart Foundation of Australia, P.O. Box 2, Woden, A.C.T. 2606. (See also Capital City telephone directory.)

Liaison Officer, CSIRO Division of Human Nutrition, Kintore Avenue, Adelaide, S.A. 5000.

Liaison Officer, CSIRO Division of Food Research, P.O. Box 52, North Ryde, N.S.W. 2113.

Department of Agriculture, State Government — see Capital City telephone directory.

The Nutrition Foundation, Inc.
Office of Education and Public Affairs,
888 Seventeenth Street, N.W.
Washington, D.C. 20006.

The British Nutrition Foundation,
15 Belgrave Square,
London SWIX 8PS.

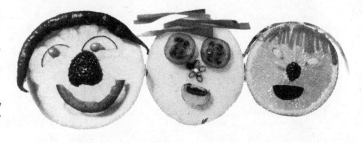

I N D E X